AF411964

COMPUTATIONAL
The Methods
NEUROANATOMY

COMPUTATIONAL NEUROANATOMY

The Methods

Moo K Chung

University of Wisconsin-Madison, USA

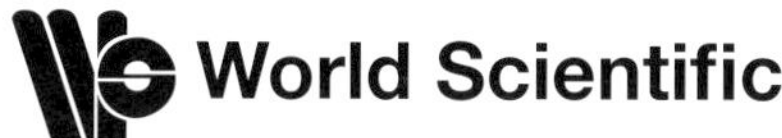

NEW JERSEY · LONDON · SINGAPORE · BEIJING · SHANGHAI · HONG KONG · TAIPEI · CHENNAI

Published by

World Scientific Publishing Co. Pte. Ltd.

5 Toh Tuck Link, Singapore 596224

USA office: 27 Warren Street, Suite 401-402, Hackensack, NJ 07601

UK office: 57 Shelton Street, Covent Garden, London WC2H 9HE

British Library Cataloguing-in-Publication Data
A catalogue record for this book is available from the British Library.

COMPUTATIONAL NEUROANATOMY
The Methods

ISBN 978-981-4335-43-0

Printed in Singapore by Mainland Press Pte Ltd.

To the memory of my teacher

Keith J. Worsley

Preface

The brain morphology across the span of human aging is not uniform. Brain growth spurts during childhood are followed by a brief period of morphological stability as loss of brain volume begins in middle age. The advancement of magnetic resonance imaging (MRI) gives us a new computational tool for the characterization of such temporally varying brain morphology and this is emerging as the new field of *computational neuroanatomy*. The computational neuroanatomy utilizes various non-invasive brain imaging modalities such as MRI and diffusion tensor imaging (DTI) in quantifying the spatiotemporal dynamics of the human brain structures in both normal and clinical populations in macroscopic level.

This discipline emerged about twenty years ago and has made substantial progress in the past decades. It usually deals with computational problems arising from the quantification of within- and between-subject variations associated with the structure and the function of the human brain. Major challenges are caused by the massive amount of nonstandard high dimensional non-Euclidean imaging data that are difficult to analyze using standard techniques. This requires new computational solutions in addressing more complex scientific hypotheses.

The main goals of the book are to provide an overview of various mathematical, statistical and computational methods used in the field to a wide range of researchers and students, and to address important yet technically challenging topics in further details. Although there are abundant research papers scattered in various journals and research monographs, there are not many research books that cover many quantitative techniques used in the field in a unified fashion. I intend to cover various diverging techniques using in a coherent manner.

Although I am indebted to many colleagues and students for writing this book, I would particularly like to thank David DeMets, the former chair of the department of Biostatistics and Medical Informatics, and Richard Davidson, the director of the Waisman Laboratory for Brain and Behavior, at the University of Wisconsin-Madison for providing endless guidance and support over the years. The book is mainly derived from research done in the brain imaging lab since 2001.

The parts of the book was written between September 2009 to December 2012 while teaching brain image analysis courses in the newly created Department of Brain and Cognitive Sciences at the Seoul National University (SNU) as a visiting professor. I would like to thank Dong Soo Lee, the chair of the Department of Nuclear Medicine, and Jae Sung Lee and Sang-Hun Lee of the Department of Brain and Cognitive Sciences at the SNU for hosting my enjoyable stay there.

This book could not have existed without the dedicated collaborators who tirelessly interacted with me. I would like to especially thank Andrew Alexander, Kim Dalton, Houri Vorperian and Seth Pollak of the Waisman Center at the University of Wisconsin-Madison for providing most of imaging data used as an illustrations in this book. Lastly I owe a special thanks to my PhD advisor Keith Worsley, who recently passed away, for introducing me to this wonderful research area.

Although most figures are produced by myself using `MATLAB`, few figures are generated by students and postdocs. Those figures are identified in the figure legend.

Moo K. Chung
April 29, 2012
Madison, Wisconsin

Contents

Chapter 1

Statistical Preliminary

In the usual structural image analysis, images are segmented and registered to a template. Then various individual imaging characteristics relative to the template are feed into general linear models. The resulting statistical parametric maps are used to quantify and localize signal while accounting for multiple comparisons across different voxels. In this chapter, the basics on general linear models and random field theory based multiple comparisons correction are presented.

1.1 General Linear Models

The effect of age, sex, brain size and possibly IQ can have severe confounding effects on the final outcome in neuroanatomical studies. For example, older population's reduced functional activation could be the consequence of age-related atrophy of neural systems (Mather *et al.*, 2004). Brain volumes is also significantly larger for children with autism 12 years old and younger compared with normally developing children (Aylward *et al.*, 1999). Therefore, it is desirable to account for various nuisance covariates in population studies. One way of factoring out the confounding effects is to use the general linear model.

The general linear model (GLM) is a very flexible and general statistical framework encompassing a wide variety of fixed effect models such as the multiple regressions, the analysis of variance (ANOVA), the multivariate analysis of variance (MANOVA), the analysis of covariance (ANCOVA) and the multivariate analysis of covariance (MANCOVA) (Timm and Mieczkowski, 1997). Note that the term linear is misleading in a sense that the model can also include mathematically nonlinear model terms such as higher degree polynomials. The GLM provides a framework

1

for testing various associations and hypotheses while accounting for nuisance covariates in the model in a straightforward fashion. The parameters of the GLM are mainly estimated by the least squares estimation and has been implemented in many statistical packages such as R (`http://www.r-project.org`) or Splus (Pinehiro and Bates, 2002) and brain imaging packages such as SPM (`http://www.fil.ion.ucl.ac.uk/spm`) and fMRI-STAT (`http://www.math.mcgill.ca/keith/fmristat`). Few important statistical issues listed below can be handled within the GLM framework.

(1) Outlier removal: We can determine outliers by checking if the measurements deviate too much from the model fit (Han *et al.*, 2006; Hodge and Austin, 2004). Outliers exceeding a certain multiple of standard deviation from the model fit might be removed and the GLM is then refitted without outliers.

(2) Multicollinearity: The multicollinearity can be remedied by the stepwise variable selection techniques (Belsley *et al.*, 2004). Note that multicollinearity does not impact the reliability of prediction, but rather makes the parameter estimation biased.

(3) Missing data: In modeling more than two variables, more observations can be excluded due to missing data value. Missing values can be imputed by replacing the missing value with the model fit (Allison, 2000).

(4) Model selection: The best model selection among all possible combination of linear models can be done using variable selection techniques (Rao and Toutenburg, 1999).

Let y_i be the response variable, which is mainly coming from images and $\mathbf{x}_i = (x_{i1}, \cdots, x_{ip})$ be the variables of interest and $\mathbf{z}_i = (z_{i1}, \cdots, z_{ik})$ to be nuisance variables corresponding to the i-th subject. We assume there are n subjects. We are interested in testing the significance of the group variable while accounting for age and gender. In a more general setting, we have a GLM

$$y_i = \mathbf{z}_i \boldsymbol{\lambda} + \mathbf{x}_i \boldsymbol{\beta} + \epsilon_i$$

where $\boldsymbol{\lambda} = (\lambda_1, \cdots, \lambda_k)'$ and $\boldsymbol{\beta} = (\beta_1, \cdots, \beta_p)'$ are unknown parameter vectors to be estimated. We assume ϵ to be the usual zero mean Gaussian noise.

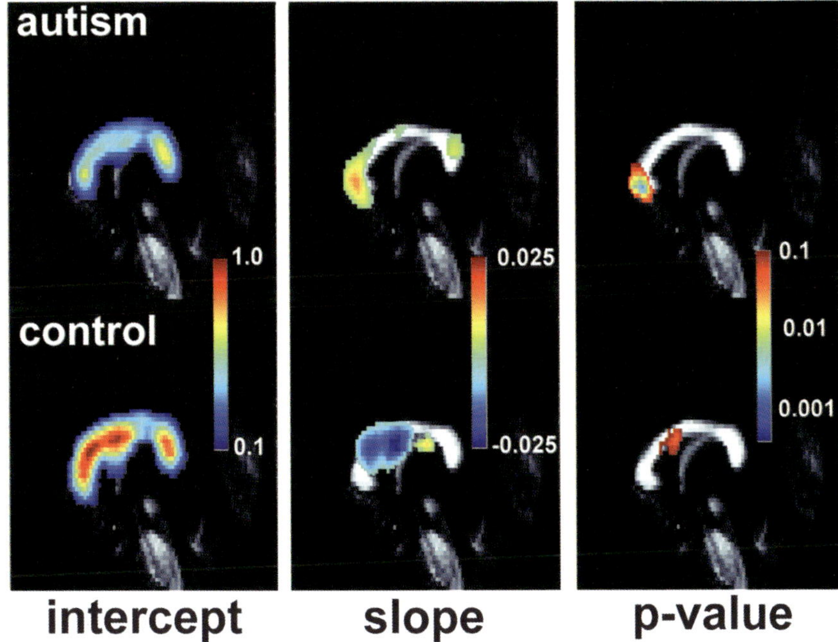

Fig. 1.1   GLM fit of the white matter density over age and group: $\texttt{density} = \lambda_1 + \lambda_2 \cdot \texttt{age} + \beta_1 \cdot \texttt{group}$. The intercept and slopes of the linear regression is for each group. The autistic group shows relatively lower white matter density compared to the control at lower age but gains white matter over time while the control group shows decreasing white matter density with age. The control group shows 2.5% per year decrease of white matter in the midbody while the autistic group shows 2.5% per year increase of white matter in the genu (Chung *et al.*, 2004).

Example. A simple example of GLM is the usual two-sample t-test setting. Given two groups, we are interested in testing the significance of group difference on tissue density, which will be covered in Chapter 4. So we consider the following GLM:

$$\texttt{density}_i = \lambda_1 + \beta_1 \cdot \texttt{group}_i + \epsilon, \tag{1.1}$$

where the dummy variable $\texttt{group}$ is 1 for autism and 0 for control. This is the case for $k = 1$, $z_{i1} = 1$ and $p = 1$. Another example is the case of liner regression for two groups, which can be combined into a single GLM:

$$\texttt{density}_i = \lambda_1 + \lambda_2 \cdot \texttt{age}_i + \beta_1 \cdot \texttt{group}_i$$

This is the case for $k = 2$ and $p = 1$ (Figure 1.1).

The significance of the variable of interests $\mathbf{x}_i$ is determined by testing the null hypothesis

$$H_0 : \boldsymbol{\beta} = 0 \text{ vs. } H_1 : \boldsymbol{\beta} \neq 0.$$

The fit of the reduced model corresponding to $\beta = 0$, i.e.

$$y_i = \mathbf{z}_i \boldsymbol{\lambda}, \qquad (1.2)$$

is measured by the sum of the squared errors (SSE):

$$\text{SSE}_0 = \sum_{i=1}^{n} (y_i - \mathbf{z}_i \widehat{\boldsymbol{\lambda}}_0)^2,$$

where $\widehat{\boldsymbol{\lambda}}_0$ is the least squares estimation obtained from the reduced model. The reduced model (1.2) can be written in a matrix form

$$\underbrace{\begin{pmatrix} y_1 \\ \vdots \\ y_n \end{pmatrix}}_{\mathbf{y}} = \underbrace{\begin{pmatrix} z_{11} & \cdots & z_{1k} \\ \vdots & \ddots & \vdots \\ z_{n1} & \cdots & z_{nk} \end{pmatrix}}_{\mathbf{Z}} \underbrace{\begin{pmatrix} \lambda_1 \\ \vdots \\ \lambda_n \end{pmatrix}}_{\boldsymbol{\lambda}}. \qquad (1.3)$$

By multiplying $\mathbf{Z}'$ on the both sides, we obtain

$$\mathbf{Z}'\mathbf{y} = \mathbf{Z}'\mathbf{Z}\boldsymbol{\lambda}.$$

Now the matrix $\mathbf{Z}'\mathbf{Z}$ is a full rank and can be invertible if $n \geq k$, which is the usual case in brain imaging. If $n < k$, we have more parameters than the number of subjects. In this case, some sort of regularization or sparse regression framework is needed. Therefore, the matrix equation can be solved by performing a matrix inversion

$$\widehat{\boldsymbol{\lambda}}_0 = (\mathbf{Z}'\mathbf{Z})^{-1}\mathbf{Z}'\mathbf{y}.$$

Similarly the fit of the full model corresponding to $\boldsymbol{\beta} \neq 0$, i.e.

$$y_i = \mathbf{z}_i \boldsymbol{\lambda} + \mathbf{x}_i \boldsymbol{\beta} \qquad (1.4)$$

is measured by

$$\text{SSE}_1 = \sum_{i=1}^{n} (y_i - \mathbf{z}_i \widehat{\boldsymbol{\lambda}}_1 - \mathbf{x}_i \widehat{\boldsymbol{\beta}}_1)^2,$$

where $\widehat{\boldsymbol{\lambda}}_1$ and $\widehat{\boldsymbol{\beta}}_1$ are the least squares estimation from the full model. The full model can be written in a matrix form by concatenating the row vectors $\mathbf{z}_i$ and $\mathbf{x}_i$ into a larger row vector $(\mathbf{z}_i, \mathbf{x}_i)$, and the column vectors $\boldsymbol{\lambda}$ and

$\boldsymbol{\beta}$ into a larger column vector $(\boldsymbol{\lambda}', \boldsymbol{\beta}')'$. Then the full model can be also written in a matrix form and solved by the matrix inversion.

Note that

$$\mathrm{SSE}_1 = \min_{\boldsymbol{\lambda}_1, \boldsymbol{\beta}_1} \sum_{i=1}^{n} (y_i - \mathbf{z}_i \boldsymbol{\lambda}_1 - \mathbf{x}_i \boldsymbol{\beta}_1)^2$$

$$\leq \min_{\boldsymbol{\lambda}_0} \sum_{i=1}^{n} (y_i - \mathbf{z}_i \boldsymbol{\lambda}_0)^2$$

$$= \mathrm{SSE}_0.$$

So the larger the value of $\mathrm{SSE}_0 - \mathrm{SSE}_1$, more significant the contribution of the coefficients $\boldsymbol{\beta}$ is. Under the assumption of the null hypothesis H_0, the test statistic is the ratio

$$F = \frac{(\mathrm{SSE}_0 - \mathrm{SSE}_1)/p}{\mathrm{SSE}_0/(n - p - k)} \sim F_{p, n-p-k}, \tag{1.5}$$

F-distribution with p and $n - p - k$ degrees of freedom. The larger the F value, it is more unlikely to accept H_0.

When $p = 1$, the test statistic F is distributed as $F_{1, n-1-k}$, which is the square of Student t-distribution with $n - 1 - k$ degrees of freedom, i.e. t^2_{n-1-k}. In this particular case, it is better to use t-statistic. The advantage of using the t-statistic is that unlike the F-statistic, it has two sides so we can actually use it to test for one sided alternative hypothesis $H_1 : \beta_1 > 0$ or $H_1 : \beta_1 < 0$. Therefore, the t-statistic map can provides the direction of the group difference that the F-statistic map cannot provide.

1.2 Random Fields

In many other brain imaging studies, it is necessary to model measurements at each voxel as a random field. The generalization of a continuous stochastic process defined in $\mathbb{R}$ to a higher dimensional abstract space $\mathcal{M}$ is called a *random field*. For the introduction to random fields, see Adler and Taylor (2007), Dougherty (1999) and Yaglom (1987).

For example, deformation fields obtained through image registration are usually modeled as continuous random fields. In the usual random field assumption, functional measurement $Y(x)$ at position $x \in \mathcal{M}$ is modeled as

$$Y(x) = \mu(x) + \epsilon(x)$$

where μ is the unknown signal to be estimated and ϵ is the measurement error. If we use a general linear model at each voxel, we can have

$$Y(x) = X\beta(x) + \epsilon(x),$$

where X is the uniform design matrix that over all voxels and β is spatially dependent parameters of the general linear model. The error ϵ and the measurement $Y(x)$ at each fixed x are random variables. Then the collection of random variables over the whole space $\{Y(x) : x \in \mathcal{M}\}$ is called a stochastic process or *random field*. The more formal measure-theoretic definition can be found in Adler and Taylor (2007). Beyond the usual Euclidean space, random field models are applied to curved cortical and subcortical surfaces (Joshi, 1998; Chung *et al.*, 2003c).

1.2.1   *Covariance Functions*

Given a probability space, a random field $T(x)$ defined is a function such that for every fixed x, $T(x)$ is a random variable on the probability space. The *covariance function* $R(x, y)$ of a random field T is defined as

$$R(x, y) = \mathbb{E}\big[T(x) - \mathbb{E}T(x)\big]\big[T(y) - \mathbb{E}T(y)\big].$$

Consider a random field T. If the joint distribution of $T(x_1), \cdots T(x_m)$ given by

$$F_{x_1, \cdots, x_m}(z_1, \cdots, z_m) = P\big[T(x_1) \le z_1, \cdots, T(x_m) \le z_m\big]$$

is invariant under the translation

$$(x_1, \cdots, x_m) \to (x_1 + \tau, \cdots, x_m + \tau),$$

T is said to be *stationary* or homogeneous. For a stationary random field T, we can show $\mathbb{E}T(x) = \mathbb{E}T(0)$ and $R(x, y) = f(x - y)$ for some function f. Although the converse is not always true, such a case is not often encountered in practical applications (Yaglom, 1987) so we may equate the stationarity with the condition

$$\mathbb{E}T(x) = \mathbb{E}T(0), \ \ R(x, y) = f(x - y).$$

A special case of stationary fields is an isotropic field which requires the covariance function to be rotation invariant, i.e.

$$R(x, y) = f(\|x - y\|)$$

for some function f. $\| \cdot \|$ is the geodesic distance in the underlying manifold.

1.2.2 *Gaussian Random Fields*

An important class of random fields is Gaussian fields. A random vector $T = (T_1, \cdots, T_m)$ is multivariate normal if $\sum_{i=1}^{m} c_i T_i$ is Gaussian for every possible choice of c_i. Similarly, a random fields T is a Gaussian random field if $T(x_1), \cdots, T(x_m)$ is multivariate normal for every $(x_1, \cdots, x_m) \in \mathbb{R}^m$.

An equivalent definition is as follows. T is a Gaussian random field if the finite joint distribution $F_{x_1, \cdots, x_m}(z_1, \cdots, z_m)$ is a multivariate normal for every $(x_1, \cdots, x_m)$. T is a mean zero Gaussian field if $\mathbb{E}T(x) = 0$ for all x. Because any mean zero multivariate normal distribution can be completely characterized by its covariance matrix, a mean zero Gaussian random field T can be similarly determined by its covariance function R. Two fields T and S are independent if $T(x)$ and $S(y)$ are independent for every x and y. For mean zero Gaussian fields T and S, they are independent if and only if the cross-covariance function

$$R(x, y) = \mathbb{E}\big[T(x)T(y)\big]$$

vanishes for all x and y.

Example. Consider the following field $T(x) = A\cos x + B$, where A and B are independent $N(0, 1)$ random variables. Note that $T(x_1), \cdots, T(x_m)$ is a multivariate normal since $\sum_{j=1}^{m} c_j T(x_j)$ is Gaussian with mean 0 and variance $\sum_{j=1}^{m} \cos^2 x_j$. Hence, $T(x)$ is a Gaussian random field with the covariance $R(x, y) = \cos x \cos y + 1$.

The Gaussian white noise is a Gaussian random field with the Dirac-delta function δ as the covariance function. Note the Dirac delta function is defined as

$$\delta(x) = \infty, x = 0,$$
$$\delta(x) = 0, x \neq 0$$
$$\int \delta(x) = 1.$$

Numerically we can simulate the Dirac delta function as the limit of the sequence of Gaussian kernel K_σ when $\sigma \to \infty$. The Gaussian white noise is simulated as independent and identical Gaussian random variable at each voxel.

1.2.3 *Differentiation and Integration of Fields*

Let $\mathcal{G}$ be a collection of Gaussian random fields. For given $X, Y \in \mathcal{G}$, we have $c_1 X + c_2 Y \in \mathcal{G}$ again for all c_1 and c_2. Therefore, $\mathcal{G}$ forms an infinite-dimensional vector space. Not only the linear combination of Gaussian fields is again Gaussian but also the derivative and integration of random fields are Gaussian. To see this, we define mean-square convergence. A sequence of random fields T_h, indexed by h converges to T as $h \to 0$ in mean-square if

$$\lim_{h \to 0} \mathbb{E}\left|T_h - T\right|^2 = 0.$$

We will denote the convergence as

$$\lim_{h \to 0} T_h = T.$$

Note that the convergence in mean-square implies the convergence in mean. This can be seen from

$$\mathbb{E}\left|T_h - T\right|^2 = \mathbb{V}\left[T_h - T\right]^2 + \left(\mathbb{E}|T_h - T|\right)^2.$$

Now let $T_h \to T$ in mean square. Each term in the right hand side should also converges to zero proving the statement. Now we define the derivative of field in mean square as

$$\frac{dT(x)}{dx} = \lim_{h \to 0} \frac{T(x+h) - T(x)}{h}.$$

Note that if $T(x)$ and $T(x+h)$ are Gaussian random fields, $T(x+h) - T(x)$ is again Gaussian, and hence the limit on the right hand side is again Gaussian. If R is the covariance function of the mean zero Gaussian field T, the covariance function of its derivative field is given by

$$\mathbb{E}\left[\frac{dT(x)}{dx}\frac{dT(y)}{dy}\right] = \frac{\partial^2 R(x, y)}{\partial x \partial y}.$$

We define the integration of a random field as the limit of Riemann sum. Let $\cup_{i=1}^{n} \mathcal{M}_i$ be a partition of $\mathcal{M}$, i.e.

$$\mathcal{M} = \cup_{i=1}^{n} \mathcal{M}_i \text{ and } \mathcal{M}_i \cap \mathcal{M}_j = \emptyset \text{ if } i \neq j.$$

Let $x_i \in \mathcal{M}_i$ and $\mu(\mathcal{M}_i)$ be the volume of $\mathcal{M}_i$. Then we define the integration of field T as

$$\int_{\mathcal{M}} T(x) \, dx = \lim \sum_{i=1}^{n} T(x_i)\mu(\mathcal{M}_i),$$

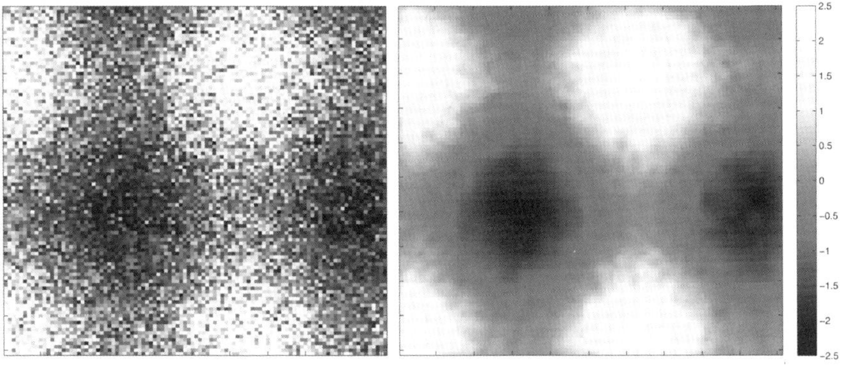

Fig. 1.2 To signal $\mu(t_1, t_2) = \cos(10t_1) + \sin(10t_2)$, Gaussian white noise $\epsilon \sim N(0, 0.4^2)$ is added. It is smoothed using Gaussian kernel with bandwidth $\sigma = 1$.

where the limit is taken as $\mu(\mathcal{M}_j) \to 0$ for all j. When we integrate a Gaussian field, it is the limit of a linear combination of Gaussian random variables so it is again a Gaussian random variable. In general, any linear operation on Gaussian fields will result in Gaussian fields. Therefore, for smooth kernel K_σ, kernel smoothing $K_\sigma * T$ will be Gaussian if T is Gaussian (Figure 1.2).

As in the case of Gaussian random variables, we can use Gaussian fields to construct new random fields such as χ^2, t, F and Hotelling's T^2 fields, all of which are extensively studied (Cao and Worsley, 1999b; Worsley *et al.*, 2004, 1996b; Worsley, 1994). For example, the χ^2-field with m degrees of freedom is defined as

$$T(x) = \sum_{i=1}^{m} X_i^2(x),$$

where $X_1, \cdots, X_m$ are independent, identically distributed Gaussian fields with zero mean and unit variance. Similarly, we can define t and F fields as well as Hotelling's T^2 field. The Hotelling's T^2-statistic has been widely used in detecting morphological changes in DBM (Cao and Worsley, 1999b; Collins *et al.*, 1998; Gaser *et al.*, 1999; Joshi, 1998; Thompson *et al.*, 1997). In particular, Cao and Worsley (1999b) derived the excursion probability of the Hotelling's T^2-field and applied it to detect gender specific morphological differences.

1.2.4 *Statistical Inference on Fields*

Statistical inferences on random fields have been traditionally based on the series expansion of the form:

$$T(x) = \sum_{i=1}^{\infty} Z_i \phi_i(x), \qquad (1.6)$$

where $\phi_i(x)$ are basis functions and Z_i are random variables. For a Gaussian random field, the most well known series expansion is called the *Karhunen-Loeve expansion* (Dougherty, 1999; Kwapien and Woyczynski, 1992; Yaglom, 1987). The inference on the expansion (1.6) is usually done on the realizations of coefficients Z_i (Basawa and Rao, 1980). On the other hand, in brain imaging, inference is based on the extrema distributions of T (Adler and Taylor, 2007; Leadbetter *et al.*, 1982) which is given by

$$P\left(\sup_{x \in \mathcal{M}} T(x) > h \right).$$

This gives a localized inference in a sense that the thresholded region is identified as signal. On the other hand, the global inference can be done by integrating the field over the region of interest $\mathcal{M}$, i,e.

$$\int_{\mathcal{M}} T(x) \, d\mu(x),$$

which collapses the random field into a single random variable. Details on the statistical inference will be given in later sections.

1.3 Multiple Comparisons

For determining the statistical significance of correlated test statistic over the whole brain, we need to account for multiple comparisons. In this section, we explain the concept in detail.

Given functional measurement Y, we have model

$$Y(x) = \mu(x) + \epsilon(x)$$

where μ is unknown signal to be estimated and ϵ is a zero mean unit variance Gaussian field. We further assume $x \in \mathcal{M} \subset \mathbb{R}^n$. In brain imaging, one of the most important problem is that of signal detection, which can be stated as the problem of identifying the regions of statistically significance. So it can be formulated as an inference problem

$$H_0 : \mu(x) = 0 \text{ for all } x \in \mathcal{M} \text{ vs. } H_1 : \mu(x) > 0 \text{ for some } x \in \mathcal{M}.$$

Let

$$H_0(x) : \mu(x) = 0$$

at a fixed point x. Then the null hypothesis H_0 is a collection of multiple hypotheses $H_0(x)$ over all x. Therefore, we have

$$H_0 = \bigcap_{x \in \mathcal{M}} H_0(x).$$

We may assume that $\mathcal{M}$ is the region of interest consisting of the finite number of voxels. We also have the corresponding point-wise alternate hypothesis

$$H_1(x) : \mu(x) > 0$$

and the alternate hypothesis H_1 is constructed as

$$H_1 = \bigcup_{x \in \mathcal{M}} H_0(x).$$

If we use Z-statistic as a test statistic, for instance, we will reject each $H_0(x)$ if $Z > h$ for some threshold h. So at each fixed x, for level $\alpha = 0.05$ test, we need to have $h = 1.64$. However, if we threshold at $\alpha = 0.05$, 5% of observations are false positives (Figure 1.3). Note that the false positives are pixels where we are incorrectly rejecting $H_0(x)$ when it is actually true. In Figure 1.3, 506 pixels are false positives. However, this is the false positives related to testing $H_0(x)$. For determining the true false positives associated with testing H_0, we need to account for multiple comparisons. The type-I error is the probability of rejecting the null hypothesis (there is no signal) when the alternate hypothesis (there is signal) is true. The type-I error is also called the *family-wise error rate* (FWER) and given by

$$
\begin{aligned}
\alpha &= P(\text{reject } H_0 \mid H_0 \text{ true}) \\
&= P(\text{reject some } H_0(x) \mid H_0 \text{ true}) \\
&= P\left(\bigcup_{x \in \mathcal{M}} \{Y(x) > h\} \,\middle|\, \mathbb{E}Y = 0 \right).
\end{aligned}
\tag{1.7}
$$

Unfortunately, $Y(x)$ is correlated over x and it makes the computation of type-I error almost intractable for random fields other than Gaussian.

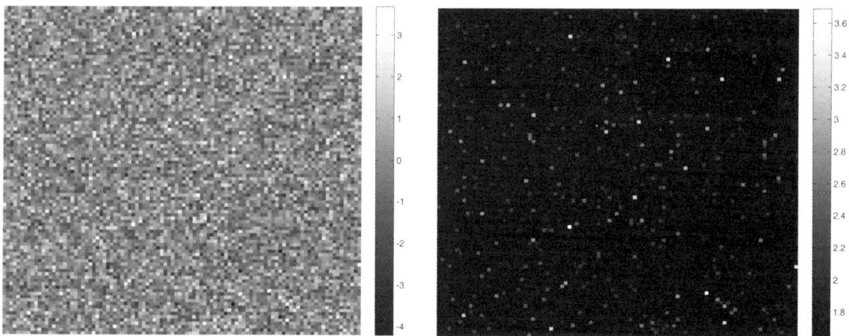

Fig. 1.3   Left: $N(0,1)$ Gaussian white noise in 100×100 image. Right: 5% of pixels are false positives at $\alpha = 0.05$ level tests. However, the Bonferroni corrected thresholding at 4.42 will not produce any false positives.

1.3.1   *Bonferroni Correction*

One standard method for dealing with multiple comparisons is to use the Bonferroni correction. Note that the probability measure is additive so that for any event E_j, we have

$$P\left(\bigcup_{j=1}^{\infty} E_j\right) \le \sum_{j=1}^{\infty} P(E_j).$$

This inequality is called Bonferroni inequalities and it has been used in the construction of simultaneous confidence intervals and multiple comparisons when the number of hypotheses are small. From (1.7), we have

$$\alpha = P\left(\bigcup_{x \in \mathcal{M}} \{Y(x) > h\} \,\Big|\, \mathbb{E}Y = 0\right) \tag{1.8}$$

$$\le \sum_{x \in \mathcal{M}} P\big(Y(x_j) > h \mid \mathbb{E}Y = 0\big) \tag{1.9}$$

So by controlling each type-I error separately at

$$P\big(Y(x_j) > h \mid \mathbb{E}Y = 0\big) < \frac{\alpha}{\#\mathcal{M}}$$

we can construct the correct level α test. Here $\#\mathcal{M}$ is the number of voxels.

For image of size 100×100 (Figure 1.3), there are 10000 hypotheses to test. So $\alpha/\#\mathcal{M} = 0.05/10000 - 0.000005$ is the corresponding point-wise p-value and the corresponding threshold is 4.42. By setting $h = 4.33$, any Y value larger than the threshold is taken as statistically significant. In the example given Figure 1.3, there is no pixel that is significant as expected.

The problem with the Bonferroni correction is that it is too conservative. The Bonferroni inequality (1.9) becomes exact when the measurements across voxels are all independent, which is unrealistic. Since the measurements are expected to be strongly correlated across voxels, we have highly correlated statistics. So in a sense, we have less number of comparisons to make.

1.3.2 *Random Fields Theory*

We can obtain less conservative estimate for (1.7) using the random field theory. Assuming $\mathbb{E}Y = 0$, we have

$$
\begin{aligned}
\alpha(h) &= P\Big(\bigcup_{x \in \mathcal{M}} \{Y(x) > h\} \Big) \\
&= 1 - P\Big(\bigcap_{x \in \mathcal{M}} \{Y(x) \le h\} \Big) \\
&= 1 - P\Big(\sup_{x \in \mathcal{M}} Y(x) \le h \Big) \\
&= P\Big(\sup_{x \in \mathcal{M}} Y(x) > h \Big).
\end{aligned}
\tag{1.10}
$$

In order to construct the α-level test corresponding to H_0, we need to know the distribution of the supremum of the field Y. The corresponding p-value based on the supremum of the field, i.e. $\sup_{x \in \mathcal{M}} Y$, is called the *corrected p-value* to distinguish it from the usual p-value obtained from the statistic Y. Note that the p-value is the smallest α-level at which the null hypothesis H_0 is rejected.

Analytically computing the exact distribution of the supremum of random fields is hard. If we denote $Z = \sup_{x \in \mathcal{M}} Y(x)$ and F_Z to be the cumulative distribution of Z, for the given given $\alpha = 0.05$, we can compuate $h = 1 - F_Z^{-1}(\alpha)$. Then the region of statistically significant signal is localized as $\{x \in \mathcal{M} : Y(x) > h\}$.

The distribution of supremum of Brownian motion is somewhat simple due to its independent increment properties. However, for smooth random field, it is not so straightforward. Read Adler (2000) for an overview of computing the distribution of the supremum of smooth fields.

Consider 1D smooth stationary Gaussian random process $Y(x), x \in \mathcal{M} = [0, 1] \subset \mathbb{R}$. Let N_h to be the number of times Y crosses over h from below (called upcrossing) in $[0, 1]$. Then we have

$$P\left(\sup_{x \in [0,1]} Y(x) > h\right) = P(N_h \geq 1 \text{ or } Y(0) > h)$$

$$\leq P(N_h \geq 1) + P(Y(0) > h)$$

$$\leq \mathbb{E}N_h + P(Y(0) > h).$$

If R is the covariance function of the field Y, we have

$$R(0) = \sigma^2 = \mathbb{E}Y^2(x).$$

It can be shown that from Rice formula (Adler *et al.*, 1993; Rice, 1944),

$$\mathbb{E}N_h = \frac{1}{\pi}\left(\frac{-R''(0)}{R(0)}\right)^{1/2} \exp\left(\frac{h^2}{2\sigma^2}\right).$$

Also note that $P(Y(0) > h) = 1 - \Phi(\frac{h}{\sigma})$ where Φ is the cumulative distribution function of the standard normal. Then from the inequality that bounds the cumulative distribution of the standard normal (Feller, 1968), we have

$$\left(1 - \frac{\sigma^2}{h^2}\right)\frac{\sigma}{\sqrt{2\pi}h}e^{-h^2/2\sigma^2} \leq 1 - \Phi\left(\frac{h}{\sigma}\right) \leq \frac{\sigma}{\sqrt{2\pi}h}e^{-h^2/2\sigma^2}$$

So

$$P\left(\sup_{x \in [0,1]} Y(x) > h\right) \leq \left[c_1 + \frac{c_2}{\sqrt{2\pi}h}\right]e^{-h^2/2\sigma^2}$$

for some c_1 and c_2. In fact we can show that

$$P\left(\sup_{x \in [0,1]} Y(x) > h\right) = \left[c_1 + \frac{c_2}{h} + O(h^{-2})\right]e^{-h^2/2\sigma^2}.$$

1.3.3 *Poisson Clumping Heuristic*

To extend the Rice formula to higher dimension, we need a different mathematical machinery. For this method to work, the random field Y to be sufficiently smooth and isotropic. The smoothness of a random field corresponds to the random field being differentiable. There are very few cases for which exact formulas for the excursion probability (1.10) is known (Adler, 1990). For this reason, approximating the excursion probability is necessary for most cases.

From the *Poisson clumping heuristic* (Aldous, 1989),

$$P\left(\sup_{x \in \mathcal{M}} Y(x) < h\right) \approx \exp\left(-\frac{\|\mathcal{M}\|}{\mathbb{E}\|A_h\|}P\big(Y(x) \geq h\big)\right),$$

where $\|\cdot\|$ is the Lebesgue measure of a set and the random set

$$A_h = \{x \in \mathcal{M} : Y(x) > h\}$$

is called the *excursion set* above the threshold h. This approximation involves unknown $\mathbb{E}\|A_h\|$, which is the mean clump size of the excursion set. The distribution of $\|A_h\|$ has been estimated for the case of Gaussian (Aldous, 1989), χ^2, t and F fields (Cao, 1999) but for general random fields, no approximation is available yet.

1.3.4 *Euler Characteristic Method*

An alternate method using the expected Euler characteristic (EC) of A_h is also available. The Euler characteristic approach reformulates the geometric problem as a topological problem. Read Adler (1981), Cao and Worsley

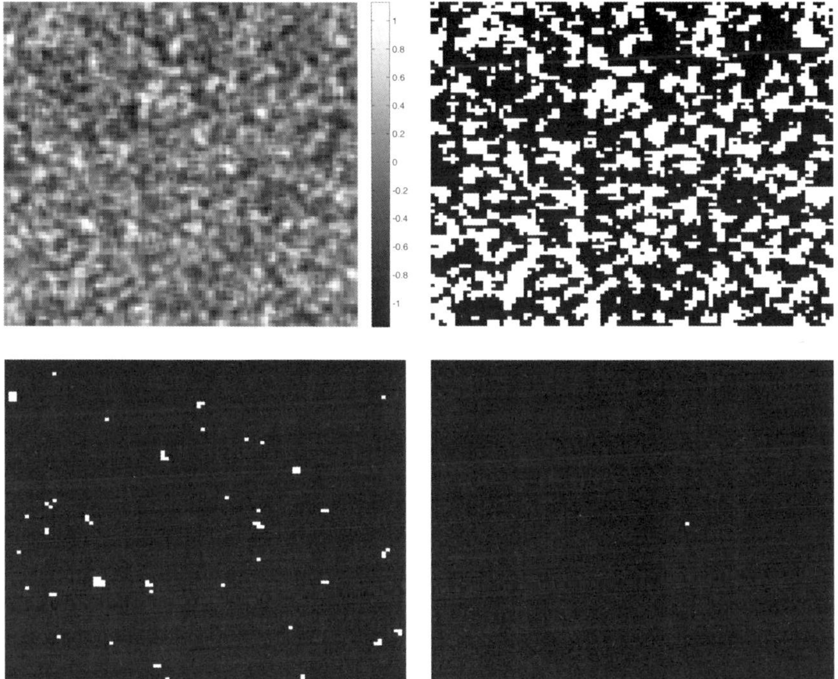

Fig. 1.4   A Gaussian random field $K_\sigma * N(0,1)$ at each pixel with $\sigma = 5$ FWHM and the corresponding excursion sets thresholded at $h = 0.1, 0.8, 1.3$ respectively. The corresponding Euler characteristics are 165, 37 and 1. As the threshold increases, only a single component remains.

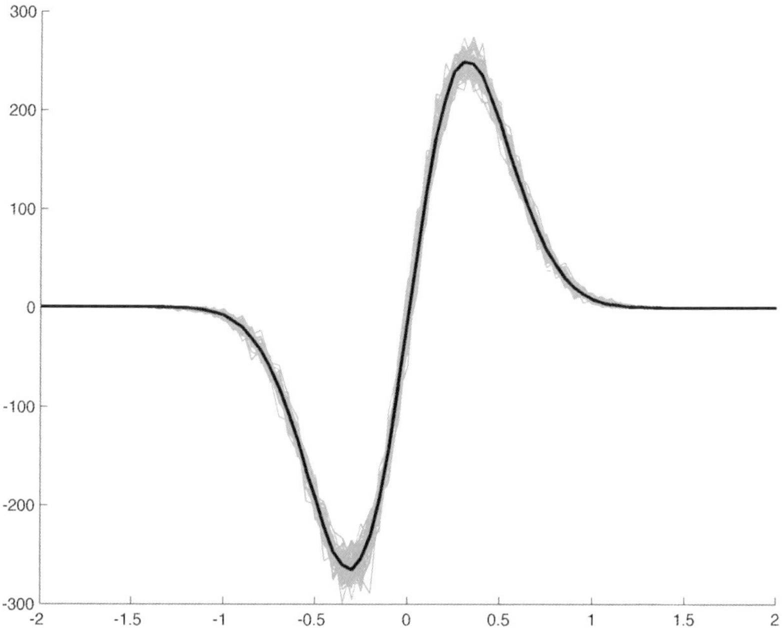

Fig. 1.5   The plot of $\chi(A_h)$ over threshold h is given in gray. The excursion set A_h is randomly generated 50 times by convolving Gaussian white noise image with Gaussian kernel. The plot of $\mathbb{E}\chi(A_h)$ over threshold h is given in black. It is estimated by averaging 50 plots of $\chi(A_h)$ over h.

(2001), Cao and Worsley (1999a), Taylor and Worsley (2007) and Worsley (2003) for an overview of the Euler characteristic method.

For sufficiently high threshold h, it is known that

$$P\left(\sup_{x \in \mathcal{M}} Y(x) > h\right) \approx \mathbb{E}\chi(A_h) = \sum_{d=0}^{N} \mu_d(\mathcal{M})\rho_d(h) \tag{1.11}$$

where $\mu_d(\mathcal{M})$ is the d-th Minkowski functional or *intrinsic volume* of $\mathcal{M}$ and ρ_d is the d-th Euler characteristic (EC) density of Y (Worsley *et al.*, 1998). For details on intrinsic volume, read Schmidt and Spodarev (2005). The expansion (1.11) also holds for non-isotropic fields but we will not pursue it any further. Compared to other approximation methods such as the Poisson clump heuristic and the tube formulae, the advantage of using the Euler characteristic formulation is that a simple exact expression can be found for $\mathbb{E} \chi(A_h)$. Figure 1.4 and Figure 1.5 show how $\chi(A_h)$ and $\mathbb{E} \chi(A_h)$ change as h increases.

1.3.5 *Intrinsic Volume*

The d-th intrinsic volume of $\mathcal{M}$ is a generalization of d-dimensional volume. Note that $\mu_0(\mathcal{M})$ is the Euler characteristic of $\mathcal{M}$. $\mu_N(\mathcal{M})$ is the volume of $\mathcal{M}$ while $\mu_{N-1}(\mathcal{M})$ is half the surface area of $\mathcal{M}$. There are various techniques for computing the intrinsic volume (Taylor and Worsley, 2007). The methods depend on the smoothness of the underlying manifold $\mathcal{M}$. For a solid sphere with radius r, the intrinsic volumes are

$$\mu_0 = 1, \ \mu_1 = 4r, \ \mu_2 = 2\pi r^2, \ \mu_3 = \frac{4}{3}\pi r^3.$$

For a 3D box of size $a \times b \times c$, the intrinsic volumes are

$$\mu_0 = 1, \ \mu_1 = a + b + c, \ \mu_2 = ab + bc + ac, \ \mu_3 = abc.$$

In general, the intrinsic volume can be given in terms of a curvature matrix. Let $K_{\partial\mathcal{M}}$ be the curvature matrix of $\partial\mathcal{M}$ and $\mathrm{detr}_d(K_{\partial\mathcal{M}})$ be the sum of the determinant of all $d \times d$ principal minors of $K_{\partial\mathcal{M}}$. For $d = 0, \cdots, N-1$ the Minkowski functional $\mu_d(\mathcal{M})$ is defined as

$$\mu_d(\mathcal{M}) = \frac{\Gamma(\frac{N-i}{2})}{2\pi^{\frac{N-i}{2}}} \int_{\partial\mathcal{M}} \mathrm{detr}_{N-1-d}(K_{\partial\mathcal{M}}) \, dA,$$

and $\mu_N(\mathcal{M}) = \|\mathcal{M}\|$, the Lebesgue measure of $\mathcal{M}$.

For nonregular jagged shapes such as the 2D corpus callosum shape $\mathcal{M}$, the intrinsic volume can be estimated in the following fashion. Treating pixels inside $\mathcal{M}$ as points on a lattice, let V be the number of vertices that forms the corners of pixels, E be the number of edges connecting each adjacent lattice points and F be the number of faces formed by four connected edges. We assume the distance between the adjacent lattice points is δ in all directions. Then

$$\mu_0 = V - E + F, \ \mu_1 = (E - 2F)\delta, \ \mu_2 = F\delta^2.$$

See Worsley *et al.* (1996a) and Chung *et al.* (2004) for details. To find the number of edges and pixels contained in $\mathcal{M}$, we start from an initial face (pixel) somewhere in the corpus callosum and add one face at a time while counting the additional edges and faces. In this fashion, we can grow a graph that will eventually contains all the pixels that form the corpus callosum. Figure 1.6 shows few possible configurations of adding a pixel (black) to the existing graph (gray pixels). A similar approach for computing the intrinsic volume for jagged irregular shapes has been implemented in FMRISTAT package (`http://www.math.mcgill.ca/keith/fmristat`).

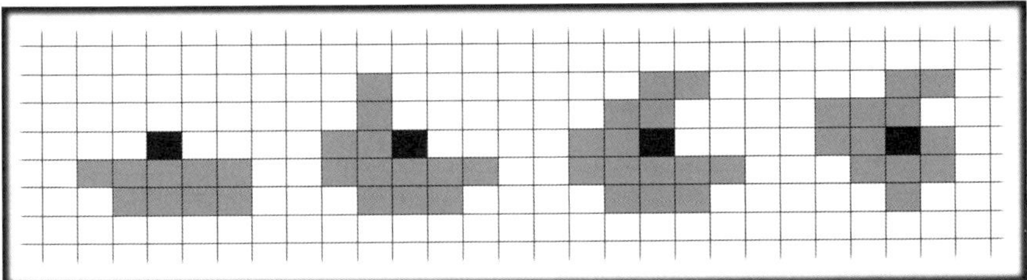

Fig. 1.6   Few possible configurations of adding additional face (black pixel) to the existing graph (collection of gray pixels). Each case corresponds to adding 3, 2, 1 and 0 edges, and 2, 1, 0 and 0 vertices. Using a region growing algorithm, each time we add a pixel to the existing graph, we can update the Euler characteristic.

1.3.6   *Euler Characteristic Density*

The d-th EC-density is given by

$$\rho_d(h) = \mathbb{E}\big[(Y > h)\det(-\ddot{Y}_d)|\dot{Y}_d = 0\big]P(\dot{Y}_d = 0),$$

where dot notation indicates partial differentiation with respect to the first d components. The subscript d represents the first d components of Y. Computation of this conditional expectation is nontrivial other than Gaussian fields. For zero mean and unit variance Gaussian field Y, we have for instance

$$\rho_0 = P(Y > h) = 1 - \Phi(h)$$

$$\rho_1 = \lambda^{1/2}\frac{e^{-h^2/2}}{\sqrt{2\pi}}$$

$$\rho_2 = \lambda h \frac{e^{-h^2/2}}{\sqrt{2\pi}}$$

$$\rho_3 = \lambda^{3/2}(h^2 - 1)\frac{e^{-h^2/2}}{\sqrt{2\pi}},$$

where λ measures the smoothness of fields, defined as the variance of the derivative of component of Y. The exact expression for the EC density ρ_d is available for other random fields such as t, χ^2, F fields (Worsley, 1994), Hotelling's T^2 fields (Cao and Worsley, 1999b) and scale-space random fields (Siegmund and Worsley, 1996). In each case, the EC density ρ_d is proportional to $c^{\frac{d}{2}}$ and it changes depending on the smoothness of the field.

If $X_1, \cdots, X_\alpha, Y_1, \cdots, Y_\beta$ are i.i.d. stationary zero mean unit variance Gaussian fields. Then F-field with α and β degrees of freedom is given by

$$F(x) = \frac{\sum_{j=1}^{\alpha} X_j^2(x)/\alpha}{\sum_{j=1}^{\beta} Y_j^2(x)/\beta}.$$

To avoid singularity, we need to assume the total degrees of freedom $\alpha + \beta \gg N$ to be sufficiently larger than the dimension of space (Worsley, 1994). The EC-density for F-field is then given by

$$\rho_0 = \int_h^\infty \frac{\Gamma(\frac{\alpha+\beta}{2})}{\Gamma(\frac{\alpha}{2})\Gamma(\frac{\beta}{2})} \frac{\alpha}{\beta} \left(\frac{\alpha x}{\beta}\right)^{\frac{(\alpha-2)}{2}} \left(1 + \frac{\alpha x}{\beta}\right)^{-\frac{(\alpha+\beta)}{2}} dx,$$

$$\rho_1 = \lambda^{1/2} \frac{\Gamma(\frac{\alpha+\beta-1}{2}) 2^{\frac{1}{2}}}{\Gamma(\frac{\alpha}{2})\Gamma(\frac{\beta}{2})} \left(\frac{\alpha h}{\beta}\right)^{\frac{(\alpha-1)}{2}} \left(1 + \frac{\alpha h}{\beta}\right)^{-\frac{(\alpha+\beta-2)}{2}},$$

$$\rho_2 = \lambda \frac{\Gamma(\frac{\alpha+\beta-2}{2})}{\Gamma(\frac{\alpha}{2})\Gamma(\frac{\beta}{2})} \left(\frac{\alpha h}{\beta}\right)^{\frac{(\alpha-2)}{2}} \left(1 + \frac{\alpha h}{\beta}\right)^{-\frac{(\alpha+\beta-2)}{2}}$$
$$\times \left[(\beta - 1)\frac{\alpha h}{\beta} - (\alpha - 1)\right].$$

If the random field Y is given as the convolution of a smooth kernel

$$K_h(x) = K(x/h)/h^N$$

with a white Gaussian noise (Siegmund and Worsley, 1996; Worsley *et al.*, 1992), the covariance matrix of $\dot{Y} = dY/dx$ is given by

$$\mathbf{Var}(\dot{Y}) = \frac{\int_{\mathbb{R}^N} \dot{K}(\frac{x}{h})\dot{K}^t(\frac{x}{h}) \, dx}{h^2 \int_{\mathbb{R}^N} K^2(\frac{x}{h}) \, dx}.$$

Applying it to a Gaussian kernel $K(x) = (2\pi)^{-n/2} e^{-\|x\|^2/2}$ gives

$$c = \mathbf{Var}(\dot{Y}_1) = 1/(2h^2).$$

In terms of the full width at half maximum (FWHM) of the kernel K_h,

$$c = \frac{4\ln 2}{\text{FWHM}^2}.$$

1.4 Statistical Power Analysis

In this section, we show how to compute the type-II error under multiple comparisons. Computation for the type-II error is slightly more involved than the type-I error computation (Hayasaka *et al.*, 2007).

Suppose, we are given the null hypothesis H_0 and the alternate hypothesis H_1 on parameters of an underlying statistical model. The probabilities of type-I (α) and type-II (β) errors are defined respectively as:

$$\alpha = P(\text{Type I error})$$
$$= P(\text{reject } H_0 \mid H_0 \text{ true})$$

and

$$\beta = P(\text{Type II error})$$
$$= P(\text{not reject } H_0 \mid H_0 \text{ false})$$
$$= 1 - P(\text{reject } H_0 \mid H_1 \text{ true}).$$

Then the *power of* the test is defined as $1 - \beta$, i.e.

$$\text{Power} = P(\text{reject } H_0 \mid H_1 \text{ ture}).$$

When the test procedure has the power of 0.8, it implies that we can correctly reject the null hypothesis H_0 80% of the time when the alternate hypothesis H_1 is true. So by counting the number of simulations that we have to reject H_0, we can numerically estimate the power as well. But here let us derive the analytic expression for the power under the Gaussian noise assumption.

1.4.1 *Statistical Power at a Voxel*

Consider two samples

$$X_1, \cdots, X_{n_1} \sim N(\mu_1, \sigma^2)$$

and

$$Y_1, \cdots, Y_{n_2} \sim N(\mu_2, \sigma^2).$$

We are interested in testing

$$H_0 : \mu_2 - \mu_1 = 0 \quad \text{vs.} \quad H_1 : \mu_2 - \mu_1 = c\sigma > 0.$$

The constant c represent the mean difference with respect to the standard deviation. As an illustration, we will only consider one sided test. As a test statistic, we use the t-statistic with the equal variance assumption:

$$T = \frac{\bar{Y} - \bar{X}}{S_p\sqrt{1/n_1 + 1/n_2}}, \tag{1.12}$$

where $\bar{X}$ and $\bar{Y}$ are the sample means and S_p^2 is the pooled sample variance. If the sample variance of the i-th group is denoted by S_i^2, the pooled sample variance is given by

$$S_p^2 = \frac{(n_1 - 1)S_1^2 + (n_2 - 1)S_2^2}{n_1 + n_2 - 2}.$$

For computing the power, the α-level has to be specified first. Under H_0,

$$T \sim t_{n_1+n_2-2}$$

and the rejection region corresponding to the α-level is given by

$$T = \frac{\bar{Y} - \bar{X}}{S_p\sqrt{1/n_1 + 1/n_2}} > t_{n_1+n_2-2,\alpha},$$

where $t_{n_1+n_2-2,\alpha}$ is the quantile satisfying

$$P(T \geq t_{n_1+n_2-2,\alpha}) = \alpha.$$

Here we assumed $\sigma \approx S_p$. This assumption simplifies the subsequent computations dramatically. Once we determined the threshold $t_{n_1+n_2-2,\alpha}$ corresponding to the α-level, we compute the power.

Under H_1, $X_i \sim N(\mu_1, \sigma^2)$ and $Y_i \sim N(\mu_1 + c\sigma, \sigma^2)$. So it follows that

$$T' = T - \frac{c}{\sqrt{1/n_1 + 1/n_2}} \sim t_{n_1+n_2-2}. \tag{1.13}$$

We cancelled out σ and S_p in (1.13). Note that our test statistic T becomes the non-central t-statistic under H_1. Then the power is simply given by

$$\text{Power} = P\left(T > t_{n_1+n_2-2,\alpha} \middle| H_1\right)$$
$$= P\left(T' > t_{n_1+n_2-2,\alpha} - \frac{c}{\sqrt{1/n_1 + 1/n_2}}\right).$$

For sufficiently large n_1 and n_2, we may assume $T' \sim N(0,1)$. Let Φ be the cumulative distribution for the standard normal distribution. Then our power is approximated as

$$\text{Power}(n_1, n_2) = 1 - \Phi\left(t_{n_1+n_2-2,\alpha} - \frac{c}{\sqrt{1/n_1 + 1/n_2}}\right). \tag{1.14}$$

For two sided α-level test, computation can be done similarly.

The sample size computation is based on the power formula (1.14). We are usually interested in how many samples we need to obtain a specific power level. Assuming $n = n_1 = n_2$, we can plot the power as a function of the sample size. For example, in order to obtain power of 0.8 for a two-sided $\alpha = 0.05$ test, in differentiating the difference $\mu_1 - \mu_2 = 0.2\sigma$, we need $n = n_1 = n_2 = 393$. See Figure 1.7 for the power vs. sample size plot.

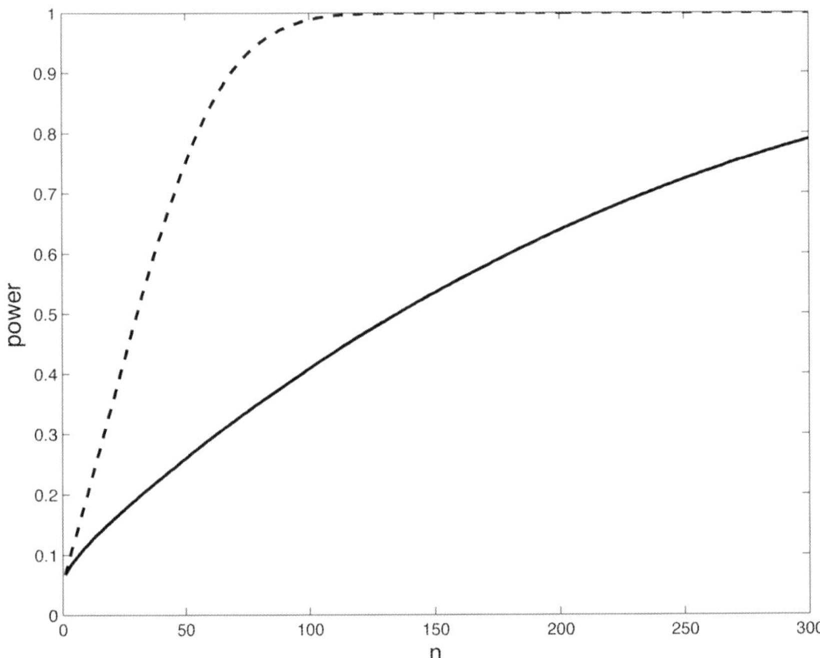

Fig. 1.7   Power vs. sample size for the two sample t test. Solid line is for at each voxel and the doted line is for whole brain surface accounting under multiple comparisons. To obtain power of 0.8 at significance $\alpha = 0.05$, in differentiating the group difference 0.2σ, we need significantly smaller sample size under multiple comparisons. This is the reason why we usually need smaller sample sizes in imaging studies.

1.4.2   *Statistical Power under Multiple Comparisons*

Up to now the power computation is based on measurements at each voxel. Assume we have two imaging measurements $X_1(t), \cdots, X_{n_1}(t)$ and $Y_1(t), \cdots, Y_{n_2}(t)$ over the brain region $t \in \mathcal{M}$. X_i and X_j can then be modeled as random fields over $\mathcal{M}$. At each fixed t, we have the same test statistic $T(t)$ given in (1.12):

$$T(t) = \frac{\bar{Y}(t) - \bar{X}(t)}{S_p(t)\sqrt{1/n_1 + 1/n_2}}.$$

The usual point-wise hypotheses are given by

$$H_0(t) : \mu_2(t) - \mu_1(t) = 0 \text{ vs. } H_1(t) : \mu_2(t) - \mu_1(t) = c\sigma > 0$$

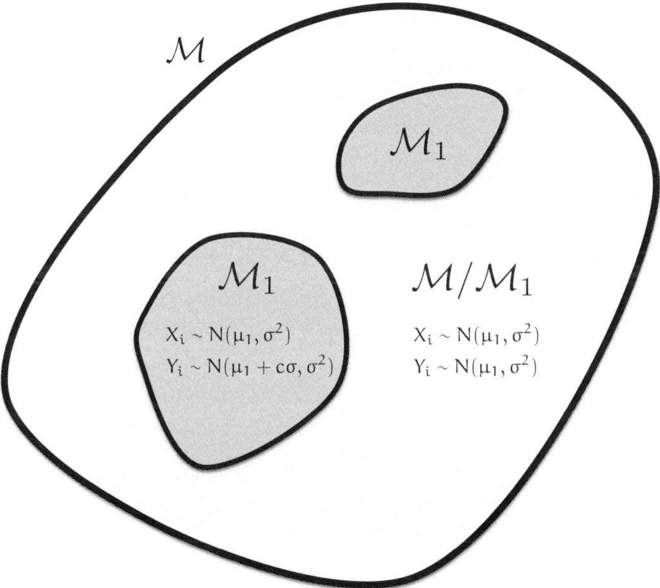

Fig. 1.8 Under J_1, there exists a nonempty rejection region $\mathcal{M}_1$ where the means of X_i and Y_i are different.

for each fixed t. Instead of the point-wise inference, what we need is a global inference for the whole parameter space $\mathcal{M}$. The usual global hypotheses accounting for multiple comparisons are then given by

$$J_0 : \mu_2(t) - \mu_1(t) = 0 \text{ for all } t \in \mathcal{M}$$

$$\text{vs.}$$

$$J_1 : \mu_2(t) - \mu_1(t) = c\sigma > 0 \text{ for some } t \in \mathcal{M}_1 \subset \mathcal{M}.$$

See Figure 1.8 for illustration of the rejection region.

The relationship between the point-wise hypotheses $H_0(t), H_1(t)$ and the global hypotheses J_0, J_1 are

$$J_0 = \bigcap_{t \in \mathcal{M}} H_0(t), \ J_1 = \bigcup_{t \in \mathcal{M}} H_1(t).$$

In order to compute the power over $\mathcal{M}$, it is necessary to determine the type-I error first. Note that we reject J_0 if $T(t) > h$ for some thresholding h for all $t \in \mathcal{M}$. This is equivalent to the event $\sup_{t \in \mathcal{M}} T(t) > h$. The type-I error over $\mathcal{M}$ is given by

$$\alpha = P\left(\sup_{t \in \mathcal{M}} T(t) > t_\alpha^* \right),$$

where t_α^* is the quantile corresponding to the random variable $\sup_{t\in\mathcal{M}} T(t)$, i.e.

$$P\left(\sup_{t\in\mathcal{M}} T(t) > t_\alpha^*\right) = \alpha.$$

Hence, the type-I error computation requires knowing the distribution of the random variable $\sup_{t\in\mathcal{M}} T(t)$ which we discussed in the previous section. It is possible to determine the quantile numerically using the permutation test but we will not pursue the issue here.

Under J_0, $T(t)$ this is a t-random field with $n_1 + n - 2$ degrees of freedom. The rejection region of J_0 corresponding to the α level is given by $\sup_{t\in\mathcal{M}} T(t) > t_\alpha^*$. Under J_1, we have

$$X_i(t) \sim N(\mu_1, \sigma^2) \text{ and } Y_i(t) \sim N(\mu_1 + c\sigma, \sigma^2)$$

at $t \in \mathcal{M}_1$. In the other region $\mathcal{M}/\mathcal{M}_1$, we have

$$X_i(t), Y_i(t) \sim N(\mu_1, \sigma^2).$$

Figure 1.8 shows the schematic view of when J_1 is true. Therefore, in $\mathcal{M}_1$, we have

$$T'(t) = T(t) - \frac{c}{\sqrt{1/n_1 + 1/n_2}} \sim t_{n_1+n_2-2}$$

pointwisely. Note that T' is not t-field in $\mathcal{M}/\mathcal{M}_1$. Then the over all power over $\mathcal{M}$ is given as

$$\begin{aligned}
\text{Power} &= P\left(\sup_{t\in\mathcal{M}} T(t) > t_\alpha^* \,\Big|\, J_1\right) \\
&= P\left(\sup_{t\in\mathcal{M}_1} T'(t) > t_\alpha^* - \frac{c}{\sqrt{1/n_1 + 1/n_2}}\right).
\end{aligned}$$

Since the analytic derivation of the exact probability is intractable, we will approximate the power using the first order term in the Euler characteristic method. For sufficiently large n_1 and n_2, we approximate the t-field T' using the Gaussian field Z with zero mean and unit variance.

Let Ψ be the tail distribution of the supremum of Z field in $\mathcal{M}$:

$$\Psi(h, \mathcal{M}) = P\left(\sup_{t\in\mathcal{M}} Z(t) > h\right).$$

If $\mathcal{M}$ is a 2D surface, Ψ is dominated by

$$\Psi(h, \mathcal{M}) \approx \frac{\mu(\mathcal{M})}{\text{FWHM}^2} \frac{4\ln 2}{(2\pi)^{3/2}} h \exp(-h^2/2), \tag{1.15}$$

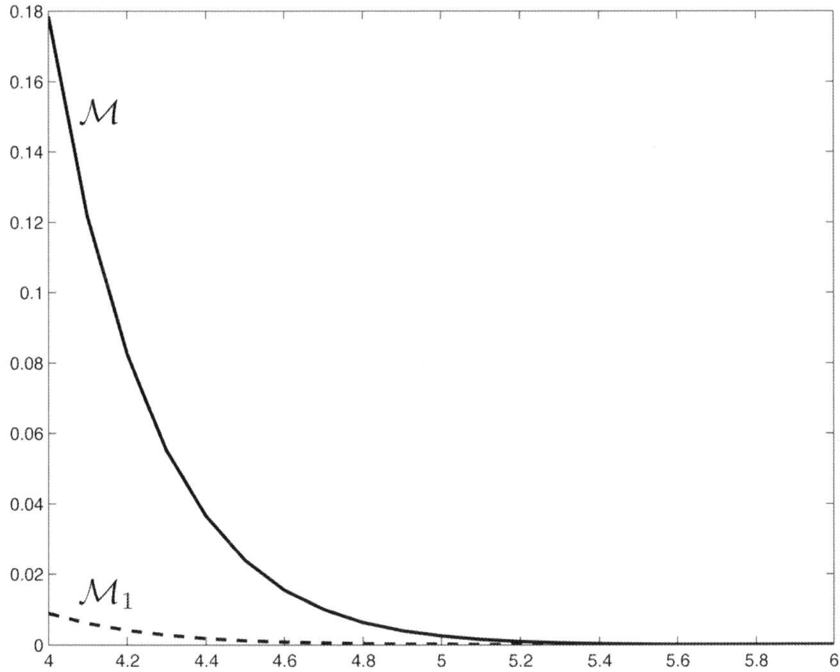

Fig. 1.9   The excursion probability $\Psi(h, \mathcal{M}) = P\left(\sup_{t \in \mathcal{M}} Z(t) > h\right)$ and $\Psi(h, \mathcal{M}_1)$ over h. $\mathcal{M}_1$ is taken as the 5% of the area of $\mathcal{M}$.   In a smaller region of interest, significantly smaller corrected threshold h is needed to achieve the same level of statistical significance.

where $\mu(\mathcal{M})$ is the surface area of $\mathcal{M}$ and FWHM is the full-width-at-half-maximum of signal or smoothing kernel (Worsley *et al.*, 1996b). Figure 1.9 shows how the excursion probability changes for different size of $\mathcal{M}$. Since Ψ is a really small number for high threshold h, the Taylor expansion

$$\exp\left[-\Psi(h, \mathcal{M})\right] \approx 1 - \Psi(h, \mathcal{M})$$

is a very good approximation for high h. Then we can write

$$P\left(\sup_{t \in \mathcal{M}} T'(t) > h\right) \approx 1 - \exp\left[-\Psi(h, \mathcal{M})\right].$$

This transformation guarantees the power estimation to be bound between 0 and 1 for any h value (Hayasaka *et al.*, 2007). Without the transformation, we can possibly get the power estimate larger than 1 for small h value. Subsequently, the power is given by

$$\text{Power} = 1 - \exp\left[-\Psi\left(t_\alpha^* - \frac{c}{\sqrt{1/n_1 + 1/n_2}}, \mathcal{M}_1\right)\right].$$

Suppose we use 5mm FWHM of smoothing kernel and the outer cortical surface area of 302180mm^2 in cortical thickness analysis (Chung *et al.*, 2003c). Assuming $n = n_1 = n_2$, we can plot the power as a function of the sample size (Figure 1.7). In order to obtain the power of 0.8 for a $\alpha = 0.05$ (corrected) test in differentiating $\mu_1 - \mu_2 = 0.2\sigma$, we need significantly smaller n compared to the power computation at each voxel.

Chapter 2

Deformation-Based Morphometry

The advancement of magnetic resonance imaging (MRI) gives us a new computational tool for the characterization of temporally varying brain morphology and this is emerging as the new field of *computational neuroanatomy*. MRI depends on the response of magnetic fields to produce digital images that provide structural information about brain tissue noninvasively. Compared to the computed tomography (CT), MRI has been mainly used for *in vivo* imaging of brain due to due to much greater image contrast in soft tissues. The T1-weighted MRI use a gradient echo sequence and it is more often used in anatomical studies compared to the T2-weighted MRI. This noninvasive but somewhat expensive procedure has become a standard brain imaging modality in examining the structure of the brain since it provides a good image contrast between soft tissues.

In computational neuroanatomy, mathematical models that try to model deformations and shapes in a continuous fashion is more often used compared to point distribution models (Cootes *et al.*, 1995, 1993). Point distribution models rely on preselected finite number of landmarks so it has an additional burden of identifying landmarks. Anatomical landmarks are points usually identified by experts or automated expert systems that corresponds between structures in a biologically meaningful way (Dryden and Mardia, 1998). The point distribution models do not provide finer details at a voxel level. In point distribution models, principal component analysis (PCA) is often used for shape quantification and there is no room for more flexible continuos models (Jolliffe, 2002). The main focus of this book is on continuous models and point distribution models will be not be covered.

There are three main components in computational neuroanatomy (Csernansky *et al.*, 2004):

(1) the computation of deformation maps between images

(2) the computation of metrics for quantifying anatomical variations

(3) the construction of statistical inference procedure.

Consider an example of comparing the shape of brains in two populations: a clinical population and normal controls. We need to build mathematical representations corresponding to brain images. Then a goal is to build general rules or models that take such representations as inputs and discriminate between the groups. Another goal is to localize the regions of brain that gives the maximum discrimination. Based on the optimal discriminating model, the clinical population can be quantified statistically with respect to the normal controls.

The main focus of this book is on the computation of metrics and the subsequent statistical inference procedures. We will not cover the topic of the deformation computation in detail. The detailed exposition of image registration is given in Toga (1999).

2.1   Image Registration

The objective of the image registration is to deform as smoothly as possible from one image to another image and obtain the deformation map between the two images. The tremendous amount of anatomical variations in the human brain presents substantial technical challenges. It is essential to be able to compare different individual functional and structural images taken at different times via image registration. For the overview of various image registration techniques, see Toga (1999) and Lester and Simon (1999).

Brain images are usually transformed into a standardized stereotactic space via a global affine transformation followed by a nonlinear deformation to match the *atlas* or *template*, which is a fixed reference coordinate system of the brain (Zijdenbos *et al.*, 1998). Mapping structural and functional brain images into the atlas is required for most brain imaging research because it provides a common coordinate system in which different subjects and imaging modalities can be compared and quantified (Figure 2.1). The atlas can be a single subject image or the population average. One of widely used atlas is the Talairach stereotaxic system which uses affine trransformations in 12 rectangular regions in a piecewise fashion (Talairach and Tournoux, 1988). The Talairach stereotaxic system is based on the postmortem sections of a 60-year-old French female brain and may not well represent developing children and other clinical populations. The Talairach coordinates provide an easy reference for comparing different study results

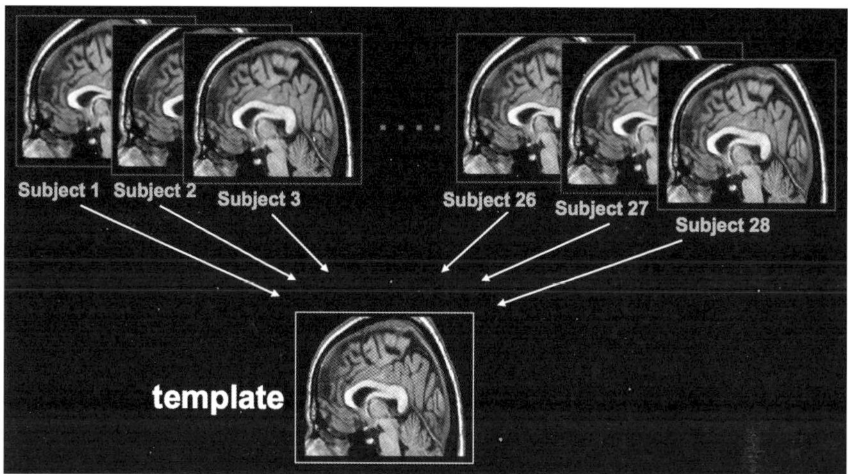

Fig. 2.1 Given multiple MRI, individual brain is registered to a template brain. The resulting deformation field or its derivative fiend is then used as inputs of a statistical inference in deformation-based morphometry or tensor-based morphometry.

and still often used. However, a more widely used approach is based on the population average atlas from the Montreal Neurological Institute. It was constructed by averaging the image intensity of the 239 male and 66 female brains at age 23.4 ± 4.1 years (Collins and Evans, 1999).

The global affine transformation to the template removes most of the within- and between-subject global differences in brain size; adult brains are approximately 5% larger than those of five year old children (Dekaban and Shadowsky, 1978). Because global brain size difference does not provide much biological information, these global morphological variabilities should be removed via global affine transform before any localized shape analysis is performed. One of the most widely used registration method has been the intensity-based matching, which tries to align one image to another in such a way that the similarity of the image intensity is maximized (Collins and Evans, 1999; Collins *et al.*, 1995). Also intensity-based basis function methods (Ashburner *et al.*, 1997) or an intensity-based multiscale approach (Collins *et al.*, 1994) are available. Alternate methods based on physical models such as elastic deformation and fluid dynamics models are also available (Christensen *et al.*, 1993; Davatzikos, 1999; Gee and Bajcsy, 1999; Thompson *et al.*, 1997; Thompson and Toga, 1999) as well as a recently popular diffeomorphic framework (Avants *et al.*, 2008; Joshi *et al.*, 2004; Vailant *et al.*, 2007).

Unlike other registration algorithms that assume a certain fluid dynamics or an elastic deformation model, the intensity-based registration does not assume any explicit physical model in which the deformation from the subject brain to the atlas brain should follow (Gee and Bajcsy, 1999; Thompson *et al.*, 2000). So the deformation fields obtained from these registration processes can be considered as free of any explicit physical model assumption although there might be some intensity-based model assumption, which somehow relates to a physical model.

2.2   Deformation-Based Morphometry

Morphological differences in brain have been examined primarily by MRI-volumetry before the development of voxel-wise morphometries. The classical MRI-volumetry requires segmentation of anatomically corresponding regions of interest (ROI), either manually or automatically in MR images. Then the total volumes V_1 and V_2 of the homologous ROIs are calculated by counting the total number of voxels. Afterwards, the volume difference $\Delta V = V_2 - V_1$ is used as an index of morphological changes (Giedd *et al.*, 1996; Rajapakse *et al.*, 1996; Riess *et al.*, 1996; Thirion and Calmon, 1999). On the other hands, *deformation-based morphometry* (DBM), which utilizes spatial position difference of corresponding voxels, does not require segmentation of *a priori* regions of interest (Davatzikos, 1997; Ashburner and Friston, 2000). The advantage of DBM over the classical MRI-volumetry is that it does not require the *a priori* knowledge of the ROI to perform the morphological analysis and structural differences can be detected at a voxel level. For example, using DBM, it is possible to detect local structural differences within the hippocampus and identify exactly what part of hippocampus is responsible for the most anatomical variation in a group of subjects. The second advantage is that it does not require a priori knowledge of the ROI to perform the morphological analysis. Moreover, DBM improves the power of detecting the regions of volume change within the limits of the accuracy of registration algorithm, which is usually the size of voxels.

Unlike classical shape analysis (Bookstein, 1989, 1991; Dryden and Mardia, 1998; Kendall, 1989; Small, 1996), DBM tries to avoid anatomical landmarks in characterizing morphological changes. Since it is hard to identify multitude of anatomical landmarks in brain images systematically, DBM is advantageous over the traditional landmark-based techniques. Since its introduction of deformation-based morphometry by Ashburner and Friston in 2000 (Ashburner and Friston, 2000), there has been an explosion of morphometric studies that utilizes DBM. For an overview, see Chung *et al.* (2001a).

2.3 Displacement Vector Fields

Through image registration, biologically homologous points in two different images are identified and the mathematical transformation between these two points, called *deformation*, can be computed. The deformation is given as a 3-dimensional vector $d(x)$ at each voxel position $x = (x_1, x_2, x_3)'$. Mathematically the deformation can be represented as a transformation from a point x to a homologous point $x + u(x)$ in the Lagrangian coordinate system:

$$d(x) = x + u(x).$$

The 3-dimensional vector $u = (u_1, u_2, u_3)'$ is called the *displacement* vector field in elastic deformation theory and it measures a relative movement of the point x (Marsden and Hughes, 1983). Although the idea of deformation originates from the elastic theory and continuum mechanics (Chandrasekharaiah and Debnath, 1994; Marsden and Hughes, 1983), perhaps the first scientist to apply this concept to deform one biological structure to another closely related structure is D'arcy Thompson in his classical book "On Growth and Form" (Thompson, 1961), where he deformed the skulls of human and primates, and other biological structures using deformable grids.

Once we obtain the deformation from nonlinear image registration techniques such as a popular diffeomorphic image registration (Zhang *et al.*, 2006), we build a statistical model. Instead of modeling on deformation, it is easier to model on the displacement:

$$u(x) = \mu(x) + \Sigma^{1/2}(x)\epsilon(x), \tag{2.1}$$

where $\Sigma(x)$ is the 3×3 symmetric positive-definite covariance matrix, which allows for correlations between components of the deformation and depends on the spatial coordinates x only (Worsley *et al.*, 1996b; Cao and Worsley, 1999b; Chung *et al.*, 2001a). Since Σ is symmetric positive-definite, the square-root of Σ always exists. The components of the error vector ϵ are assumed to be independent and identically distributed as smooth stationary Gaussian random fields with zero mean and unit standard deviation. The model has been widely used in localizing the regions of abnormal displacement differences.

2.3.1   *Dynamic Model on Displacement*

Unlike most of cross-sectional studies that try to characterize the structural variabilities among different individuals of similar age groups, morphological studies of temporally varying brain structure have an extra temporal dimension. Therefore, a slightly different model from (2.1) is needed to fully characterize the spatio-temporal complexity of brain development. Let $u(x, t) = (u_1, u_2, u_3)$ be the 3D displacement vector field required to move the structure at position x and at the reference time 0 of a subject brain to the corresponding position after time t. This model was first introduced in Chung *et al.* (2001a) for developmental studies. The structure at x deforms to $x + u(x, t)$ with respect to fixed reference coordinates. The displacement field $u(x, t)$ at fixed time t is usually estimated via volume-based non-linear registration techniques on two images taken at time 0 and at time t. Then the static model (2.1) can be changed to incorporate longitudinal change:

$$\frac{\partial u}{\partial t}(x, t) = L(u) + \Sigma^{1/2}(x)\epsilon(x), \tag{2.2}$$

where L is a partial differential operator involving spatial components. An equation of the type (2.2) is called a *stochastic evolution equation* and it models how the structure evolves over time. Any smooth morphological change can be completely described by (2.2) within a bounded domain by the error term $\Sigma^{1/2}\epsilon$. Modeling the rate of change as a differential equation originates from Newton. If the deformation is assumed to follow a diffusive behavior, then L can be chosen as the Laplacian

$$L = \sigma^2 \left(\frac{\partial^2}{\partial x_1^2} + \frac{\partial^2}{\partial x_2^2} + \frac{\partial^2}{\partial x_3^2} \right)$$

with some constant σ. If the morphological changes are assumed to follow a fluid dynamics model, L becomes a Navier-Stokes operator (Landau and Lifshitz, 1989).

Longitudinal analysis base on the model (2.2) can be viewed as the inverse problem of image registration. In longitudinal analysis, we tries to determine the partial differential operator L when the displacement fields u is given. On the other hand, in image registration, the objective is to find the displacement field u that matches homologous points between two images based on minimizing a cost function or actually solving partial differential equations. The often used physical models for brain image registration have been elastic deformations and fluid dynamics models (Christensen *et al.*, 1993; Thompson and Toga, 1999; Davatzikos, 1997; Gee and Bajcsy, 1999). Suppose that the displacement field U is obtained as a solution of the elastic deformation equation given by (2.2), where the elastic operator

$$L(u) = \lambda_1 \nabla^2 u + \lambda_2 \nabla(\nabla \cdot u) + F$$

is defined in Warfield *et al.* (1999). Then using this displacement field U as given data, we try to estimate (2.2) which minimizes a certain error criterion. The best estimator of L is heavily biased toward the prior operator L. It indicates that the estimation of (2.2) should be based on an image registration method that does not assume an *a priori* physical model or on an empirical Bayesian framework. Few such methods are image intensity-based registration algorithms that do not have explicit physical model assumptions to warp one brain to another (Collins *et al.*, 1994; Ashburner *et al.*, 1997), but there should be further comparative studies of the different image registration methods to draw any general conclusions.

It can be assumed that, in the case of morphological changes occurring in a healthy brain over a relatively short period of time, deformation occurs continuously and smoothly, so the higher order temporal derivatives of the displacement u are relatively small compared to the displacement itself. In such a case, the first-order approximation to $L(u)$ is sufficient to capture most of the morphological variabilities over time. Therefore, we can approximate $\partial u/\partial t$ with only a first-order term $\mu_0(x)$ which is constant over time. If one wishes to see the convexity of the growth curve, an additional second-order term is needed. Then we model $\partial u/\partial t$ as

$$\frac{\partial u}{\partial t} = \mu_0(x) + \mu_1(x)t.$$

Unlike estimating the first-order linear term μ_0, the problem of estimating the second-order term requires a large amount of data to have a statistically stable result due to large between-subject variabilities across spatial and temporal dimensions.

2.3.2 *Local Inference via Hotelling's T^2-Field*

We are interested in detecting local regions of statistically significant changes in displacement using the linear model (2.1). This is a standard multivariate statistical inference problem and can be solved using the

Hotelling's T^2 statistic (Thompson *et al.*, 1997; Joshi, 1998; Cao and Worsley, 1999b; Gaser *et al.*, 1999; Chung *et al.*, 2001a). Under the assumption (2.1), we test if the two groups have the same displacement with respect to the template:

$$H_0 : \mu_1(x) = \mu_2(x) \text{ for all } x \text{ vs. } H_1 : \mu_1(x) \neq \mu_2(x) \text{ for some } x, \quad (2.3)$$

where μ_i is the unknown mean vector field for the i-th group. The inference is based on the Hotelling's T^2 statistic. Let us rewrite (2.1) for an individual subject using the group index i and the subject index j:

$$u^{ij}(x) = \mu^i(x) + \Sigma^{1/2}(x)\epsilon^{ij}(x),$$

where μ^{ij} are the i-th group mean vector and ϵ^{ij} are independent and identically distributed Gaussian random vector field. Let n_i be the number of subjects in the i-th group. The unknown i-th group mean μ^i is estimated as

$$\overline{\mu}^i = \frac{1}{n_i} \sum_{j=1}^{n_i} u^{ij}.$$

Testing hypotheses (2.3) is done by checking the significance of the mean difference $\overline{\mu}^2 - \overline{\mu}^1$.

The Hotelling's T^2 field framework is fairly flexible and can be applicable to wide variety of situations. If we only have one group, we can simply assume μ_2 to be a known vector field and treat the problem as a one sample problem. In the case of a longitudinal study, where two scans per subject are available, we can take μ_1 as the growth velocity by dividing the displacement difference by the scan interval. Then we are testing if there is any significant growth over time. For instance, arrows in Figure 2.2 indicate the principal direction of the brain growth in normally developing children.

The significance of the group difference can be tested using the Hotelling's T^2 statistic

$$H(x) = \frac{n_1 n_2 (n_1 + n_2 - 4)}{3(n_1 + n_2)(n_1 + n_2 - 2)} (\overline{\mu}^2 - \overline{\mu}^1)' \widehat{\Sigma}^{-1} (\overline{\mu}^2 - \overline{\mu}^1)$$

with the pooled sample covariance matrix

$$\widehat{\Sigma} = \frac{1}{n_1 + n_2 - 2} \left[\sum_{j=1}^{n_1} (u^{1j} - \overline{\mu}^1)(u^{1j} - \overline{\mu}^1)' + \sum_{j=1}^{n_2} (u^{2j} - \overline{\mu}^2)(u^{2j} - \overline{\mu}^2)' \right].$$

At each x, under the null hypothesis of $\mu_1(x) = \mu_2(x)$, H is distributed as a F-statistic with 3 and $n_1 + n_2 - 4$ degrees of freedom. This is for two samples but a one-sample case is similar (Chung *et al.*, 2001a, 2008c).

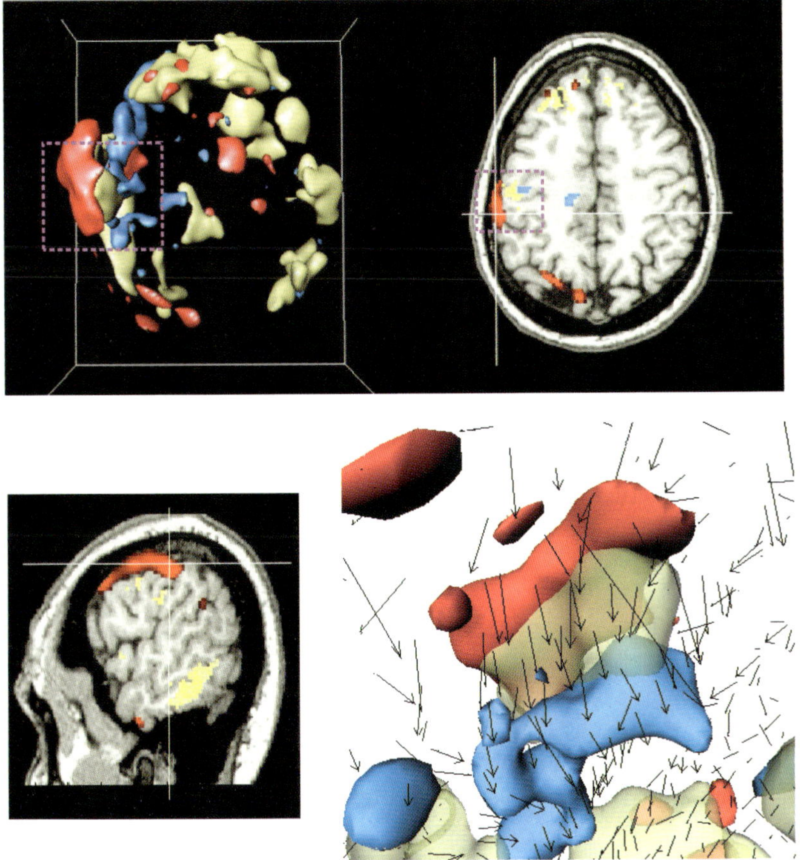

Fig. 2.2 The *p*-value maps of local volume increase (red), volume decrease (blue), and structural displacement (yellow) thresholded at 0.025, 0.025 and 0.05 (corrected) for normally developing children (Chung *et al.*, 2001a). The *p*-value maps are superimposed on the template. The arrows represent the mean displacement difference over time (growth rate). The direction of the growth velocity suggests how the local volume expansion (red) causes the translational movement of the structure (yellow) toward the region of atrophy (blue).

For the one-sample case, we assume μ_2 is a known vector field and the corresponding Hotelling's T^2 statistic is given by

$$H(x) = \frac{n_1(n_1 - 3)}{3(n_1 - 1)} (\overline{\mu}^1 - \mu_2)' \widehat{\Sigma}^{-1} (\overline{\mu}^1 - \mu_2), \qquad (2.4)$$

where the sample covariance is given by

$$\widehat{\Sigma} = \frac{1}{n_1 - 1} \sum_{j=1}^{n_1} (u^{1j} - \overline{\mu}^1)(u^{1j} - \overline{\mu}^1)'.$$

At each voxel x, under the hypothesis, $H(x)$ is distributed as a F-statistic with 3 and $n_1 - 3$ degrees of freedom.

As pointed out in Ashburner and Friston (2000), the Hotelling's T^2 statistic does not directly localize regions within different structures, but rather identifies brain structures that have translated to different positions. It measures relative position of two particular voxels before and after the deformation. In the context of temporally varying brain morphology, where the brain tissue growth is an important concern, the statistic based on the displacement field should be taken as an indirect measure of brain growth (Chung *et al.*, 2001a). A more direct morphological criterion that corresponds to the actual brain tissue growth is the Jacobian of the deformation field, which we will look at in the next chapter.

2.3.3   *Detecting Local Brain Growth*

In this section, we illustrate how DBM can be used to localize the regions of brain growth in detail. The study detail can be found in Chung *et al.* (2001a). Twenty eight normal subjects were selected based on the physical, neurological and psychological criteria described in Giedd *et al.* (1996). Two T1-weighted MR scans were acquired for each subject at different times on the same GE Sigma 1.5 T superconducting magnet system. The first scan was obtained at the age 11.5 ± 3.1 years (min. 7.0 year, max. 17.8 year) and the second scan was obtained at the age 16.1 ± 3.2 years (min. 10.6 year, max. 21.8 year). The time difference between the first and the second scan was 4.6 ± 0.9 years (min. time difference 2.2 year , max. time difference 6.4 year). Using the automatic image-processing pipeline (Zijdenbos *et al.*, 1998), a total of 56 MR images were transformed into standardized stereotactic space via a global affine transformation followed by a nonlinear deformation to match the atlas brain. The global affine transformation removes most of the intra- and inter-subject global differences in brain size; adult brains are approximately 5% larger than those of five year old children (Dekaban, 1977; Dekaban and Shadowsky, 1978). Because we are only interested in finding local morphological changes, these global morphological variabilities should be removed via global affine transform in order to improve the power of detection. These registration procedures

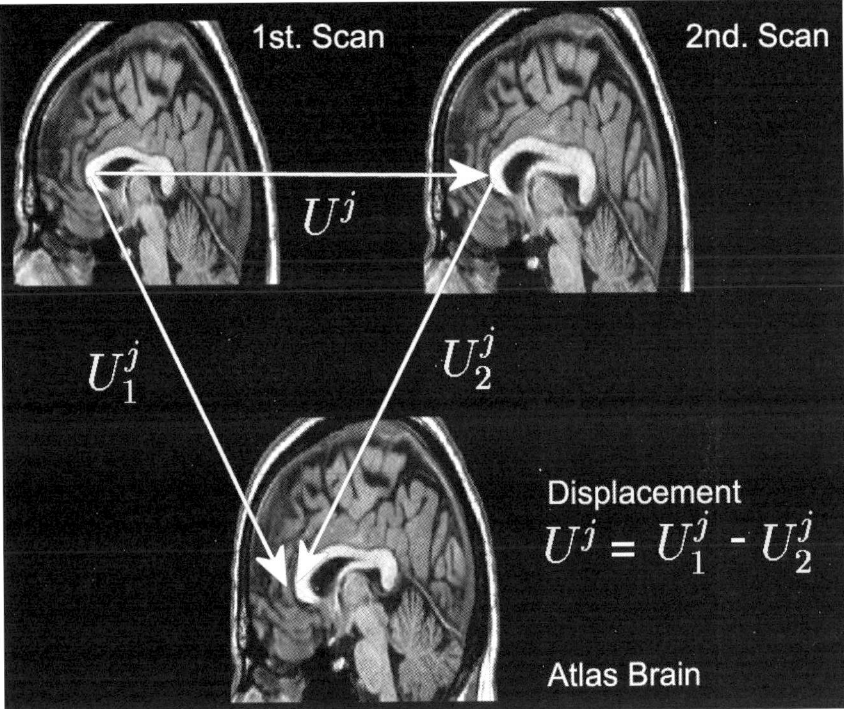

Fig. 2.3   Schematic of registration for longitudinally collected images. If u_1^j and u_2^j are the displacements obtained from registering the first and the second scan of subject j to the atlas brain, the actual displacement u^j between the two scans is $u^j = u_1^j - u_2^j$.

are based on an automatic multi-resolution intensity matching algorithm (Collins and Evans, 1999; Collins *et al.*, 1994). Unlike other registration algorithms that assume a certain fluid dynamics or an elastic deformation model, the intensity-based registration does not assume any explicit physical model in which the deformation from the subject brain to the atlas brain should follow (Gee and Bajcsy, 1999; Thompson *et al.*, 2000). So the deformation fields obtained from these registration processes can be considered free of any explicit physical model assumption although there might be some intensity-based model assumption,which somehow relates to a physical model.

If u_1^j and u_2^j are the displacements obtained from the non-linear registration of the first and the second scan of subject j to the atlas brain $\mathcal{M}$ at time t_1^j and t_2^j, the actual displacement u^j between the first and the second scan is $u^j = u_1^j - u_2^j$ and the time difference is $t_j = t_2^j - t_1^j$ (Figure 2.3). It is true that if the first scan were directly registered to the second scan without going through the template, the registration error would be smaller. However, the displacement fields obtained by the direct registration method still have to be registered onto the atlas brain in order to form statistical parametric maps. The reason for such statistical treatment to analyze the structural data is obvious considering that the displacement field obtained from image registration algorithms for brain development contains a fairly large component of error. The length of the displacement velocity we have observed for the spatially normalized MR scans of 28 normal subjects is usually less than 1mm/year, i.e.

$$\mu_0 = \mathbb{E}\left(\frac{du}{dt}\right) \leq 1 \text{ mm/year}$$

in average. Optimistically assuming that the image registration algorithm is accurate to within one voxel distance (usually 1 or 2 mm), the registration error seems to be relatively large in brain development. So one may be skeptical about whether the deformation-based morphometry can possibly detect such small changes. Nevertheless it is still possible to pick out the signal when there are enough data (Chung *et al.*, 2001a).

Before the test statistic is constructed, image smoothing is usually necessary to guarantee Gaussianness of the displacement field and smooth out possible registration error. Without the smoothing, it may be difficult to detect morphological patterns that may be masked by anatomical noise. However, Gaussian kernel smoothing sometimes tends to blur the fine details of deformation pattern. So the care should be taken in choosing proper amount of smoothing. The standard method for smoothing is to convolve images with Gaussian kernel with predetermined bandwidth that usually ranges from 5-15mm FWHM (full width at half maximum). Given the Gaussian kernel

$$K_\sigma(x) = \frac{1}{(4\pi\sigma)^{3/2}} e^{-\frac{(x-y)^2}{4\sigma}},$$

FWHM of kenrel is given by $4(\ln 2\sigma)^{1/2}$. Gaussian kernel smoothing of image f is then given by the convolution

$$K_\sigma * f = \int_{\mathbb{R}^3} K_\sigma(x-y)f(y)\, dy.$$

Unlike the usual point-wise inference for Hotelling's T^2 statistic, the inference on vector fields needs to account for multiple comparisons across different spatial positions. This is done by determining the threshold for the supremum of the test statistic (Cao and Worsley, 1999b):

$$P\left(\sup_{x \in \mathcal{M}} H(x) > 60.0\right) = 0.05.$$

This determines the statistically significant regions that gives the over all p-value of 0.05 for testing over $\mathcal{M}$. Yellow regions in Figure 2.2 are the thresholded regions showing significant displacement over time. The multiple comparison correction issues are further discussed in Section 1.3. The overall significance computed using the supremum of H field is called the multiple comparisons correction and it will be cored in the next section.

Most of the structural movements were observed in the frontal lobe without any accompanying significant change in local volume. This may indicate that there are continued readjustments of the exact position of brain structures in the frontal lobe without any brain tissue growth or loss in adolescence. Also note that the statistically significant displacement occurs evenly and shows some degree of symmetry between the left and the right hemispheres. Because the local translation statistic measures the relative displacement of brain structure, it does not truly reflect the brain tissue growth process. However, it does indicate the principal direction of the brain growth as shown in the purple box and enlarged in Figure 2.2. Hence, the local translation statistic should be used in conjunction with the local volume change statistic to fully understand the complex dynamics of temporally changing morphological pattern.

2.4 Global Inference via Integral Statistic

Instead of testing the significance of local displacement difference at a specific voxel, we can also test difference in a specific region of interest (ROI) $\mathcal{M}$. We will consider a more general setting where the displacement in (2.1) is defined in d-dimension so that the error term has d components:

$$\epsilon(x) = (\epsilon_1, \cdots, \epsilon_d)'.$$

We will assume further that the covariance matrix Σ is known or can be estimated using the sample covariance.

We are interested in testing

$$H_0 : \mu(x) = 0 \text{ for all } x \in \mathcal{M} \text{ vs. } H_1 : \mu \neq 0 \text{ for some } x \in \mathcal{M}. \quad (2.5)$$

Similar to the Hotelling's T^2 field, we define W-field as

$$W(x) = u'(x)\Sigma^{-1}(x)u(x).$$

Under the null hypothesis, $W(x) = \sum_{i=1}^{d} \epsilon_i^2(x)$ is distributed as a stationary χ_d^2 random field (Worsley, 1994). Consider another null hypothesis

$$H_0' : \int_{\mathcal{M}} \|\mu\|^2(x)\, dx = 0, \qquad (2.6)$$

where $\mathcal{M}_0$ is the ROI. The two hypotheses H_0 and H_0' are equivalent over the equivalent class of a function g which satisfies

$$\int_{\mathcal{M}} |g|^2(x)\, dx = 0.$$

Therefore, instead of testing the null hypothesis H_0, we will test H_0'. Under H_0', the exact distribution of the random variable $\int_{\mathcal{M}} W(x)\, dx$ can be found using the Karhunen-Loève expansion (Adler, 1990; Dougherty, 1999; Kwapien and Woyczynski, 1992; Yaglom, 1987).

2.4.1   *Karhunen-Loève Expansion*

Let $\mathcal{G}$ be the space of zero mean Gaussian random fields in $\mathcal{M} \subset \mathbb{R}^d$ with inner product

$$\langle X, Y \rangle = \mathbb{E} \int_{\mathcal{M}} X(x)Y(x)\, dx$$

with $\|X\| < \infty$. This is basically the integral of cross-covariance function between fields X and Y. $\mathcal{G}$ can be shown to be a separable Hilbert space. This can be shown by finding countable orthonormal basis in $\mathcal{G}$ (Adler and Taylor, 2007). The Karhunen-Loéve expansion states that for a mean zero Gaussian random field $Z(x)$ in $\mathcal{G}$ with mean square continuity property over a bounded domain $\mathcal{M} \subset \mathbb{R}^d$, there exist independent mean zero Gaussian random variables $Z_i \sim N(0, \sigma_i^2)$ and orthonormal bases ψ_i such that

$$Z(x) = \sum_{i=0}^{\infty} Z_i \psi_i(x). \qquad (2.7)$$

If $\mathbb{E}Z(x) \neq 0$ for some x, we can always center the field by translating toward the sample mean. The basis ψ_i are orthonormal in $\mathcal{M}$ such that $\langle \psi_i, \psi_j \rangle = \delta_{ij}$. Let $\sigma_i^2 = \mathbb{E}Z_i^2 < \infty$. Since $\mathbb{E}Z(x) = 0$, the covariance function of $Z(x)$ is given by

$$R(x, y) = \mathbb{E} \sum_{i,j=0}^{\infty} Z_i \psi_i(x) Z_j \psi_i(y) \qquad (2.8)$$

$$= \sum_{i=0}^{\infty} \sigma_i^2 \psi_i(x) \psi_i(y). \qquad (2.9)$$

The covariance function of a zero mean Gaussian field completely characterizes the field itself. Obviously R has to be symmetric to be expressible in this fashion. This fact is related to Mercer's theorem (Conway, 1990).

If $f_j(x)$ is the realization of the random field Z, the parameters σ_i^2 can be estimated by matching the moment in the following fashion. From (2.9), we have

$$R(x,x) = \sum_{i=0}^{\infty} \sigma_i^2 \psi_i^2(x).$$

If we assume f_j are also centered, the left hand side is the variance field, which can be estimated using the sample variance field:

$$\frac{1}{n} \sum_{j=1}^{n} f_j^2(x).$$

Then we first estimate the parameter σ_0 by solving

$$\frac{1}{n} \sum_{j=1}^{n} \int_{\mathcal{M}} f_j^2(x) \, dx = \sigma_0^2 \int_{\mathcal{M}} \psi_0^2(x) \, dx.$$

Once we estimated σ_0 as $\widehat{\sigma_0}$, the next parameter σ_1 is then estimated by solving

$$\frac{1}{n} \sum_{j=1}^{n} \int_{\mathcal{M}} f_j^2(x) - \widehat{\sigma_0}^2 \int_{\mathcal{M}} \psi_0^2(x) \, dx = \sigma_1^2 \int_{\mathcal{M}} \psi_1^2(x) \, dx.$$

The process is iteratively performed until we obtain a sufficiently high degree representation.

Example. The Karhunen-Loève expansion is just one example of many possible orthonormal expansions of a function. Through the book, we will see many different types of similar expansions. Here is an example of orthonormal expansion on a displacement field. Consider a 3D MRI of size $L_1 \times L_2 \times L_3$. For instance, $L_1 \times L_2 \times L_3 = 236 \times 191 \times 171$ mm. In this 3D domain, the orthonormal basis can be computed easily. The eigenfunctions and the eigenvalues of the Laplacian

$$\Delta = \frac{\partial^2}{\partial x_1^2} + \frac{\partial^2}{\partial x_2^2} + \frac{\partial^2}{\partial x_3^2}$$

is constructed by solving

$$\Delta g + \lambda g = 0. \tag{2.10}$$

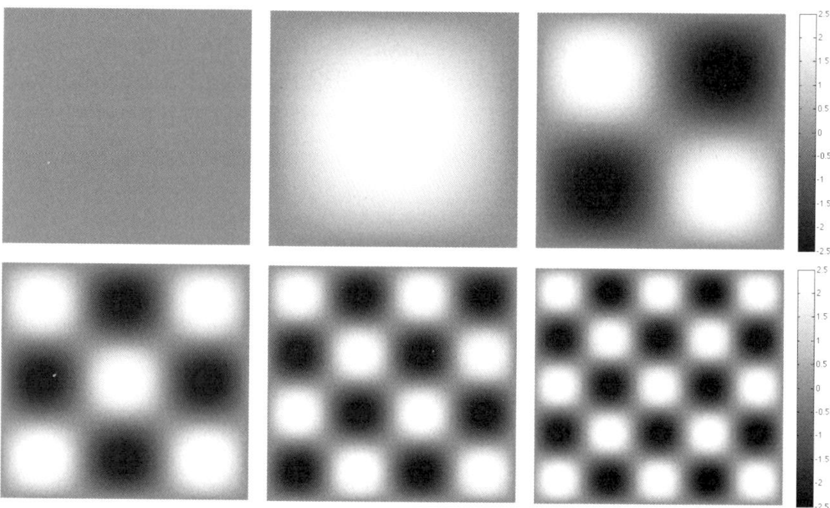

Fig. 2.4   The first six eigenfunctions ψ_l in a rectangular domain. Any sufficiently smooth random signal f can represented as $f = \sum_{l=0}^{k} f_l \psi_l$ with the Fourier coefficients f_l, which are random.

Some literatures define the Laplacian negatively, so care should be taken. With notation $l = (l_1, l_2, l_3)$, the eigenfunctions are

$$\psi_l(x) = \left(\frac{\sqrt{2}}{L_1} \sin \frac{\pi l_1 x_1}{L_1} \right) \left(\frac{\sqrt{2}}{L_2} \sin \frac{\pi l_2 x_2}{L_2} \right) \left(\frac{\sqrt{2}}{L_3} \sin \frac{\pi l_3 x_2}{L_3} \right)$$

and the eigenvalues are

$$\lambda_l = \left(\frac{l_1 \pi}{L_1} \right)^2 + \left(\frac{l_2 \pi}{L_2} \right)^2 + \left(\frac{l_3 \pi}{L_3} \right)^2.$$

An example of the first six eigenfunctions in 2D rectangular domain is given in Figure 2.4. Let $L^2(\mathcal{M})$ be the space of square integrable functions in $\mathcal{M}$ with the inner product

$$\langle g_1, g_2 \rangle = \int_{\mathcal{M}} g_1(p) g_2(p) \, dp. \tag{2.11}$$

The norm $\| \cdot \|$ is defined as $\|g\| = \langle g, g \rangle^{1/2}$. With respect to the inner product, the eigenfunctions ψ_l form orthonormal basis in $\mathcal{M}$ so that $\langle \psi_l, \psi_m \rangle = \delta_{lm}$, the Dirac-delta. Then using the orthonormal basis ψ_l, it is possible to expand a displacement field in a coordinate-wise fashion (Figure 2.5).

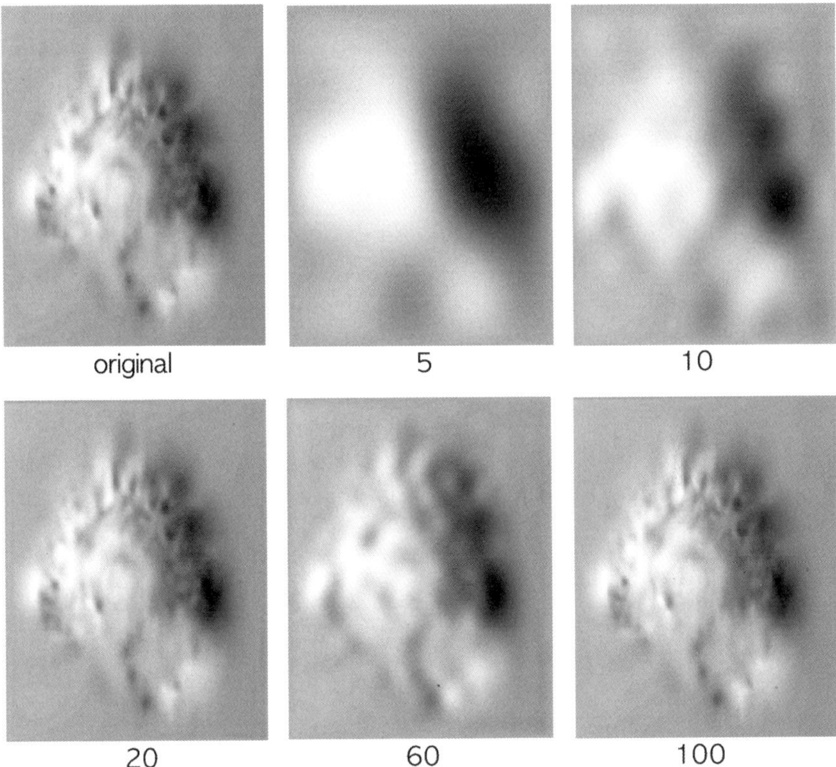

original	5	10
20	60	100

Fig. 2.5 The orthonormal expansion of displacement vector (x-coordinate) using ψ_l in the midsagittal cross section. The numbers represent the degree of expansion. For instance 100 is for $l = (100, 100)$ which uses 10000 number of basis.

2.4.2 *Mercer's Theorem*

For continuous symmetric kernel R, define linear operator $\mathcal{L} : L^2(\mathcal{M}) \to L^2(\mathcal{M})$ as

$$\mathcal{L}f(x) = \int_{\mathcal{M}} R(x, y) f(y) \, dy.$$

This is a compact self-adjoint operator. The linear operator yields unique countable eigenvalues σ_i^2 and orthonormal eigenfunctions ψ_i of the operator $\mathcal{L}$ such that

$$\mathcal{L}\psi_i = \sigma_i^2 \psi_i \tag{2.12}$$

with $\sigma_\infty^2 = 0$. Equation (2.12) is a Fredholm equation of the first kind and ψ_i and σ_i^2 can be estimated numerically if the kernel $R(x, y)$ is given

(Arfken, 2000). We will order the eigenvalues such that

$$\sigma_0^2 > \sigma_1^2 > \sigma_2^2 > \cdots .$$

Then any function $f \in L^2(\mathcal{M})$ can be represented as

$$f = \sum_{i=1}^{\infty} \langle \psi_i, f \rangle \psi_i.$$

Subsequently, the operator $\mathcal{L}$ has a spectral representation

$$\mathcal{L}f = \sum_{i=0}^{\infty} \sigma_i^2 \langle \psi_i, f \rangle \psi_i.$$

Then Mercer's theorem states that kernel R is expressed as

$$R(x,y) = \sum_{i=0}^{\infty} \sigma_i^2 \psi_i(x)\psi_i(y). \tag{2.13}$$

A special case of Mercer's theorem is when R is the heat kernel given by

$$R(x,y) = \sum_{i=0}^{\sigma} e^{-\lambda_i t}\psi_i(x)\psi_i(y).$$

The corresponding linear operator $\mathcal{L}$ is the *heat kernel smoothing* operator defined as

$$\mathcal{L}f(x) = \sum_{i=0}^{\sigma} e^{-\lambda_i t}\langle \psi_i, f \rangle \psi_i(x).$$

Mercer's theorem can be proved using the following argument given in Courant and Hilbert (1953). Suppose we fix y. Then from the Weierstrass's approximation theorem, for continuous function, $R(x, \cdot) = \sum_{i=0}^{\infty} \alpha_i(x)$ for some basis functions α_i uniformly. Now fix x and we have

$$R(x,y) = \sum_{i=0}^{\infty} \alpha_i(x) \sum_{j=0}^{\infty} \beta_j(y) \tag{2.14}$$

$$= \sum_{i,j=0}^{\infty} \alpha_i(x)\beta_j(y) \tag{2.15}$$

Again, β_j are basis functions. For basis $\alpha_1, \cdots, \alpha_p$ and $\beta_1, \cdots, \beta_p$, they can be rewritten as a linear combination of our orthonormal basis ψ using the Gram-Schmidt orthogonalization. So some algebraic manipulation can show that

$$R(x,y) = \sum_{i,j=0}^{\infty} c_{ij}\psi_i(x)\psi_j(x) \tag{2.16}$$

for some c_{ij}. Another way of looking at this problem is by noting that $\psi_i(x)\psi_j(y)$ forms a orthonormal basis for $\mathcal{M} \otimes \mathcal{M}$. Then for the covariance function $R(x,y) \in L^2(\mathcal{M} \otimes \mathcal{M})$, we immediately have the series expansion (2.16).

We will identify c_{ij}, using the definition of $\mathcal{L}$. We have

$$
\begin{aligned}
\mathcal{L}\psi_k(x) &= \sum_{i,j=0}^{\infty} c_{ij}\psi_i(x) \int_{\mathcal{M}} \psi_k(y)\psi_j(y)\,dy \\
&= \sum_{i,j=0}^{\infty} c_{ij}\psi_i(x)\delta_{kj} \\
&= \sum_{i=0}^{\infty} c_{ik}\psi_i(x).
\end{aligned}
\tag{2.17}
$$

We need to equate (2.17) to $\sigma_k^2\psi_k(x)$. The only way it is satisfied for all x and k is when $c_{kk} = \sigma_k^2$ and $c_{ik} = 0$ for $i \neq k$. Hence we proved the statement of Mercer's theorem (2.13).

2.4.3 *Integral Statistic on Displacement*

Let us continue our derivation of the distribution of $\int_{\mathcal{M}} W(x)\,dx$. The error components ϵ_i are distributed as independent and identically distributed isotropic Gaussian random fields. Using the Karhunen-Loève expansion, we represent the error components as

$$
\epsilon_i(x) = \sum_{j=0}^{\infty} \epsilon_{ij}\psi_j(x)
$$

with $\mathbb{E}(\epsilon_{ij}^2) = \sigma_j^2$ and ϵ_{ij} are independent Gaussian random variables for all i, j. Then it follows that

$$
\begin{aligned}
\int_{\mathcal{M}} W(x)\,dx &= \sum_{i=1}^{d} \langle \epsilon_i, \epsilon_i \rangle \\
&= \sum_{i=1}^{d} \sum_{j,k=0}^{\infty} \int_{\mathcal{M}} \epsilon_{ij}\epsilon_{ik}\psi_j(t)\psi_k(t)\,dt \\
&= \sum_{i=1}^{d} \sum_{j=0}^{\infty} \epsilon_{ij}^2 \\
&= \sum_{j=0}^{\infty} \sum_{i=1}^{d} \epsilon_{ij}^2.
\end{aligned}
$$

Note that

$$\sum_{i=1}^{d} \epsilon_{ij}^2 \overset{D}{\sim} \sigma_j^2 X_j,$$

where X_j are distributed as independent χ_d^2, the chi-square distribution with d degrees of freedom. Summing up the results, we have the exact distribution for global displacement change:

$$\int_{\mathcal{M}} W(x)\, dx \overset{D}{\sim} \sum_{j=0}^{\infty} \sigma_j^2 X_j. \tag{2.18}$$

This is the infinite sum of i.i.d. χ^2 random variables with different degrees of freedom. There is no close form expression for the distribution so we will approximate it with a single scaled χ^2 distribution by matching moments (Satterthwaite, 1946). Approximately we have

$$\sum_{j=0}^{\infty} \sigma_j^2 X_j \overset{D}{\sim} c\chi_\nu^2, \tag{2.19}$$

where c and degree ν need to be estimated by matching the 1st and 2nd moments.

The expectation and the variance of the left hand side in (2.19) are given by

$$\mathbb{E}\left(\sum_{j=0}^{\infty} \sigma_j^2 X_j\right) = d \sum_{j=0}^{\infty} \sigma_j^2$$

$$\mathbb{V}\left(\sum_{j=0}^{\infty} \sigma_j^2 X_j\right) = 2d \sum_{j=0}^{\infty} \sigma_j^4.$$

This is due to the fact that the mean and the variance of χ_d-distribution is d and $2d$ respectively. The variance can be directly derived by computing the 4th moment of a Gaussian random variable. Consider Gaussian random variables $Z_i \sim N(0,1)$. We have

$$\mathbb{E}\left(\sum_{j=0}^{\infty} \sigma_j^2 X_j\right)^2 = \sum_{j=0}^{\infty} \sigma_j^4 \mathbb{E}X_j^2.$$

Since X_j is chi-square with d degrees of freedom, it can be written as

$$X_j = \sum_{i=1}^{d} Z_i^2$$

and we have

$$\mathbb{E}X_j^2 = \sum_{i,k=1}^{d} \mathbb{E}(Z_i^2 Z_k^2)$$
$$= d\mathbb{E}Z_1^4 + (d^2 - d)\mathbb{E}Z_1^2 \mathbb{E}Z_2^2$$
$$= d^2 + 2d.$$

The first term $\mathbb{E}Z_1^4$ is computed iteratively (Janssen and Stoica, 1988):

$$\mathbb{E}[Z_1 Z_2 Z_3 Z_4] = \mathbb{E}[Z_1 Z_2]\mathbb{E}[Z_3 Z_4] + \mathbb{E}[Z_1 Z_3]\mathbb{E}[Z_2 Z_4]$$
$$+\mathbb{E}[Z_1 Z_4]\mathbb{E}[Z_2 Z_3].$$

Now let $Z_1 = Z_2 = Z_3 = Z_4$. Then $\mathbb{E}Z_1^4 = 3$. The higher order moment of zero mean Gaussian random variable can be also obtained by differentiating the moment generating function $e^{-t^2/2}$ which yields Hermite polynomials. The variance $\mathbb{V}X_i^2$ is then given by $2d$.

The mean and the variance of the right hand side of (2.19) are $c\nu$ and $2c^2\nu$. Now by matching the mean and variance on both sides of (2.19), we obtain

$$c\nu = d\sum_{j=0}^{\infty} \sigma_j^2, \ c^2\nu = d\sum_{j=0}^{\infty} \sigma_j^4.$$

Solving the equations simultaneously we obtain

$$c = \frac{\sum_{j=0}^{\infty} \sigma_j^4}{\sum_{j=0}^{\infty} \sigma_j^2}, \ \nu = d\frac{(\sum_{j=0}^{\infty} \sigma_j^2)^2}{\sum_{j=0}^{\infty} \sigma_j^4}.$$

Based on this approximate distribution, a statistical inference on ROI can be done.

Chapter 3

Tensor-Based Morphometry

Another very promising technique for non-ROI based morphometry is tensor-based morphometry (TBM), which uses the spatial derivatives of deformation fields (Ashburner and Friston, 2000; Thompson *et al.*, 2000; Chung *et al.*, 2001a). Similar to DBM, TBM does not require segmentation of *a priori* regions of interest (Ashburner and Friston, 2000; Davatzikos, 1999). The morphological tensor maps are computed at each voxel level and used to quantify the variations in length, area, volume, the cortical thickness and surface curvature (Thompson *et al.*, 2000; Chung *et al.*, 2003c). From these tensor maps, 3D statistical parametric maps (SPM) are created for a group of subjects to quantify the variations in length, area, volume and surface curvature and to visualize these variations in the 3D is whole brain volume (Chung *et al.*, 2001a), on the 2D cortical surface (Thompson *et al.*, 2001; Andrade *et al.*, 2001; Chung *et al.*, 2003c) and on the surface of the brain substructures such as the hippocampus and amygdala (Wang *et al.*, 2003). In TBM, the Jacobian determinant of the deformation field, which is required to register one brain to another, is mainly used to quantify volumetric changes at voxel level. By definition, the Jacobian determinant of the deformation is the volume of the unit-cube after the deformation. Assuming that one can find the deformation field at each voxel, tissue growth or loss can be quantified at a voxel level.

Davatzikos *et al.* used the Jacobian determinant of the 2D deformation field as a measure of local area-change in 2D cross-sections of the corpus callosum to test gender-specific shape differences (Davatzikos *et al.*, 1996) . Thompson and Toga applied the Jacobian of 3D deformations as a measure of the regional growth of the corpus callosum (Thompson and Toga, 1999). Also dilatation, which is the first order approximation of the Jacobian determinant, has been used instead of the Jacobian itself to measure local

49

volume change (Chung *et al.*, 2001a). Thirion *et al* (Thirion and Calmon, 1999) used the divergence of the displacement vector field, which is equivalent to the dilatation, for detecting growth of brain tumors. Thompson *et al* (Thompson *et al.*, 2000) used local rates of dilatation, contraction and shearing from the deformation field to detect morphological changes in brain development. In particular, Chung *et al.* (2001a) showed the unified modeling framework for combining DBM and TBM in a single general linear modeling framework rather than two separate linear models for each techniques. Although it seems that there are many different ways of detecting morphological changes in DBM or TBM, a translation, a rotation and a strain are sufficient for detecting a relatively small displacement and, in turn, for characterization of morphological changes over time.

3.1   Jacobian Determinant

Let $u(x) = (u_1, u_2, u_3)$, $x \in \mathbb{R}^3$ be the displacement vector field of warping the template to an individual image. The actual deformation is given by $d(x) = x + u(x)$. The *Jacobian matrix J* of the deformation d is then defined as the spatial derivative of d:

$$ J = \frac{\partial d}{\partial x'} = I + \nabla u, $$

where I is a 3×3 identity matrix and ∇u is the *displacement gradient matrix* given by

$$ \nabla u = \frac{\partial u}{\partial x'} = \begin{pmatrix} \frac{\partial u_1}{\partial x_1} & \frac{\partial u_1}{\partial x_2} & \frac{\partial u_1}{\partial x_3} \\ \frac{\partial u_2}{\partial x_1} & \frac{\partial u_2}{\partial x_2} & \frac{\partial u_2}{\partial x_3} \\ \frac{\partial u_3}{\partial x_1} & \frac{\partial u_3}{\partial x_2} & \frac{\partial u_3}{\partial x_3} \end{pmatrix}. $$

The nine components of the gradient matrix ∇u are called the *displacement tensor* and are used to measure the second-order morphological variabilities (Ashburner *et al.*, 2000; Chung *et al.*, 2001a). Note that the displacement u, which can be viewed as local translation at each voxel, captures the first-order morphological variability. A statistical model for the displacement gradient is directly derived from (2.1) by taking the partial derivative with respect to the spatial coordinates x. This avoids having two separate possibly incompatible statistical models for deformation and the Jacobian determinant of the deformation (Chung *et al.*, 2001a). In this unified statistical framework, all possible statistical distributions of morphological test criteria can be directly derived and easily manipulated from (2.1).

The *Jacobian determinant* det J is then given by

$$\det J(x) = \det(I + \nabla u).$$

The Jacobian determinant det J measures the volume of the deformed unit-cube. In brain imaging, a voxel can be considered as the unit-cube; therefore, the Jacobian determinant essentially measures the change in the volume of voxel at the voxel position x after the deformation. Expanding the Jacobian determinant det J, we get

$$\det J = \det(I + \nabla u)$$
$$= 1 + \mathrm{tr}\ \nabla u + \mathrm{detr}_2 \nabla u + \det \nabla u,$$

where $\mathrm{detr}_2 \nabla u$ is the sum of 2×2 principal minors of ∇u. For sufficiently small displacements, we may neglect the higher order terms and get

$$\det J \approx 1 + \mathrm{tr}\ \nabla u.$$

In the elastic theory (Marsden and Hughes, 1983), the *volume dilatation* is defined as

$$\nabla \cdot u = \ \mathrm{tr}\nabla u. \tag{3.1}$$

Therefore, the Jacobian determinant difference with respect to the unit-cube, i.e. $\det J - 1$ is then linearly approximated by the volume dilation (Chung *et al.*, 2001a).

3.2   Distributional Assumptions

The Jacobian determinant has been widely used as the major morphometric measure for quantifying the amount of brain tissue locally at each voxel. Traditionally a normal distribution has been assumed in the Jacobian determinant (Chung *et al.*, 2001a; Davatzikos *et al.*, 1996; Thompson and Toga, 1999; Thompson *et al.*, 2000). In particular, a unified Gaussian noise model for a deformation field and its Jacobian determinant is proposed in (Chung *et al.*, 2001a) using the dilatation rate, which is the trace of the Jacobian determinant and linearly approximates the Jacobian determinant. Recently the lognormal distribution has been more often used in modeling the Jacobian determinant since it provides intuitively pleasurable interpretation in the inverse-consistent registration framework (Ashburner *et al.*, 1999; Leow *et al.*, 2007, 2006). The argument for log-normality is as follows.

(1) Skewness: In order to have one-to-one mapping, the Jacobian determinant $\det J$ has to be positive. Therefore, $\det J$ can not possibly be normally distributed since the normal distribution has infinite support. On the other hand, lognormal distributions are skewed and defined in $\mathbb{R}^+$.

(2) Symmetry: Given the Jacobian determinant $\det J_d$ of deformation d, the Jacobian determinant $\det J_{d^{-1}}$ of the inverse mapping d^{-1} is simply $1/\det J_d$. In the usual inverse-consistent registration framework, the distributions of $\det J_d$ and $1/\det J_d$ have to be identical. If we assume $\det J_d$ is lognormal, $\log \det J_d$ and $\log(1/\det J_d) = -\log \det J_d$ are normally distributed satisfying the inverse-consistency in statistical sense.

(3) Multiplicity: If the length measure L follows some distribution, it is reasonable to assume the volume measure L^3 will also follow a similar distribution. Lognormal distributions satisfy this multiplicity rule. In Ashburner *et al.* (1999), the Jacobian determinant is decomposed using the singular value decomposition

$$J = USV'.$$

The unitary matrices U and V represent rotations and the diagonal matrix $S = (s_{ij})$ represents the relative stretching in orthogonal directions. It is argued that length and volume changes should have similar distributions. If the diagonal elements s_{jj} follow lognormal distributions,

$$\log \det J = \log s_{11} + \log s_{22} + \log s_{33}$$

is distributed as normal and subsequently $\det J$ is lognormal as well.

On the other hand, normality of the Jacobian determinant is also proposed (Chung *et al.*, 2001a). Traditionally the displacement vector field u has been modeled to follow Gaussian. In (2.1), we have modeled the components of displacement field as correlated Gaussian with the covariance matrix Σ. Since derivatives of a Gaussian field and the sum of Gaussian field are again Gaussian, the volume dilatation is again Gaussian. Therefore, we have a linear model on the volume dilatation Λ given by

$$\Lambda(x) = \lambda(x) + \epsilon(x), \tag{3.2}$$

where λ is the mean volume dilatation rate and ϵ is a Gaussian random field with zero mean. When $\lambda(x) = 0$ in the neighborhood of x, the deformation is incompressible so there is no volume change. However, if $\lambda > 0$, the volume increases while $\lambda < 0$, the volume decreases after the deformation. In certain image registration algorithms, the Jacobian determinant is forced to be larger than a certain threshold to ensure the homologous correspondence between two brains (Christensen *et al.*, 1997). When such a registration algorithm is used, the power of detecting the region of statistically significant volume change may be reduced. The statistical inference on the dilation model (3.2) is easier than the displacement model (2.1). To detect statistically significant local volume change, a t random field can be used (Worsley, 1994). The t random field is defined as

$$T(x) = \sqrt{n}\frac{M(x)}{S(x)}, \qquad (3.3)$$

where M and S are the sample mean and standard deviation of the j-th dilatation Λ^j. Under the assumption of no local volume change at x, i.e. $\lambda(x) = 0$, t-field is distributed as t_{n-1}, the student t-distribution with $n-1$ degrees of freedom. Then the p-value of the maxima of $T(x)$, which corrects for searching across a whole brain volume, is used to localize the region of statistically significant structural displacement.

3.3 Local Volume Changes

DBM and TBM are competing but complimentary techniques providing different but related characterization of morphometric changes. Interesting relations between displacement change and volume change is illustrated in Figure 2.2, which is the close-up view of the parietal region of the left hemisphere (the purple square), showing a large local displacement from the region of local volume increase (gray matter) to a region of local volume decrease (white matter), indicating how the structure boundary (inner cortical surface) has moved from the increasing volume to the decreasing volume. This phenomenon is also schematically illustrated in Figure 3.1, where the original cartesian coordinates (a) undergoes various deformations: (b) horizontal translation from the region of volume increase on the left to the region of volume decrease on the right, (c) rotation without volume change, and (d) volume expansion in the middle causing the neighboring structures to radially translate outward.

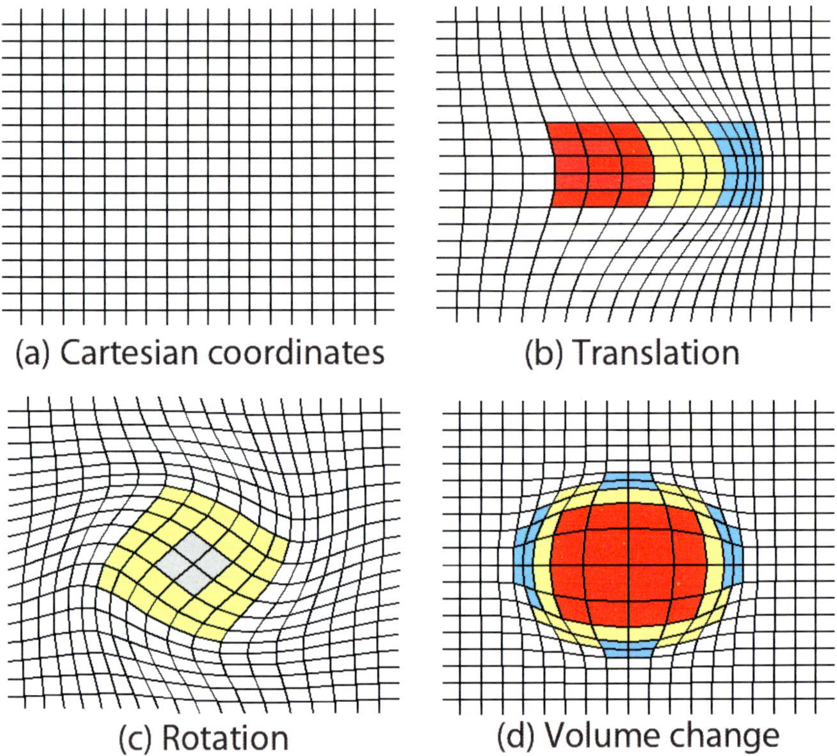

Fig. 3.1   Schematics of cartesian coordinates under translation, rotation and volume change. Red: volume increase, Blue: volume decrease, Grey: rotation, Yellow: translation. (a) Cartesian coordinates under no deformation. (b) Horizontal translation caused by local volume increase on the left side. (c) 45 degree clockwise rotation. The rotation induces the outer region of the center of the rotation to translate. (d) Volume expansion in the middle causes the grid to radially translate outward.

So far we have presented two different statistics (2.4) and (3.3), based on translation and volume changes to measure morphological changes. One might ask if these two statistics obtained from DBM and TBM are sufficient to capture morphological changes in brain and how one statistic is related to the other. Do they measure common morphological properties or different aspects of morphological changes? In this section, we will give some answers to these questions.

For relatively small displacement, neglecting higher order terms, the displacement u at $x + dx$ can be approximated using the first order Taylor expansion:

$$u(x + dx) \approx u(x) + \nabla u(x)\, dx.$$

The displacement tensor is then further decomposed into two components depending on whether it is symmetric or antisymmetric:

$$\frac{\partial u_j}{\partial x_i} = \frac{1}{2}\left(\frac{\partial u_j}{\partial x_i} - \frac{\partial u_i}{\partial x_j}\right) + \frac{1}{2}\left(\frac{\partial u_j}{\partial x_i} + \frac{\partial u_i}{\partial x_j}\right).$$

The antisymmetric first part corresponds to a rotation or vorticity of the deformation and the symmetric second part corresponds to a strain. Then the displacement at $x + dx$ can be decomposed into three parts:

$$u(x + dx) \approx u(x) - w(x) \times dx + \varepsilon(x)dx, \tag{3.4}$$

where $w = \frac{1}{2}(\nabla \times u)$ is the vorticity vector and

$$\varepsilon = (\varepsilon_{ij}) = \frac{1}{2}\left[\nabla u + (\nabla u)'\right]$$

is the strain matrix. (3.4) captures most of the variabilities of the displacement into three components: translation, rotation and and strain for relatively small displacement. The strain tensor ε_{ij} can be further separated into two parts: the diagonal elements ε_{ii} describing the length change of the volume element in each x_1, x_2 and x_3 coordinate, and the off-diagonal elements ε_{ij} describing the shearing rate of the volume element.

The *volume element* is a mathematical abstraction defined as an infinitesimally small cube, but because the smallest unit in brain imaging is a voxel, we may take the voxel as the volume element. Shearing is the deformation that preserves the volume of a voxel but distorts its shape. Note that the sum of the diagonal elements of the strain rate is the volume dilatation. It seems that we need to consider translational, rotational and strain changes for a complete morphological description. However, the most meaningful measurement of brain tissue growth or loss is the Jacobian determinant or dilation because it directly measures the volumetric changes in the brain. The local translation, the local rotation and the local shearing change can all be considered as readjustments and reorientations of the local brain structures due to the volumetric changes in the neighboring regions. In between-subject morphological studies of different clinical populations, such measurements might be useful criteria of shape differences. However, in temporally varying within-subject brain morphological studies, we are more interested in regions of brain tissue growth or loss that cause the volumetric changes so the Jacobian determinant or volume dilation would be more important measures.

The dilatation statistic that consists of spatial derivatives of the displacement field is *statistically independent* from the local translation statistic. To see this, note that any partial derivative of a stationary Gaussian random field is statistically independent from the field itself (Adler, 1981). Since the dilatation consists of spatial derivatives of the displacement, it must be statistically independent of the displacement. So the Hotelling's T^2 field of the displacement and the T-field of the dilatation measure morphologically and statistically different properties even at the same voxel. By studying these two statistics simultaneously, the complex dynamic patterns in brain morphology can be captured.

3.4 Longitudinal Modeling

Longitudinal modeling usually entails analyzing multiple image scans per subject while explicitly incorporating within-subject correlation between the scans. In general, longitudinal anatomical variation within-subject is supposed to be smaller than cross-sectional anatomical variation between-subject.

Suppose a subject has m scans $\mathcal{I}_1, \cdots, \mathcal{I}_m$ obtained at times $t_1 < \cdots < t_m$. Let d_{ij} be the deformation from $\mathcal{I}_i$ to $\mathcal{I}_j$ and d_i be the deformation from $\mathcal{I}_i$ to a template $\mathcal{T}$. We expect the variance of d_{ij} is likely to be substantially smaller than that of d_i or d_j, i.e.

$$\text{tr}\,(\mathbb{V}d_{ij}) < \text{tr}\,(\mathbb{V}d_i),$$

where $\mathbb{V}d_{ij}$ is the covariance matrix of d_{ij}. In order to minimize the total image registration error associated with registering m scans to the template $\mathcal{T}$, we usually register the within-subject scans sequentially first among them and register one of them to the template. We obtain deformation to the template sequentially as follows

$$d_2 = d_{21} \circ d_1, \tag{3.5}$$

$$d_3 = d_{32} \circ d_2 = d_{32} \circ d_{21} \circ d_1, \tag{3.6}$$

$$d_m = d_{m,m-1} \circ d_{m-1} = d_{m,m-1} \circ \cdots \circ d_{21} \circ d_1. \tag{3.7}$$

In this backward scheme, the first scan $\mathcal{I}_1$ is registered to the template and all other scans are sequentially registered in the backward direction to the first scan. In the forward scheme, scans are sequentially registered in the forward direction to the last scan $\mathcal{I}_m$ and obtain

$$d_{m-1} = d_{m-1,m} \circ d_m,$$
$$d_{m-2} = d_{m-2,m-1} \circ d_{m-1} = d_{m-2,m-1} \circ d_{m-1,m} \circ d_m,$$
$$d_1 = d_{12} \circ d_2 = d_{12} \circ d_{23} \cdots \circ d_{m-1,m} \circ d_m.$$

Alternatively, we may choose to register longitudinal scans to scan $\mathcal{I}_k$ which is somewhere in the middle of age range t_1 and t_m to even further minimize the total within-subject registration error. In this case, the total variance associated with registering to $\mathcal{I}_k$ and then to the template is

$$\mathrm{tr}\ (\mathbb{V}d_{1k}) + \cdots + \mathrm{tr}\ (\mathbb{V}d_{m,k}) + \mathrm{tr}\ (\mathbb{V}d_k),$$

which is smaller than the total variance associated with registering all m scans to the template:

$$\sum_{i=1}^{m} \mathrm{tr}\ (\mathbb{V}d_i).$$

If we denote J_{ij}, J_i be the Jacobian of the deformations d_{ij}, d_i respectively, the Jacobian determinant for the composite map (3.7) obeys the multiplicity rule:

$$\det J_2 = \det J_{21} \det J_1.$$

Then the log-Jacobian follows the addictivity rule:

$$\log \det J_2 = \log \det J_{21} + \log \det J_1.$$

Therefore, under the assumption of lognormality, longitudinal analysis on the Jacobian determinant becomes a straightforward linear modeling problem.

3.4.1 *Normal Brain Development in Children*

This study is based on the longitudinally collected MRI of children between ages 11 and 16 and published in Chung *et al.* (2001a). This is the same data set where we applied the deformation-based morphometry in Section 2.3.2). Two MR scans were acquired for each subject at about 11 and 16 years. The aim of the study is to localize the region of the brain tissue growth and atrophy using the Jacobian determinants. The longitudinal modeling is usually done via mixed effect models that account for correlation structure of the repeated scans of the same subjects. However, we will show how to set up a dynamic growth model without using the mixed effect model first. The mixed effect model will be covered in the later chapter.

Since the Jacobian J measures the volume of the deformed unit-cube after time t, the rate of the change of the Jacobian J, i.e. $\partial J/\partial t$ is the rate of the local volume change. Expanding the Jacobian J and taking the partial derivative with respect to the temporal coordinate t, we get

$$
\begin{aligned}
\frac{\partial J}{\partial t} &= \frac{1}{\partial t}\det\left(I + \frac{\partial u}{\partial x}\right) \\
&= \frac{1}{\partial t}\left(1 + \frac{\partial u_1}{\partial x_1} + \frac{\partial u_2}{\partial x_2} + \frac{\partial u_3}{\partial x_3} + \cdots\right),
\end{aligned}
$$

where the higher order terms are relatively small compared to the first order terms $\partial u_j/\partial x_j$. So neglecting the higher order terms, we can approximate the rate of the Jacobian change linearly:

$$
\begin{aligned}
\frac{\partial J}{\partial t} &\doteq \frac{\partial u_1}{\partial t \partial x_1} + \frac{\partial u_2}{\partial t \partial x_2} + \frac{\partial u_3}{\partial t \partial x_3} \\
&= \frac{1}{\partial t}(\nabla \cdot u),
\end{aligned}
$$

where $\nabla \cdot$ is the divergence operator.

Therefore, the rate of the Jacobian change is approximately the rate of the volume dilatation $K = \nabla \cdot u$ change for relatively small displacements, i.e.

$$
\frac{\partial J}{\partial t} \doteq \frac{\partial K}{\partial t}.
$$

Since derivatives of a Gaussian field and the sum of Gaussian fields are again Gaussian fields, from the equation, we have a linear model on the dilatation rate given by

$$
\frac{\partial K}{\partial t}(x, t) = \kappa(x) + \epsilon(x), \tag{3.8}
$$

where $\kappa(x)$ is the mean dilatation rate and $\epsilon(x)$ is a Gaussian random field with zero mean. When $\kappa(x) = 0$, there is no volume change over time. However, if $\kappa(x) > 0$, the volume increases while $\kappa(x) < 0$, the volume decreases.

Statistical inference on the linear model (3.8) is easier than that of (2.1) since it is a univariate Gaussian. To detect statistically significant local volume-change, the T random field with its p-value of the maximum field can be used (Worsley, 1994). Let K_j denote the dilatation rate of the j-th subject with the displacement $u^j = (u_1^j, u_2^j, u_3^j)$ after time t_j. The dilatation rate K_j is then given by

$$
K_j(x) = \frac{1}{t_j}\left(\frac{\partial u_1^j}{\partial x_1} + \frac{\partial u_2^j}{\partial x_2} + \frac{\partial u_3^j}{\partial x_3}\right)
$$

and the sample mean dilatation rate $\bar{K}$ of n subjects is

$$\bar{K}(x) = \frac{1}{n} \sum_{j=1}^{n} K_j(x).$$

In the numerical implementation, the displacement tensor $\partial u_i^j / \partial x_i$ can be computed by the finite difference method on a rectangular grid system. For example, at voxel position $x = (a, b, c)$,

$$\frac{\partial u_1^j}{\partial x_1} = \frac{u_1^j(a+1, b, c) - u_1^j(a, b, c)}{\delta x_1},$$

where δx_1 is the length of the edge of a voxel along the x_1-axis. So if the dimension of the voxel is given by $2 \times 2 \times 1$ mm^3, then $\delta x_1 = 2, \delta x_2 = 2, \delta x_3 = 1$. Also the sample standard deviation S is given by

$$S(x) = \left(\frac{1}{n-1} \sum_{j=1}^{n} (K_j - \bar{K})^2 \right)^{1/2}.$$

Subsequently, the T random field is defined as

$$T(x) = \sqrt{n} \frac{\bar{K}(x)}{S(x)}. \tag{3.9}$$

If there is no local volume change at x, i.e. $\kappa(x) = 0$, $T(x) \sim t_{n-1}$, a student t-distribution with $n - 1$ degrees of freedom. The sample mean dilatation rate $\bar{K}(x)$ does not provide accurate information about where the brain growth is dominant but the T field does (Chung *et al.*, 2001a). The result is shown in Figure 3.2. In obtaining the robust statistical result, it was necessary to smooth out the displacement velocity field with a 10mm FWHM Gaussian kernel. Without the smoothing, it may have been more difficult to detect morphological patterns. However, Gaussian kernel smoothing sometimes tends to blur the fine details of deformation pattern while boosting the statistical power (Figures 3.2 and 3.3).

The local volume change statistic $T(x)$ is computed using the formula (3.9). The t-statistic map is thresholded at

$$P(\max_x T(x) > 6.5) < 0.025,$$
$$P(\max_x T(x) < -6.5) < 0.025.$$

At these high thresholds, most of the local volume increase is observed around the corpus callosum (Figure 3.2). Pujol *et al.* (1993), Giedd *et al.* (1999) and Thompson *et al.* (2000) reported similar results of growth at the corpus callosum. However, the growth at the corpus callosum seems

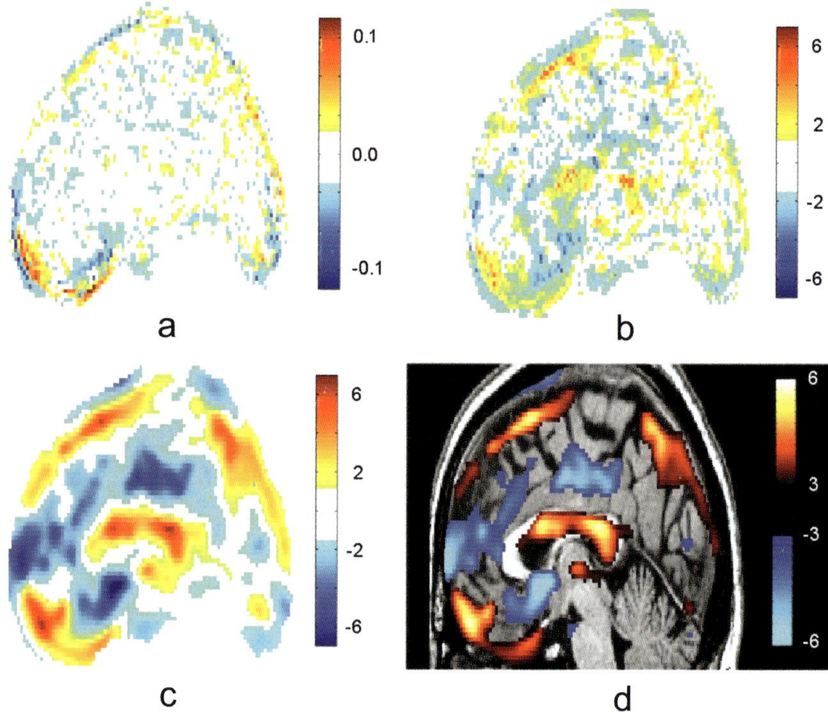

Fig. 3.2 The effects of image smoothing and statistical treatments on the Jacobian determinant on the mid-sagittal section (Chung *et al.*, 2001a). (a) The sample mean dilatation rate for 28 normal subjects. This map gives an incorrect impression that the local volume change only occurs near cortical boundaries possibly due to a registration error. (b) The division of the sample mean by the sample standard deviation gives the *t*-statistic map. The local maxima appear in the corpus callosum. A lot of noise on the cortical boundaries disappears. (c) *t*-map of the 10mm Gaussian kernel smoothing on the Jacobian determinant. The smoothing is applied directly to the displacement fields and the signal-to-noise ratio substantially improves. (d) The thresholded *t*-map superimposed on the mid-sagittal section of the template MRI. The corpus callosum shows volume increase. When the multiple comparison corrected threshold of $t > 6.5$ is applied, most of the red regions will disappear except the local peak point in the splenium of the corpus callosum.

very small when compared to that observed in the frontal and in particular parietal cortex (the largest red cluster in Figure 2.2).

We have computed the overlapping regions between the significant volume-change and the translation statistics. The volume of the overlapping regions is less than 10% of the total volume of the two statistics combined together. These two statistics are independent in statistical sense

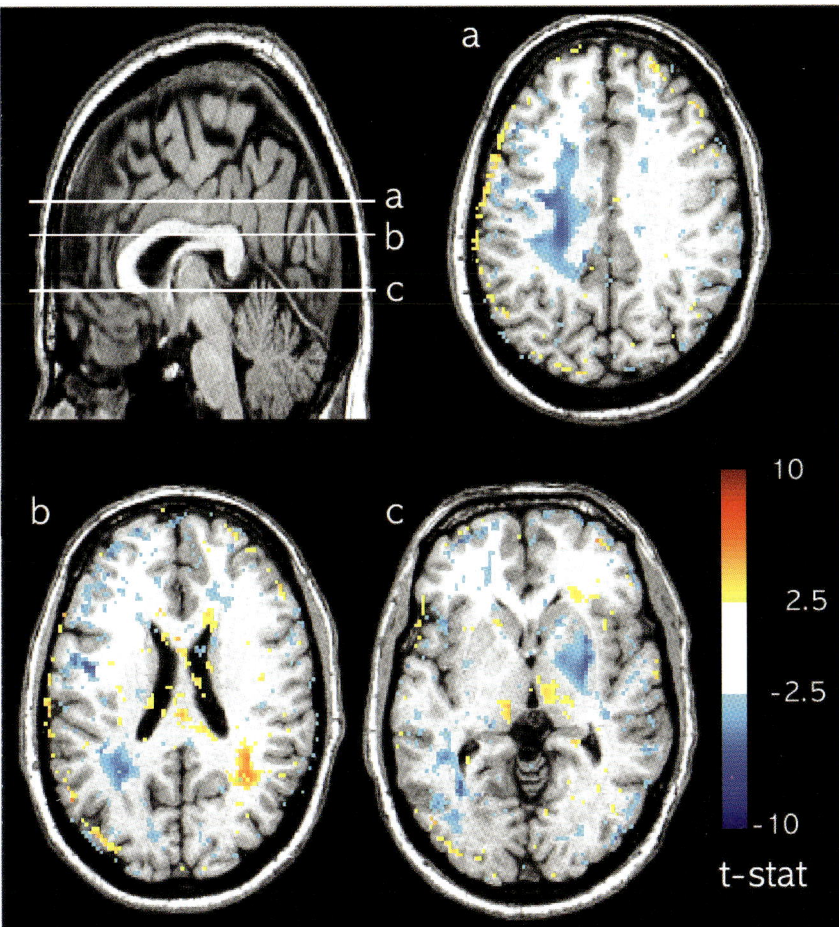

Fig. 3.3 *t*-map of local volume change without Gaussian kernel smoothing. Notice that the most of the local volume decrease is concentrated in the white matter. It may be useful as a visual aid for determining deformation patterns, but due to low *t*-value in most parts, such deformation pattern were found to be statistically insignificant. Smoothing is really necessary to boost statistical power and reduce the amount of false positives.

(Chung *et al.*, 2001a). The voxel-by-voxel computation seems to support the claim that these two statistics are indeed measuring different aspect of morphological changes. Although they measure different morphological properties, we have observed very interesting relations between these two statistics as illustrated in Figure 2.2. The figure is the close-up view of the parietal region of the left hemisphere, showing a large local displacement from the region of volume growth to a region of volume loss, indicating how the structure boundary has moved from the increasing volume to the decreasing volume. It seems that by studying these two statistical parametric maps simultaneously, the complex dynamic patterns in temporally varying brain morphology can be captured.

3.5   Global Inference via Divergence Theorem

Standard MRI-based volumetry, where we are interested in detecting volume-changes of the regions of interest, can be considered as an extension of TBM. Let $\mathcal{M}_t$ be the 3D region of interest with smooth 2D boundary $\partial\mathcal{M}_t$ at time t. The region $\mathcal{M}_0$ at reference time $t = 0$ deforms to $\mathcal{M}_t$ under the deformation $x \to x + u(x, t)$. Then the rate of volume-change of $\mathcal{M}_t$ is given by

$$\frac{d}{dt} \int_{\mathcal{M}_t} dx = \frac{d}{dt} \int_{\mathcal{M}_0} J(x, t) dx$$
$$\doteq \int_{\mathcal{M}_0} \frac{\partial K}{\partial t} dx.$$

From the linear model (3.8), $\partial K / \partial t$ is distributed as a Gaussian random field. When the Gaussian field $\partial K / \partial t$ is integrated over $\mathcal{M}_0$, we get a Gaussian random variable. So testing the hypothesis whether there is any volume change between $\mathcal{M}_0$ and $\mathcal{M}_t$, can be done by testing if

$$\frac{d}{dt} \int_{\mathcal{M}_t} dx = 1.$$

Hence the standard MRI-based volumetry can be achieved by taking the integral test statistic in TBM.

It is also possible to detect the global volume-change via surface analysis (Chung, 2001). The Gauss's divergence theorem states that

$$\int_{\mathcal{M}_0} \nabla \cdot u(x, t)\, dx = \int_{\partial\mathcal{M}_0} u \cdot \mathbf{n}\, dS, \qquad (3.10)$$

where $\mathbf{n}$ is a unit normal vector on the surface $\partial\mathcal{M}_0$ and dS is the surface area element. Hence, we have the following linear model of the global volume change of the region of interest $\mathcal{M}_t$ based on the geometry of the surface $\partial\mathcal{M}_0$:

$$\frac{d}{dt} \int_{\mathcal{M}_t} dx = \int_{\partial\mathcal{M}_0} \mu \cdot \mathbf{n}\, dS + \varepsilon, \qquad (3.11)$$

where μ is the mean displacement vector field on the surface $\partial \mathcal{M}_0$ and ε is a Gaussian random variable.

3.6 Second Order Tensor Fields

So far, our morphological descriptors are based on length, area and volume changes, which directly measure the amount of brain tissue growth or loss. However, it is possible to develop more sophisticated morphological descriptors that measure completely different morphological properties in brain deformation.

3.6.1 *Membrane Spline Energy*

Consider two geometric objects $\mathcal{M}_1$ and $\mathcal{M}_2$ in $\mathbb{R}^N$ which have slight shape variations. We are interested in identifying the regions of maximum shape differences between $\mathcal{M}_1$ and $\mathcal{M}_2$. Let

$$u = (u_1(x), \cdots, u_N(x))'$$

be the displacement vector field from $\mathcal{M}_1$ to $\mathcal{M}_2$, whose components are assumed to follow zero-mean stationary Gaussian random fields. The deformation from $\mathcal{M}_1$ to $\mathcal{M}_2$ can be assumed to minimize an associated *membrane spline energy* (Gee *et al.*, 1993) given by

$$E(u) = \int_{\mathcal{M}_1} \sum_{i,j=1}^{N} \left(\frac{du_j}{dx_i} \right)^2 dx. \tag{3.12}$$

For instance, the membrane spline energy in 2D is

$$E(u) = \int_{\mathcal{M}_1} \left[\left(\frac{\partial u_1}{\partial x_1} \right)^2 + \left(\frac{\partial u_2}{\partial x_1} \right)^2 + \left(\frac{\partial u_1}{\partial x_2} \right)^2 + \left(\frac{\partial u_2}{\partial x_2} \right)^2 \right] dx_1 \, dx_2$$

The functional inside the energy integral in (3.12) is the squared Frobenius norm of the displacement gradient matrix ∇u. Let us denote $\|\nabla u\|_F$ to be the Frobenius norm of ∇u, i.e.

$$\|\nabla u\|_F = \left[\sum_{i,j=1}^{N} \left(\frac{\partial u_j}{\partial x_i} \right)^2 \right]^{1/2}.$$

The Frobenius norm will measure the amount of local membrane spline energy associated with the deformation $x \to x + u(x)$ in the neighborhood of x and it would be interesting to compare this local energy functional to local volume change and local displacement change statistics. Other spline energy functionals such as thin-plate spline energy can be also used as morphological descriptors (Bookstein, 1989; Green and Silverman, 1994; Wahba, 1990).

3.6.2 *Vorticity Tensor Fields*

We briefly introduced the concept of vorticity tensor, which measures the amount of rotation at a given point but never studied its statistical properties. Assume an object $\mathcal{M}_1$ to be at time 0 and after a unit time, the object $\mathcal{M}_1$ goes through the viscous fluid deformation to $\mathcal{M}_2$. The vorticity vector is then defined as the curl of the velocity,

$$\mathcal{M}(x) = \frac{1}{2}\nabla \times u(x),$$

where

$$\nabla = \left(\frac{\partial}{\partial x_1}, \cdots , \frac{\partial}{\partial x_N} \right)'$$

and it completely determines infinitesimal rotation of the deformation. The obvious test procedure for detecting any local rotational change is to use the Hotelling's T^2 statistics. Since the components of $\mathcal{M}(x)$ are correlated, the random field constructed from $\mathcal{M}(x)$ is not the Hotelling's T^2 field. So it would be of interest to be able to compute the excursion probability based on this Hotelling's T^2 like random field.

The vorticity tensor $\mathcal{V}_{ij}$ is given by

$$\mathcal{V}_{ij} = \frac{1}{2}\left(\frac{\partial u_i}{\partial x_j} - \frac{\partial u_j}{\partial x_i} \right).$$

Let ϵ_{ijk} be the Levi-Civita tensor (Saffman, 1992; Marsden and Hughes, 1983), then the i-th element of $\mathcal{M}$ can be given in terms of the vorticity tensor

$$\mathcal{V}_i = -\epsilon_{ijk}\mathcal{V}_{jk}.$$

In 3D, the vorticity vector $\mathcal{W} = (\mathcal{V}_{23}, \mathcal{V}_{31}, \mathcal{V}_{12})$ is the angular velocity. Assuming that the displacement velocity components are i.i.d. mean zero isotropic Gaussian fields with smooth isotropic covariance function, we have linear model:

$$\frac{\partial \mathcal{W}}{\partial t} = w(x) + \Sigma^{1/2}\epsilon(x),$$

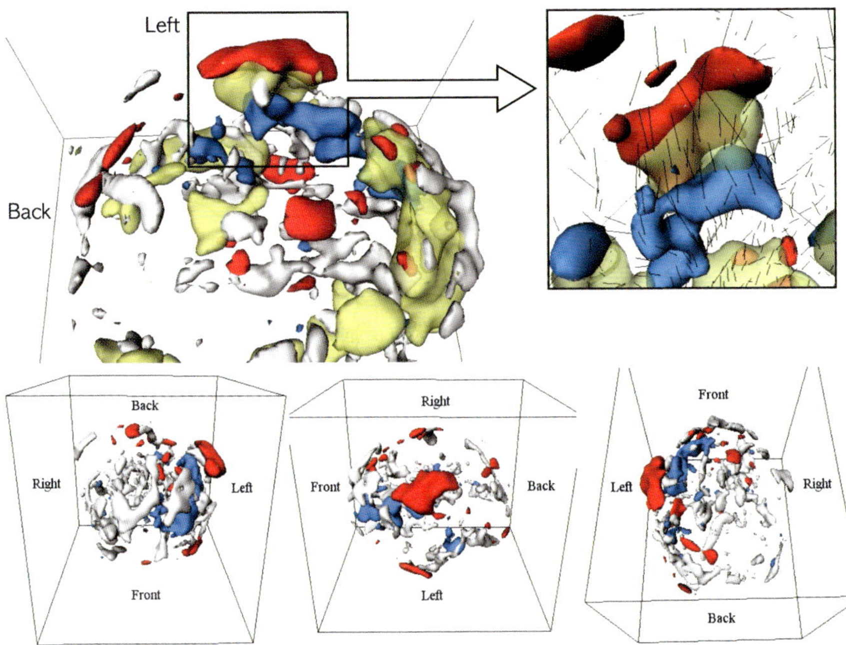

Fig. 3.4   The statistical parametric map showing large displacement (yellow) from a region of growth (red) to a region of atrophy (blue) as well as vorticity change (gray) in normal development between ages 11 and 16 (Chung *et al.*, 2001a). The smaller figure is a close up of part of the outer left hemisphere where black arrows represent mean displacement velocity subsampled every 10mm and scaled by 50mm/year.

where w is the mean vorticity rate vector, $e(x)$ is i.i.d. mean zero isotropic Gaussian field and Σ is the covariance matrix that accounts for dependency between the components. Then we are interested in testing if

$$H_0 : w(x) = 0 \text{ for all } x$$
$$H_1 : w(x) \neq 0 \text{ for some } x.$$

The test statistic is then the usual Hotelling's T^2 random field

$$H(x) = nM'(x)V^{-1}(x)M(x),$$

where $M(x)$ is the sample mean of the vorticity rate and $V(x)$ is the sample covariance matrix of the vorticity rate. The details on the Hotelling's T^2 test procedure can be found in the pervious chapter.

Figure 3.4 shows the regions of brain growth or atrophy in MRI scans of 29 subjects (age $=13.5 \pm 4.1$) over 4.5 ± 1.0 year time span (Chung *et al.*, 2001a).

The angular speed is defined as

$$\|\mathcal{V}\| = \Big(\sum_{i=1}^{N} \mathcal{V}_i^2\Big)^{1/2}.$$

The angular speed is a useful scalar morphological descriptor which measures the amount of rotation per unit time in deformation. Finding the exact statistical distribution and its p-value based on the maximum of its field is not straightforward.

3.6.3   *Generalized Variance Field*

Here we introduce a new morphological descriptor based on the determinant of the matrix. Suppose components of the displacement vector $u(x) \in \mathbb{R}^N$ are identically and independently distributed as a mean zero stationary Gaussian field with the covariance function $R(x, y) = f(x - y)$. Let

$$\nabla u_i = \Big(\frac{\partial u_i}{\partial x_1}, \cdots, \frac{\partial u_i}{\partial x_N}\Big)'.$$

The N-dimensional displacement gradient matrix ∇u is defined as

$$\nabla u = \big(\nabla u_1, \cdots, \nabla u_N\big)' = \begin{pmatrix} \frac{\partial u_1}{\partial x_1} & \cdots & \frac{\partial u_1}{\partial x_N} \\ & \ddots & \\ \frac{\partial u_N}{\partial x_1} & \cdots & \frac{\partial u_N}{\partial x_N} \end{pmatrix}.$$

The generalized variance field is defined as the determinant of

$$W = (\nabla u)'\nabla u$$
$$= \sum_{i=1}^{N} \nabla u_i (\nabla u_i)'.$$

It would be very useful to approximate the excursion probability of the generalized variance field. Unfortunately, it is not easy to compute the expected Euler characteristic of the excursion set of W.

The covariance function of the field $W^{1/2}$ can be easily computed. By expanding the determinant $W^{1/2} = \det(\nabla u)$, we obtain

$$W^{1/2} = \sum_{\sigma \in S_N} \mathrm{sgn}(\sigma) \frac{\partial u_1}{\partial x_{\sigma(1)}} \cdots \frac{\partial u_N}{\partial x_{\sigma(N)}},$$

where S_N is a symmetric group of order N and $\mathrm{sgn}(\sigma)$ is the sign function of the order of permutation σ (Harville, 1997). Since $\frac{\partial u_1}{\partial x_{\sigma(1)}}, \cdots, \frac{\partial u_N}{\partial x_{\sigma(N)}}$

are independent mean zero Gaussian fields, $\mathbb{E}W^{1/2} = 0$. The covariance function R^* of $W^{1/2}$ is

$$R^*(x,y) = \mathbb{E}[W^{1/2}(x)W^{1/2}(y)]$$

$$= \mathbb{E}\left[\sum_{\sigma,\tau \in S_N} \text{sgn}(\sigma)\text{sgn}(\tau)\frac{\partial u_1(x)}{\partial x_{\sigma(1)}}\frac{\partial u_1(y)}{\partial x_{\tau(1)}}\cdots\frac{\partial u_N(x)}{\partial x_{\sigma(N)}}\frac{\partial u_N(y)}{\partial x_{\tau(N)}}\right]$$

$$= \sum_{\sigma,\tau \in S_N} \text{sgn}(\sigma)\text{sgn}(\tau)\mathbb{E}\left[\frac{\partial u_1(x)}{\partial x_{\sigma(1)}}\frac{\partial u_1(y)}{\partial x_{\tau(1)}}\right]\cdots\mathbb{E}\left[\frac{\partial u_N(x)}{\partial x_{\sigma(N)}}\frac{\partial u_N(y)}{\partial x_{\tau(N)}}\right]$$

$$= \sum_{\sigma,\tau \in S_N} \text{sgn}(\sigma)\text{sgn}(\tau)R_{\sigma(1)\tau(1)}(x,y)\cdots R_{\sigma(N)\tau(N)}(x,y),$$

where

$$R_{ij}(x,y) = \frac{\partial^2 R(x,y)}{\partial x_i \partial y_i}.$$

There exists a permutation $\rho \in S_N$ such that

$$\tau = \rho\sigma \text{ and } \text{sgn}(\rho) = \text{sgn}(\tau)\text{sgn}(\sigma).$$

Then by summing up over the index ρ,

$$R^*(x,y) = \sum_{\sigma \in S_N}\sum_{\rho \in S_N} \text{sgn}(\rho)R_{\sigma(1)\rho\sigma(1)}(x,y)\cdots R_{\sigma(N)\rho\sigma(N)}(x,y)$$

$$= \sum_{\sigma \in S_N} \det\frac{\partial^2 R(x,y)}{\partial x \partial y'}$$

$$= N!\det\frac{\partial^2 R(x,y)}{\partial x \partial y'}$$

$$= (-1)^N \det\left[\mathbf{H}f(x-y)\right],$$

where $\mathbf{H}f = \left(\frac{\partial^2 f}{\partial x_i \partial y_j}\right)$ is the Hessian matrix of f.

If the covariance function R is isotropic with the covariance function

$$R(x,y) = g(\tau), \tau = \|x-y\|^2$$

for some function g, then the covariance function R^* can be further simplified. We can show that

$$\frac{\partial^2 g(\tau)}{\partial x_k \partial x_l} = 2\delta_{kl}g'(\tau) + 4(x_k-y_k)(x_l-y_l)g''(\tau),$$

$$\mathbf{H}g(\tau) = 2g'(\tau)I_N + 4g''(\tau)(x-y)(x-y)^t.$$

For any matrix A and any scalar c,

$$\det(cI_N + A) = \sum_{j=0}^{N} c^j \det r_{N-j}(A),$$

where $\det r_j(A)$ is the total sum of the determinant of $j \times j$ principal minors of A (Harville, 1997). Since

$$\det r_j(xx') = 0 \text{ for all } j = 2, 3, \cdots, N$$

except

$$\det r_0(xx') = 1 \text{ and } \det r_1(xx') = \text{tr}(xx') = ||x||^2,$$

by letting $c = 2g'(\tau)$ and

$$A = 4g''(\tau)(x - y)(x - y)',$$

we get

$$\det\left(\mathbf{H}g(\tau)\right) = [2g'(\tau)]^N + [2g'(\tau)]^{N-1} 4\tau g''(\tau)$$

Therefore, the covariance function can be simplified to

$$R^*(x, y) = (-1)^N 2^N N! [g'(\tau)]^{N-1} [g'(\tau) + 2\tau g''(\tau)].$$

Chapter 4

Voxel-Based Morphometry

The drawback of the deformation-based morphometry (DBM) and tensor-based morphometry (TBM) is a need for accurate nonlinear image registration technique. In this chapter, we present a radically different method called voxel-based morphometry (VBM) that can be performed even with less accurate image registration. VBM involves a voxel-wise comparison of the local concentration of gray or white matters between populations (Ashburner and Friston, 2000). It requires spatially normalizing images from all the subjects in the study to a template. This is followed by segmenting the gray and white matters and cerebrospinal fluid (CSF) from the spatially normalized images (Figure 4.1).

The tissue segmentation is based on a Gaussian mixture model that assumes the image intensity values to follow the mixture of three independent Gaussians and the unknown parameters of Gaussian distributions are estimated by maximizing the likelihood function using the expectation maximization (EM) algorithm. The widely used Statistical Parametric Mapping (SPM) package (Wellcome Department of Cognitive Neurology, London, UK. http://www.fil.ion.ucl.ac.uk/spm) is based on a Bayesian formulation of the Gaussian mixture model with a prior probability image obtained by averaging already segmented large number of images (Ashburner et al., 1997; Ashburner and Friston, 2000). Based on the prior probability of each voxel belong to a specific tissue type, the Bayesian framework is then used to get the posterior probability. This Bayesian update of the probability is iterated many times until the probability converges. The resulting probability map is interpreted as the tissue density. This is not physical density so it should be interpreted probabilistically. The tissue density is then smoothed out using sufficiently large Gaussian kernel to reduce image registration and segmentation errors. Statistical inference is subsequently

69

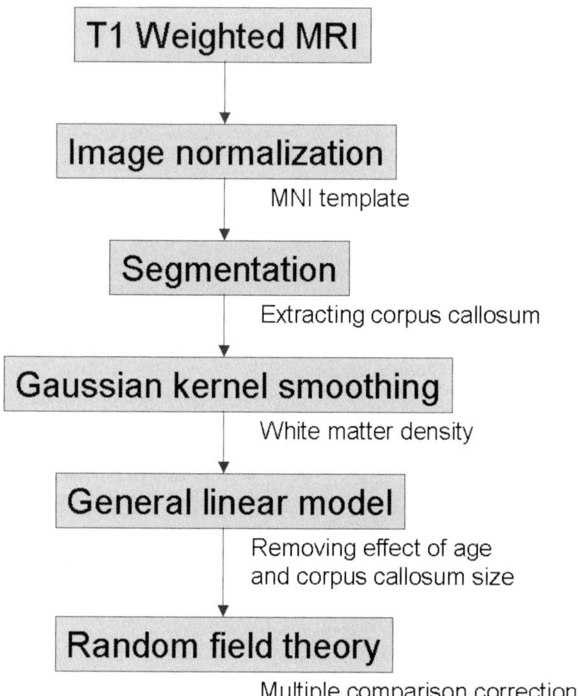

Fig. 4.1   The image processing and analysis flow in voxel-based morphometry.   It involves different processing pipelines that include image registration segmentation, smoothing.   Once we obtain the tissue density, general linear models and the random field theory are used for statistical inference and localizing signals.

done at each voxel level on the smoothed tissue densities while accounting for multiple comparisons.

The tissue densities have been often used in various structural imaging studies: normal development (Good *et al.*, 2001; Paus *et al.*, 1999), autism (Chung *et al.*, 2004), depression (Pizzagalli *et al.*, 2004), epilepsy (McMillan *et al.*, 2004) and Alzheimer's disease (Johnson *et al.*, 2004; Thompson *et al.*, 2003). In the standard VBM, the tissue density is modeled as a Gaussian mixture on image intensity values (Ashburner and Friston, 2000; Good *et al.*, 2001). In the modulated-VBM (Good *et al.*, 2001), the density obtained from the standard VBM is rescaled by the Jacobian determinant of deformation to preserve the total amount of gray matter. This is related to the RAVENS (regional analysis of volumes examined in normalized space) approach proposed by Davatzikos *et al.* (2001). There has been heated discussions about the optimal amount of image registration needed in VBM and the modulation by the the corresponding Jacobian determinant (Bookstein, 2001; Ashburner and Friston, 2001; Mehta *et al.*, 2004).

4.1 Image Segmentation

There are few variations to the VBM framework. It depends on how we define the tissue density. Paus *et al.* (1999) modeled the density as a Bernoulli random variable taking value 1 inside the gray matter segmentation and 0 outside the segmented regions. In a slightly different formulation, Thompson *et al.* (2003) computed the tissue density as the fraction of gray matter within a ball of radius 15mm along a cortical surface . This approach is equivalent to convoluting the binary mask of the gray matter with a uniform probability distribution of radius 15mm and interpolating voxel values to the cortical surface mesh. Chung *et al.* (2006) computed the gray mater density using the 3D Euclidean distance map of the outer and inner cortical surfaces that bound the gray matter. In all these studies, segmentation of tissues or tissue boundaries are crucial. So let us review few image segmentation techniques that are often used in brain imaging.

4.1.1 *Mumford-Shah Model*

The Mumford-Shah model is a widely used for image segmentation formulated as a variational problem (Mumford and Shah, 1989). Given image intensity value f defined in domain $\mathcal{M}$, we approximate f with two discrete values v_0 and v_1. $\mathcal{M}$ is segmented into two disjoint regions $\mathcal{M}_0$ and $\mathcal{M}_1$ depending on if a pixel takes value v_0 or v_1. The segmentation boundary is denoted as $\partial\mathcal{M}_0$. Then we define the associated energy as

$$E(\mathcal{M}_0, v_0, v_1) = \int_{\mathcal{M}_0} g_0(v_0, t)\, dt + \int_{\mathcal{M}_1} g_1(v_1, t)\, dt + \beta \|\partial\mathcal{M}_0\|,$$

where $\|\partial\mathcal{M}_0\|$ is the length of the segmentation boundary and g_0 and g_1 are some functions measuring the goodness-of-fit of the discrete approximation in each disjoint regions. The segmentation is mainly done by minimizing the energy or solving the corresponding partial differential equations (Darbon, 2007). When the regions are discretized as a graph, graph-cut algorithms can be used for segmentation (Boykov and Kolmogorov, 2003). The Mumford-Shah model is a basis for segmenting images into geometric and textured components in computer vision (Meyer, 2001) and it has been used in segmenting various imaging modalities including diffusion tensor images (Wang and Vemuri, 2005).

4.1.2 *Level Sets*

The level set methods (Osher and Fedkiw, 2003; Sethian, 2002) show promise in tissue boundary segmentation and has been used in segmenting simple boundary shapes such as the midsagittal cross-section of the corpus callosum (Hoffmann *et al.*, 2004) but for more complex boundaries, it tend to suffer numerical and topological instabilities. The method was originally developed by Stanley Osher and James Sethian in the 1980's (Osher and Sethian, 1988). The level set method starts with an initial surface inside the region of interest, and and propagate it with certain constraints so that an accurate estimate of the boundary of the region is found. The boundary of a closed curve in $\mathbb{R}^2$ is given as the zero level set of some function Ψ, i.e. $\Psi(x, y) = 0$. If the boundary curves moves in the normal direction with the velocity F, the evolution of propagating boundary is described using the Hamilton-Jacobi equation

$$\frac{\partial \Psi}{\partial t} + F|\nabla \Psi| = 0, \tag{4.1}$$

where $\partial \Psi / \partial t$ is the signed distance of each pixel to the boundary. $\partial \Psi / \partial t$ is positive if it is inside the boundary, and negative if it is outside of the boundary. F is the boundary propagation velocity given as, for example,

$$F(x) = \exp\left(-\alpha \nabla K_\sigma * I(x)\right),$$

a function of convolution between Gaussian kernel K_σ and image intensity $I(x)$ at x. Iteratively solving (4.1) for each time step Δt using finite differences on pixels, the boundary is updated at the $(n + 1)$-th step as

$$\Psi^{n+1} = \Psi^n - \Delta t F|\nabla \Psi|.$$

Figure 4.2 shows the level set segmentation of the courpus callosum boundary.

4.1.3 *Active Contours*

Active contour models or snakes first proposed by Kass *et al.* (1988) is a variational method for detecting object boundaries in images. This is a precursor to more general deformable surface models often used in extracting cortical surfaces. Given n points $C^0 = \{p_1^0, \cdots, p_n^0\}$ that define the initial closed contour, we deform the points to lie along the object boundary.

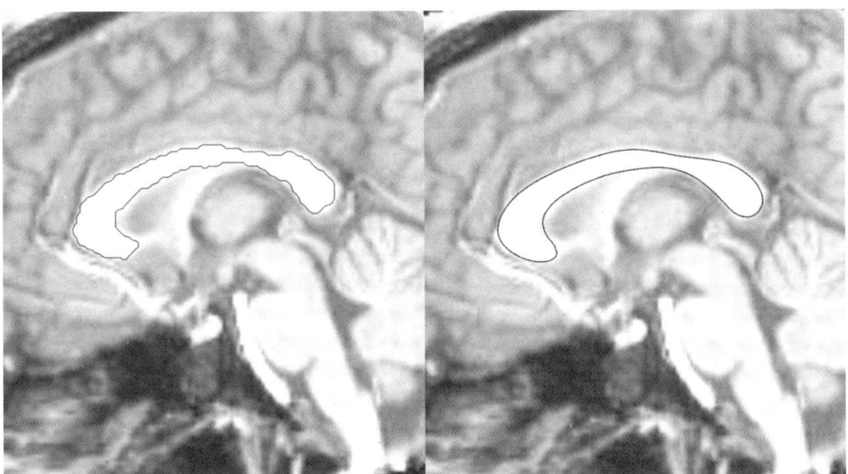

Fig. 4.2 Level set segmentation showing zigzag discretization pattern. Smoothing of the level set contour is necessary for any subsequent morphometric analysis to reduce the segmentation artifacts. Here spline smoothing was used to substantially reduces the discretization noise (Hoffmann *et al.*, 2004).

The initial contour C^0 is deformed to $C^1 = \{p_1^1, \cdots, p_n^1\}$ by minimizing a certain energy function E. We deform contour $C^i = \{p_1^i, \cdots, p_n^i\}$ to $C^{i+1} = \{p_1^{i+1}, \cdots, p_n^{i+1}\}$ by the displacement d such that

$$p_j^{i+1} = p_j^i + d(p_j^i) \text{ for all } j.$$

Hamarneh and Gustavsson (2002) used the displacement that is given in terms of some force terms

$$d(p_j^i) = -\nu(F_{internal} + F_{external}).$$

This iterative update of the position is performed until the snake C^i hits the object boundary.

In general, the displacement d is usually chosen such that it minimizes the energy function E. Let $X(p)$ be a parameterization of contour C and I be the image intensity (Sapiro, 2001). For simplicity, we may assume $p \in [0, 1]$. Many researchers incorporate different energy terms depending on applications. The energy function is often decomposed into two parts

$$E(C) = E_{internal}(C) + \lambda E_{external}(C),$$

where λ balance the two energy terms (Kass *et al.*, 1988). The internal energy term is

$$E_{internal} = \alpha \int |X'(p)|^2 \, dp + \beta \int |X''(p)| \, dp$$

while the external energy term is

$$E_{external} = - \int \|\nabla I(X(p))\| \, dp.$$

The internal energy is generated from the interaction of the snakes itself and control the smoothness of the snake while the external energy is responsible for attracting the contour toward the object boundary. For a more stable result, the image intensity is usually smoothed with Gaussian kernel K_σ so we usually have

$$E_{external} = - \int \|\nabla K_\sigma * I(X(p))\| \, dp.$$

The parameters α, β and λ are determined a priori. α and β control the snakes tension and rigidity. Smaller λ reduces the noise but can not capture the sharp corners while larger λ can effectively capture boundary but it is sensitive to the noise.

The energy corresponding to each point p_j^i is denoted as $E(p_j^i)$. The energy terms are then

$$E_{internal} = \sum_{j=1}^{n} E_{internal}(p_j^i)$$

and

$$E_{external} = \sum_{j=1}^{n} E_{external}(p_j^i).$$

The first internal energy term $\int |X'(p)|^2$ is related to the linear elastic potential of a string that is proportional to the squared distance between neighboring points, i.e.

$$E_{elastic}(p_j^i) = \|p_{j+1}^i - p_j^i\|^2 + \|p_j^i - p_{j-1}^i\|^2.$$

The second term $\int |X''(p)|^2$ measures the curvature and at each point it is estimated as

$$E_{curvature}(p_j^i) = \|p_{j+1}^i - 2p_j^i + p_{j-1}\|^2.$$

The external energy is forces the contour to move toward the extreme image gradient so it is given by

$$E_{gradient}(p_j^i) = \|\nabla K_\sigma * I(p_j^i)\|^2.$$

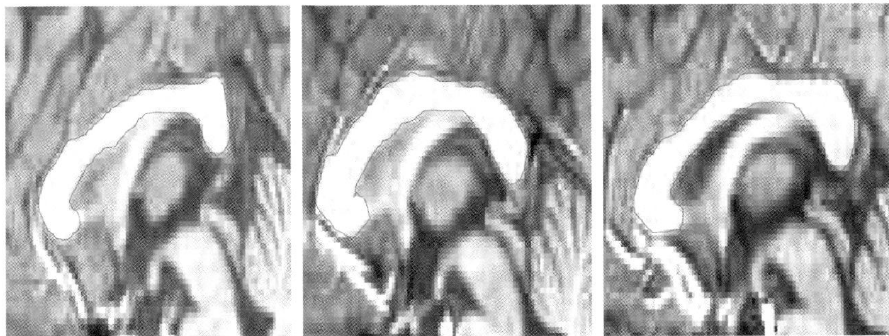

Fig. 4.3 Active contour based segmentation of corpus callosum in three subjects (Wang and Chung, 2005).

If necessary, an additional external energy term depends on the image intensity is also added:

$$E_{intensity}(p_j^i) = f\big(I(p_j^i)\big)$$

for some simple function f. $E_{intensity}$ attracts the contour to either high or low intensity regions.

Instead of directly minimizing the total energy, we can also solve equivalent differential equations. It can be shown from the calculus of variations, the contour should satisfy the Euler-Lagrange equation:

$$-\frac{d}{dp}(\alpha X') + \frac{d^2}{dp^2}(\beta X'') + \lambda \Delta I(X) = 0.$$

Figure 4.3 shows a demonstration of segmenting the boundary of the corpus callosum using the active contour method.

4.1.4 *Deformable Surface Models*

Instead of the 3D volume-based segmentation techniques, which are mainly intensity based, 2D tissue boundary segmentation techniques have been also popular in modeling highly convoluted cortical surfaces. The advantage of the boundary segmentation over the usual volume segmentation is the reduction of partial volume effect (Tohka *et al.*, 2004).

For this purpose, deformable surface models (Davatzikos and Bryan, 1995; Dale and Fischl, 1999; MacDonald *et al.*, 2000) have been used to segment tissue boundaries by either solving a partial differential equation or optimizing an objective function. The result of deformable surface modeling is usually represented as triangular meshes. The triangular meshes that represents the cortical surfaces are not constrained to lie on voxel boundaries. Instead the triangular meshes can cut through a voxel, which can be considered as correcting where the true boundary ought to be and reducing the partial volume effect.

In particular method given in MacDonald *et al.* (2000) starts with an ellipsoidal mesh that already has the topology of a sphere and deformed to match the shape of the cortex guaranteeing the same topology. The resulting triangular mesh consists of 40,962 vertices and 81,920 triangles with the average internodal distance of 3 mm.

4.1.5 *Thin-Plate Spline Thresholding*

Here we present a method for segmenting images using thin plate splines. The method is first introduced in Xie *et al.* (2006). Consider n data points $t_1, \cdots, t_n \in \mathbb{R}^d$ and the corresponding responses $y_1, \cdots, y_n$. A thin plate spline (TPS) of fitting these points, in the most general form, is the minimizer of the following optimization problem (Wahba, 1990):

$$\frac{1}{n} \sum_{i=1}^{n} \left(y_i - f(t_i) \right)^2 + \lambda J_m^d(f) \tag{4.2}$$

where the penalty function $J_m^d(f)$ is given by

$$J_m^d(f) = \sum_{\alpha_1 + \cdots + \alpha_d = m} \frac{m!}{\alpha_1! \cdots \alpha_d!} \int_{\mathbb{R}^d} \left(\frac{\partial^m f}{\partial x_1^{\alpha_1} \cdots \partial x_d^{\alpha_d}} \right)^2 dx_1 \cdots dx_d.$$

For the two dimensional TPS, when $d = m = 2$, we have

$$J_2^2(f) = \int_{-\infty}^{\infty} \int_{-\infty}^{\infty} \frac{\partial^2 f}{\partial x_1^2} + \frac{\partial^2 f}{\partial x_1 \partial x_2} + \frac{\partial^2 f}{\partial x_2^2} \, dx_1 dx_2.$$

Under some regularity conditions, we can show that the minimization problem (4.2) has a unique solution

$$f_\lambda(t) = \sum_{\nu} d_\nu \phi_\nu(t) + \sum_{i} c_i E_m(t - t_i), \tag{4.3}$$

where ϕ is a polynomial basis and $E^m(\cdot)$ is the thin plate spline radial basis.

TPS is fitted on image intensity values and thresholded to obtain the analytic representation for tissue boundaries. This results in smooth differentiable boundaries compared to other segmentation methods (Figures 4.4 and 4.5). The method can be divided into four sequential steps. Here we present a method applied to segmenting 2D image slices but it can be easily adopted to 3D.

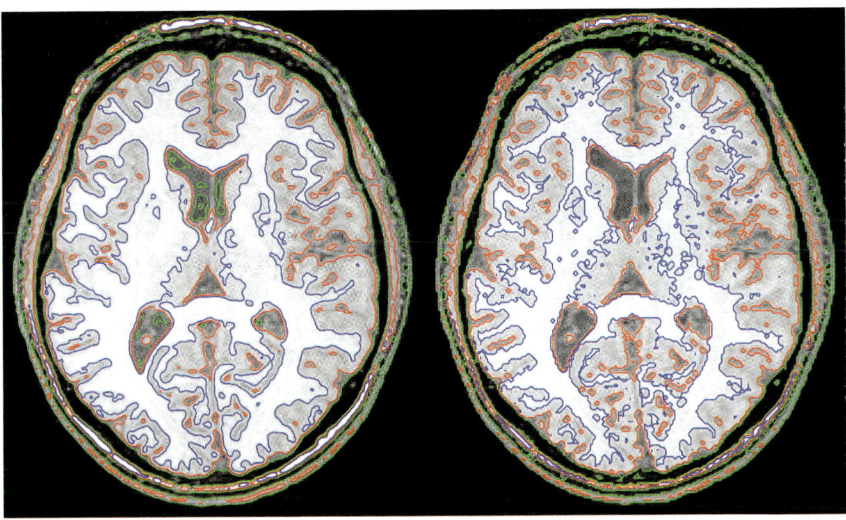

Fig. 4.4   Left: Thin plate spline segmentation (Xie *et al.*, 2006). Right: Neural network classifier. The thin plate spline segmentation shows a smoother tissue boundary.

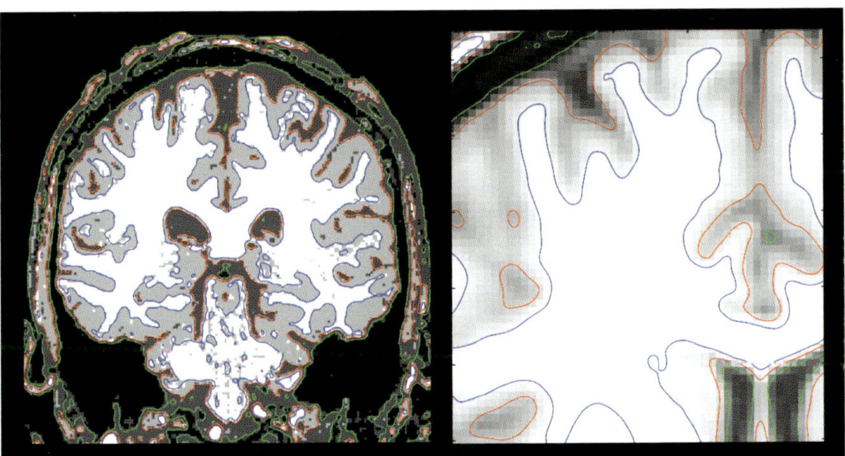

Fig. 4.5   Thin plate spline segmentation results. The tissue boundaries are obtained analytically.

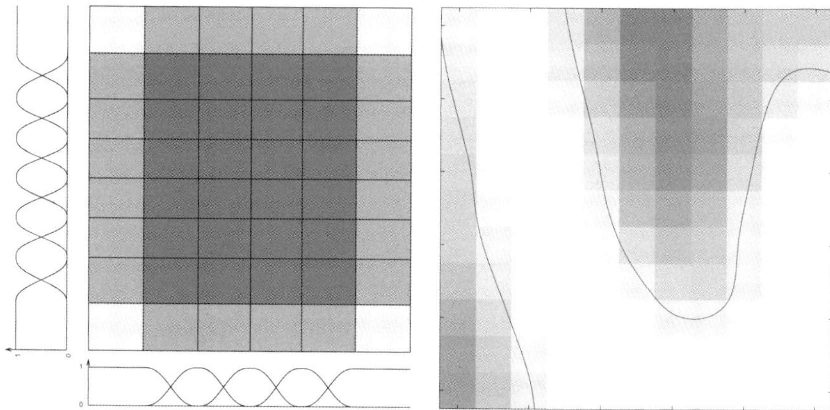

Fig. 4.6 Left: The overlapping scheme with 5 by 7 blocks. Each 4 adjacent shaded rectangles form one block. TPS is constructed at each block and connected to other blocks smoothly in a piecewise fashion. Right: Neural network classifier. Right: zoomed out thin plate spline segmentation result showing smoother tissue boundaries that pass through voxels. The detail is given in Xie *et al.* (2006).

(1) Partitioning of slice images: We divide each slice into overlapping blocks (Figure 4.6). The same idea was used in Kovacevic *et al.* (2002). Following similar line of thinking, we allow some degree of overlapping between adjacent blocks (horizontally, vertically, or diagonally). With a typical slice of size 256×256 pixels, we can divide the slice into blocks of about size 50×50.

(2) Fitting TPS in each block: We fit thin plate splines to each block with different number of knots, and search for the knots configuration that gives us the smallest general cross validation score. Even for one block of size 50×50, there are more than two thousand data points, so this fitting TPS is computation intensive.

(3) Determining TPS thresholding: We determine the thresholds on each block with the K-means algorithm. The K-means is used with 4 centers, which correspond to the background, cerebrospinal fluid, gray matter, and white matter. This is consistent with the peaks in the intensity histogram.

(4) Blending each blocks smoothly: Blend the predicted block images and the thresholds with some smooth weighting functions. The

averages of the corresponding thresholds on all the blocks and the thresholds on the blended smooth image are calculated as well.

TPS-thresholding method is an intensity based segmentation technique. It uses thin plate splines to reconstruct the image. The TPS method has the advantage of giving subpixel level results and generating smoother boundaries. The partial volume effects are addressed by the subpixel segmentation (Figure 4.6). Also, it offers the potential for more accurate estimate of distances and curvatures on the cortical surfaces. The method can also tackle the image intensity non-uniformity through local thresholding and blending.

4.2 Mixture Models

Probably the most widely used image segmentation method in brain imaging is a Bayesian Gaussian mixture model. This is the basis of the VBM implemented in SPM package. So we will devote the significant part of this chapter on this framework.

4.2.1 *Bayesian Segmentation*

The Bayesian segmentation framework utilizes the Bayes theorem in estimating the posterior probability of a voxel belong to a particular tissue type from a given prior probability. Let C be the event of a voxel belong to a particular class. We may assume there are three classes corresponding to gray, white matters and CSF. The prior probability $P(C)$ is obtained by averaging a large sample of normalized binary segmentation and dividing the average by the total number of sample. Let T be the event that a voxel has a particular image intensity value. This is what we usually observe in T_1-weighted MRI. Then we wish to obtain the conditional probability $P(C|T)$ of the voxel belong to the class C given that we have observed T:

$$P(C|T) = \frac{P(C \cap T)}{P(T)}. \tag{4.4}$$

$P(C|T)$ is interpreted as the probability of the voxel belong to a specific class when the voxel has a particular intensity value. This is what we likely to determine in the Bayesian segmentation framework and it is termed as tissue density in VBM. The numerator can be written as

$$P(C \cap T) = P(T|C)P(C)$$

while, from the law of total probability, the total probability $P(T)$ can be decomposed as

$$P(T) = \sum_C P(T \cap C)$$

$$= \sum_C P(T|C)P(C).$$

The conditional probability (4.4) can be written in terms of the prior probability as

$$P(C|T) = \frac{P(T|C)P(C)}{\sum_C P(T|C)P(C)}. \tag{4.5}$$

The likelihood term $P(T|C)$ is interpreted as the probability of a voxel obtaining a particular intensity value given the voxel belong to a particular tissue type, and it can be estimated from mixture models. The likelihood term is given by evaluating the probability density for the class C at each voxel intensity value (Ashburner and Friston, 2000).

4.2.2 *Mixture Models*

To estimate the likelihood term, it is necessary to introduce mixture models and the expectation-maximization algorithm. Mixture models have been widely used for segmenting various images. The image intensity value at a given voxel can come from different tissue classes with specific proportions p_j. We will assume

$$\sum_j p_j = 1 \ (0 < p_j < 1).$$

We may assume that image intensity values for each class to follow a certain distribution f_j. This is the likelihood term $P(T|C)$. Then the k-component mixture model on image intensity values assume image intensity values Y to come from k different distributions $f_1, \cdots, f_k$ with mixing proportions $p_1, \cdots, p_k$. This can be modeled by conditioning on a multinomial distribution. Another way of saying this is that the the k-component mixture model can be obtained by mixing samples obtained from distributions f_j with p_j proportions.

Let X_j be an indicator variable for the j-th class such that

$$P(X_j = 1) = p_j, \ P(X_j = 0) = 1 - p_j.$$

X_j is a Bernoulli random variable. The collection of variables $X = (X_1, \cdots, X_k)$ form a multinomial distribution with parameters $(p_1, \cdots, p_k)$

if we have the additional constraint $X_1 + \cdots + X_k = 1$. The probability mass function of X is given by

$$f(x_1, \cdots, x_k) = P(X_1 = x_1, \cdots, X_k = x_k)$$
$$= p_1^{x_1} \cdots p_k^{x_k}.$$

Now we define a random variable Y conditionally on the event $X_j = 1$ such that $Y \sim f_j$ if $X_j = 1$. The conditional density $f(y|x_j = 1) = f_j$ is the distribution for the j-th class. The joint density between X_j and Y is then given by

$$f(x_j = 1, y) = p_j f_j(y),$$

which can be compactly written as

$$f(x, y) = \left[p_1 f_1(y) \right]^{x_1} \cdots \left[p_k f_k(y) \right]^{x_k}$$

for all j. The marginal density of Y is subsequently given as

$$f(y) = \sum_x f(x, y) = \sum_{i=1}^{k} p_i f_i(y). \tag{4.6}$$

The unknown parameters in (4.6) will be denoted as Θ. The unknown parameters include the mixing proportions p_j as well as parameters of the distribution f_i. Then we write the *k-component mixture model* as

$$f(y|\Theta) = \sum_{i=1}^{k} p_i f_i(y). \tag{4.7}$$

to indicate the dependence of the model on the parameters Θ. The most widely used technique for estimating Θ in (4.7) is the *maximum likelihood estimation* (MLE). Suppose we have a sample $Y = \{Y_1, \cdots, Y_n\}$ drawn from the distribution $f(y|\Theta)$. The likelihood estimation of Θ is given by maximizing the loglikelihood:

$$\widehat{\Theta} = \arg\max_{\Theta} \prod_{i=1}^{n} f(y_i|\Theta) = \arg\max_{\Theta} \sum_{i-1}^{n} \ln f(y_i|\Theta).$$

For most mixture models, the optimization cannot be done analytically and it requires an iterative approximation technique called the expectation maximization (EM) algorithm.

4.2.3 *Expectation Maximization Algorithm*

The expectation maximization (EM) algorithm was first introduced by Dempster *et al.* (1977). For the introductory overview on the algorithm, see Robert and Casella (2004) and Flury (1997). The EM-algorithm proceeds as follows.

Following the argument in Robert and Casella (2004), we augment the observed data Y with latent (unobserved or missing) data Y^m. The complete complete data is then denoted as $Y^c = (Y, Y^m)$. The latent data is introduced as an artifice to make the problem tractable. The probability density of the complete data Y^c is denoted as $f(y^c) = f(y, y^m)$. The conditional density for the latent data Y^m, condition on the observation Y, is

$$f(y^m|y, \Theta) = \frac{f(y, y^m|\Theta)}{f(y|\Theta)}.$$

Again we introduced Θ to indicate the dependency of the probability on the parameters. Taking the logarithm on the both sides, we get the loglikelihood for the observed data

$$\ln f(Y|\Theta) = \ln f(Y^c|\Theta) - \ln f(Y^m|Y, \Theta).$$

Since the logarithm is a strictly increasing function, the value that maximizes $f(Y|\Theta)$ also maximizes $\ln f(Y|\Theta)$. Now taking the expectation with respect to $f(y^m|y, \Theta_0)$ for some fixed Θ_0 on the both sides, we have

$$\mathbb{E}[\ln f(Y|\Theta)|Y, \Theta_0] = \mathbb{E}[\ln f(Y^c|\Theta)|Y, \Theta_0] - \mathbb{E}[\ln f(Y^m|Y, \Theta)|Y, \Theta_0]. \quad (4.8)$$

Now denote the expected loglikelihood for the complete data as

$$Q(\Theta|\Theta_0, Y) = \mathbb{E}[\ln f(Y^c|\Theta)|Y, \Theta_0].$$

We then maximize the likelihood in iterative two-steps:

(1) E-step: compute the expectation $Q(\Theta|\widehat{\Theta}_{j-1}, Y)$.

(2) M-step: maximize $Q(\Theta|\widehat{\Theta}_{j-1}, Y)$ and take

$$\widehat{\Theta}_j = \arg\max_{\Theta} Q(\Theta|\widehat{\Theta}_{j-1}, Y). \quad (4.9)$$

Starting with the initial estimate $\widehat{\Theta}_0$, we have a sequence of estimators $\widehat{\Theta}_1, \widehat{\Theta}_2, \cdots$ and it can be shown to converges to the true MLE $\widehat{\Theta}$. However, the proof is beyond the scope of the book and we will only show that the Q function monotonically increases. The argument is as follows. By the definition (4.9), we have

$$Q(\widehat{\Theta}_j|\widehat{\Theta}_j, y) \le Q(\widehat{\Theta}_{j+1}|\widehat{\Theta}_j, y).$$

Now let

$$R(\Theta|\Theta_0, Y) = \mathbb{E}[\ln f(Y^m|Y, \Theta)|Y, \Theta_0].$$

This is the second term in (4.8).

The Jensen's inequality states that for a convex function ψ,

$$\psi(\mathbb{E}X) \leq \mathbb{E}\psi(X).$$

If ψ is a concave function, $-\psi$ is convex and we obtain

$$\psi(\mathbb{E}X) \geq \mathbb{E}\psi(X).$$

Then from the Jensen's inequality, we have

$$
\begin{aligned}
R(\Theta|\Theta_0, y) - R(\Theta_0|\Theta_0, y) &= \mathbb{E}\left[\ln \frac{f(Y^m|Y, \Theta)}{f(Y^m|Y, \Theta_0)}\Big|\Theta_0, y\right] \\
&\leq \ln \mathbb{E}\left[\frac{f(Y^m|Y, \Theta)}{f(Y^m|Y, \Theta_0)}\Big|\Theta_0, y\right] \\
&= \ln \int \frac{f(y^m|y, \Theta)}{f(y^m|y, \Theta_0)} f(y^m|y, \Theta_0)\, dy^m = 0.
\end{aligned}
$$

Hence we have $R(\widehat{\Theta}_{j+1}|\widehat{\Theta}_j, y) \leq R(\widehat{\Theta}_j|\widehat{\Theta}_j, y)$. Consequently

$$
\begin{aligned}
\ln f(y|\widehat{\Theta}_j) &= Q(\widehat{\Theta}_j|\widehat{\Theta}_j, y) - R(\widehat{\Theta}_j|\widehat{\Theta}_j, y) \\
&\leq Q(\widehat{\Theta}_{j+1}|\widehat{\Theta}_j, y) - R(\widehat{\Theta}_{j+1}|\widehat{\Theta}_j, y) \\
&\leq \ln f(y|\widehat{\Theta}_{j+1}).
\end{aligned}
$$

The inequality guarantees the the sequence of estimators $\widehat{\Theta}_j$ monotonically increase the likelihood function. Further, since the monotonically increasing sequence is bounded, i.e. $\ln f(y|\widehat{\Theta}_j) \leq \ln f(y|\widehat{\Theta})$, the sequence must be converging to a constant, but it is not clear if the limit is in fact $\ln f(y|\widehat{\Theta})$. To guarantee that the limit converges to the true maximum likelihood estimator, additional conditions are needed (Boyles, 1983; Wu, 1983).

The difficulty of implementing the EM-algorithm is at the E-step where we need to compute the conditional expectation $Q(\Theta|\widehat{\Theta}_{j-1}, y)$. The Monte Carlo version of the EM algorithm overcome this problem by simulating the missing data Y^m from the conditional density $f(y^m|y, \Theta)$ so that

$$\widehat{Q}(\Theta|\Theta_0, y) = \frac{1}{k}\sum_{j=1}^{k} \ln f(Y, Y^m|\Theta).$$

4.2.4   *Two Components Gaussian Mixtures*

As an illustration, two components Gaussian mixture model is shown. The three components model implemented in the SPM package simply add one more component to the model.

The image intensity will be modeled as a Gaussian mixture of the form

$$f(y) = p_1 f_1(y) + p_2 f_2(y)$$

where $p_1 + p_2 = 1$ and $f_1 \sim N(\mu_1, \sigma_1^2)$ and $f_2 \sim N(\mu_2, \sigma_2^2)$ are all known. There are 5 unknown parameters $\Theta = \{p_1, \mu_1, \mu_2, \sigma_1^2, \sigma_2^2\}$ to be estimated. Once p_1 is estimated, p_2 is automatically given as $1 - p_1$. The likelihood function is given by

$$f(\Theta|y) = \prod_{i=1}^{n} \left[p_1 f_1(y_i) + p_2 f_2(y_i) \right].$$

The loglikelihood is

$$L(\Theta|y) = \sum_{i=1}^{n} \ln \left[p_1 f_1(y_i) + p_2 f_2(y_i) \right].$$

The loglikelihood is maximized by solving

$$\frac{\partial L(\Theta|y)}{\partial p_i} = 0, \quad \frac{\partial L(\Theta|y)}{\partial \mu_i} = 0, \quad \frac{\partial L(\Theta|y)}{\partial \sigma_i^2} = 0$$

but this is not tractable. So we argument the data with the latent data and apply the EM-algorithm.

Let X be a Bernoulli random variable with

$$P(X = 1) = p, \ \ P(X = 0) = q = 1 - p.$$

This choice of latent random variable makes the subsequent EM-aglorithm tractable. Now define the conditional distribution $Y \sim f_1$ if $X = 1$ and $Y \sim f_2$ if $X = 0$. This defines the conditional density $f(y|x)$. The joint density $f(x, y)$ is

$$f(1, y) = p f_1(y), \ \ f(0, y) = q f_2(y).$$

This can be compactly written as

$$f(x, y) = \left[p f_1(y) \right]^{x} \left[q f_2(y) \right]^{1-x}.$$

The marginal density of Y is obviously

$$f(y) = \sum_{x=0,1} f(x, y) = p f_1(y) + q f_2(y).$$

The conditional density of X given Y is then

$$f(x|y) = \frac{[pf_1(y)]^x [qf_2(y)]^{1-x}}{pf_1(y) + qf_2(y)}.$$

The conditional expectation of X with respect to $f(x|y)$ is then

$$\mathbb{E}(X|y,p) = \frac{pf_1(y)}{pf_1(y) + qf_2(y)}. \tag{4.10}$$

The likelihood for the complete data (x,y) is

$$f(\Theta|x,y) = \prod_{i=1}^{n} \left[pf_1(y_i)\right]^{x_i} \left[qf_2(y_i)\right]^{1-x_i}$$

and the corresponding loglikelihood is given by

$$L(\Theta|x,y) = \sum_{i=1}^{n} x_i \ln\left[\frac{pf_1(y_i)}{qf_2(y_i)}\right] + \ln\left[qf_2(y_i)\right].$$

Take the expectation with respect to the latent variable X to get the Q-function

$$Q(\Theta|\Theta_0,y) = \mathbb{E}\left[\ln L(\Theta|X,Y)\big|y,\Theta_0\right]$$
$$= \sum_{i=1}^{n} \mathbb{E}(X_i|y,\Theta_0) \ln\left[\frac{pf_1(y_i)}{qf_2(y_i)}\right] + \ln\left[qf_2(y_i)\right]. \tag{4.11}$$

From (4.10), we have

$$\mathbb{E}(X_i|y,\Theta_0) = \frac{p_0 f_1(y_i)}{p_0 f_1(y_i) + q_0 f_2(y_i)} = \pi_{1i}$$

is the posterior probability of the i-th observation coming from the first class. Hence the expression (4.11) can be written as

$$Q(\Theta|\Theta_0,y) = \sum_{i=1}^{n} \pi_i \ln\left[\frac{pf_1(y_i)}{qf_2(y_i)}\right] + \ln\left[qf_2(y_i)\right]. \tag{4.12}$$

Maximize Q with respect to p by solving $\partial Q/\partial p = 0$. Then we obtain

$$p = \frac{1}{n}\sum_{i=1}^{n} \pi_{1i}. \tag{4.13}$$

(4.13) states that the prior probability for the 1st class is estimated as the average of the posterior probabilities in the 1st class. Note that we did not

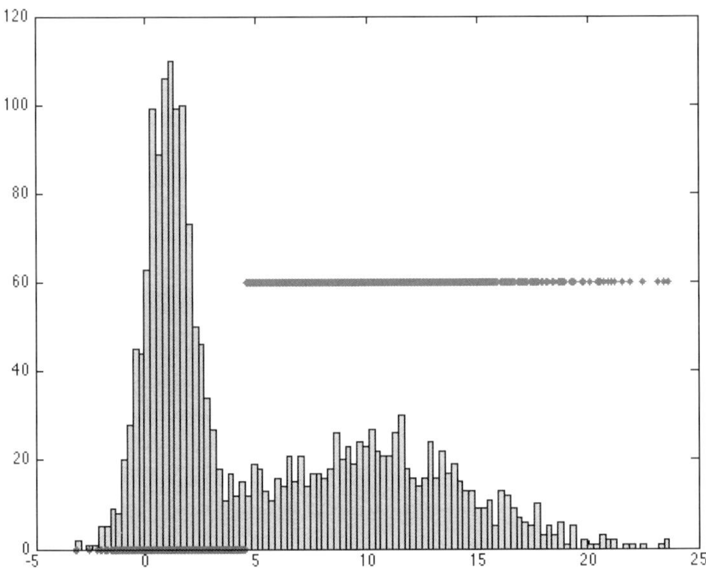

Fig. 4.7   Simulated two component Gaussian mixture with parameters $\mu_1 = 10, \sigma_1 = \sqrt{5}, \mu_2 = 1, \sigma_2 = 1, p_1 = 0.5, p_2 = 0.5$. The parameters are then estimated using the EM-algorithm. Using the estimated model, we can segment data depending on $f_1(x) < f_2(x)$ or $f_1(x) \geq f_2(x)$.

use the explicit forms for f_1 and f_2 so this result is general for any type of mixture distributions. Based on (4.13), we set up the iteration

$$\widehat{p}_{j+1} = \frac{1}{n} \sum_{i=1}^{n} \frac{\widehat{p}_j f_1(y_i)}{\widehat{p}_j f_1(y_i) + (1 - \widehat{p}_j) f_2(y_i)}$$

with any arbitrary initial $\widehat{p}_0 \in (0, 1)$. For other parameters, we obtain similar iterative formulas:

$$\mu_j = \frac{\sum_i \pi_{ji} y_i}{\sum_i \pi_{ji}}$$

and

$$\sigma_j^2 = \frac{\sum_i \pi_{ji}(y_i - \mu_j)^2}{\sum_i \pi_{ji}}.$$

Figure 4.7 shows the results of the two components model of simulated 1D data.

4.3   Voxel-Based Morphometry

All brain images are inherently noisy due to errors associated with image acquisition. Compounding the image acquisition errors, there are errors caused by image registration and segmentation. So it is necessary to smooth out the segmented images before VBM is performed. Among many possible image smoothing methods (Kovačič and Bajcsy, 1999; Perona and Malik, 1990), *Gaussian kernel smoothing* has emerged as a de facto smoothing technique in VBM due to its simplicity. Consider a n-dimensional Gaussian kernel

$$K(x) = \frac{1}{(2\pi)^{n/2}} \exp\left(-\frac{\|x\|^2}{2}\right),$$

where $\| \cdot \|$ is the Euclidean norm of $x \in \mathbb{R}^n$. The rescaled kernel K_σ is defined as

$$K_\sigma(x) = \frac{1}{\sigma^n} K\left(\frac{x}{\sigma}\right). \tag{4.14}$$

Then an integral version of Gaussian kernel smoothing in n-dimension is defined as

$$F(x, \sigma) = \int_{\mathbb{R}^n} K_\sigma(x - y) f(y) \, dy,$$

where $F(x, \sigma)$ is the scale-space representation of image $f(x)$ first introduced in Witkin (1983). Each $F(x, \sigma)$ for different values of σ produces a blurred copy of its original. The resulting scale-space representation from coarse to fine resolution can be used in multiscale approaches such as hierarchical searches and image segmentation. See Lindeberg (1994), Poline and Mazoyer (1994), Poline *et al.* (1995), Siegmund and Worsley (1996), and Worsley *et al.* (1996a) for the review of the major problems in scale-space and multiscale descriptions of images.

4.3.1   *ROI Volume Estimation in VBM*

Let $p(x)$ be the obtained tissue density of a region of interest (ROI) $\mathcal{M}$. For example, Figure 4.8 shows the white matter density of the corpus callosum. Let $\mathbf{1}_{\mathcal{M}}$ be an indicator function defined as

$$\mathbf{1}_{\mathcal{M}}(x) = \begin{cases} 1 \text{ if } x \in \mathcal{M}, \\ 0 \text{ otherwise.} \end{cases}$$

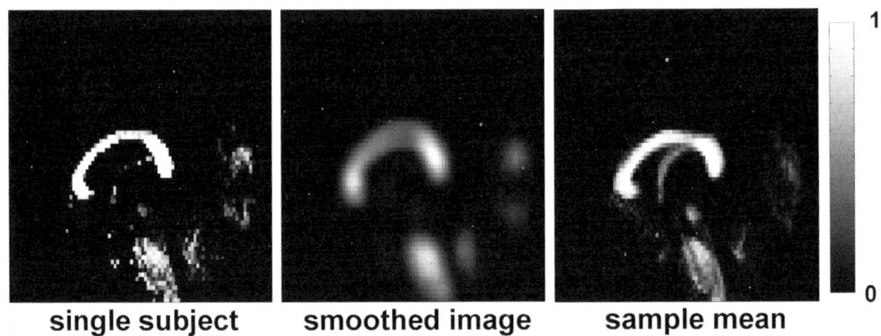

Fig. 4.8   Left: white matter segmentation of an individual midsagittal MRI using the three component Gaussian mixture model. Middle: 2D Gaussian kernel smoothing of the white matter segmentation. Right: the average of the smoothed white matter density of 12 normal subjects.

We may assume that the shape of $\mathcal{M}$ is random and we associate it with probability $p(x)$:

$$P(x \in \mathcal{M}) = p(x),$$
$$P(x \notin \mathcal{M}) = 0.$$

Then the volume of $\mathcal{M}$ is given by

$$\mu(\mathcal{M}) = \int \mathbf{1}_{\mathcal{M}}(x)\, dx. \tag{4.15}$$

Since the shape of $\mathcal{M}$ is random, the volume is random as well. By taking the expectation in (4.15), we obtain the estimate for the volume given by

$$\widehat{\mu}(\mathcal{M}) = \int \mathbb{E}\mathbf{1}_{\mathcal{M}}(x)\, dx \tag{4.16}$$

$$= \int p(x)\, dx. \tag{4.17}$$

So the sum of the white matter density over all voxels can be used as an estimate for the volume of the corpus callosum. In order to compute the volume of ROI, we do not need to identify the boundary of ROI. In this probabilistic context, ROI-based volumetry (Piven *et al.*, 1997; Hardan *et al.*, 2000; Manes *et al.*, 1999) can be viewed as a subset of the VBM framework.

Let us investigate the effect of smoothing on the volume estimate (4.17). Let K_σ be a Gaussian kernel given in (4.14). Kernel smoothing of scalar function p is given by

$$\int K_\sigma * p(x)\, dx = \int \int K_\sigma(x-y)p(y)\, dy\, dx \tag{4.18}$$

$$= \int p(y)\, dy. \tag{4.19}$$

From equation (4.17) and (4.19) it can be seen that the volume estimate

$$\widehat{\mu}(\mathcal{M}) = \int K_\sigma * p(x)\, dx \qquad (4.20)$$

is invariant under the scale change. This can be used to estimate the corpus callosum area from VBM white matter density maps for instance (Chung *et al.*, 2004). The corpus callosum area estimate does not differ by more than 0.6% in average when scales differ by 10 times. The numerical difference is due to the truncation of the Gaussian kernel. Assuming normality for the smoothed image $K_\sigma * p$, $\widehat{\mu}(\mathcal{M})$ is again normal so the usual statistical tests based on normality is applicable.

The tissue density (after smoothing) is a probability ranging between 0 and 1 so it is not exactly normally distributed. In order to set up a general linear model (GLM) which assumes Gaussian noise model, it is necessary to make the tissue density more normal. One way of doing this is to apply the Fisher or logit transform. However it is not necessary to perform the Fisher and logit transforms if we perform Gaussian kernel smoothing with relatively large bandwidth. The Gaussian kernel smoothing tend to make data more Gaussian due to the central limit theorem. For detailed distributional assumptions in VBM, see Ashburner and Friston (2000) and Salmond *et al.* (2002).

4.3.2 *Limitations of Witelson Partition*

In subsequent sections, we will use VBM in differentiating the amount of white matter in the corpus callosum for the group of 16 high functioning autistic and 12 normal subjects. Traditionally morphometric technique on the corpus callosum relied on the Witelson partition. We will review traditional corpus callosum morphometric studies in relation to autism.

Autism is a neurodevelopmental disorder affecting behavioral and social cognition but there is little understanding about the link between the functional deficit and its underlying neuroanatomy. Autism began to attract *in vivo* structural magnetic resonance imaging (MRI) studies in the region of the corpus callosum (Piven *et al.*, 1996, 1997; Egaas *et al.*, 1995; Hardan *et al.*, 2000; Manes *et al.*, 1999). These studies use the Witelson partition or a similar partition scheme of the corpus callosum (Witelson, 1989). Witelson partitioned the midsagittal cross-sectional images of the corpus callosum along the maximum anterior-posterior line (Talairach and Tournoux, 1988) and defined the region of the genu, rostrum, midbodies, isthmus and splenium from the anterior to posterior direction. Based on the

Witelson partition, there has been a consistent finding in abnormal reduction in anterior, midbody and posterior of the corpus callosum (Brambilla *et al.*, 2003).

Piven *et al.* (1997) compared 35 autistic individuals with 36 normal control subjects controlling for total brain volume, gender and IQ and detected a statistically significant smaller midbody and posterior regions of the corpus callosum in the autistic group. Manes *et al.* (1999) compared 27 low functioning autistic individuals with 17 normal controls adjusting for the total brain volume. They found a smaller corpus callosum compared to the control group in genu, rostrum, anterior midbody, posterior midbody and isthmus but did not find statistically significant differences in the rostrum and the splenium although the sample mean of the rostrum and splenium size are smaller than that of the control group. Hardan *et al.* (2000) compared 22 high functioning autistic to 22 individually matched control subjects and showed smaller genu and rostrum of the corpus callosum adjusting for the total brain volume based on the Witelson partition. The smaller corpus callosum size was considered as an indication of a decrease in interhemispheric connectivity. They did not detect other regions of significant size difference. For an extensive review of structural MRI studies for autism that have been published between 1966 and 2003, one may refer to Brambilla *et al.* (2003).

The shortcoming of the Witelson partition is the artificial partitioning. The Witelson partition may dilute the power of detection if the anatomical difference occurs near the partition boundary. Alternative voxel-wise approaches that avoid predefined regions of interests (ROI) have begun to be used in structural autism studies. Vidal *et al.* (2003) used the tensor-based morphometry (TBM) to show reduced callosal thickness in the genu, midbody and splenium in autistic children. Hoffmann *et al.* (2004) used a similar TBM to show curvature difference in the midbody. Abell *et al.* (1999) used voxel-based morphometry (VBM) (Wright *et al.*, 1995; Ashburner and Friston, 2000, 2001; Good *et al.*, 2001) in high functioning autism to show decreased gray matter volume in the right paracingulate sulcus, the left occipito-temporal cortex and increased amygdala and periamygdaloid cortex.

The advantage of the VBM framework over the Witelson partition approach is that it is completely automated and does not require the artificial partitioning of the corpus callosum that introduces undesirable bias. Further it is not restricted to *a priori* ROI enabling us to perform the statistical analysis at each voxel level and to pinpoint the exact location of the anatomical differences within ROI even if there is no ROI size differences. Although VBM was originally developed for whole brain 3D morphometry, our study concentrates on the midsagittal cross sectional corpus callosum regions to be able to compare the result with the previous 2D Witelson partition studies such as Hardan *et al.* (2000), Manes *et al.* (1999) and Piven *et al.* (1997). Hence we will mainly apply the 2D version of VBM over 3D VBM for corpus callosum.

4.3.3 *General Linear Models on Tissue Densities*

Since individuals are usually different in age, brain size and IQ, there might be confounding effects of age, brain size and IQ on the white matter density. Previous anatomical studies in the corpus callosum suggest this (Brambilla *et al.*, 2003). On the other hand, deformation-based morphometry and tensor-based morphometry in the normal developmental studies in children show that there is relative brain tissue growth in the corpus callosum over time (Chung *et al.*, 2001a; Thompson *et al.*, 2000). In particular, Chung *et al.* (2001a) showed white matter local volume increase in the midbody, isthmus and splenium of the corpus callosum in 28 normal subjects from 12 to 16 years.

To evaluate any possible effect of age on tissue density, we can fit the linear model

$$\texttt{density} = \lambda_1 + \lambda_2 \cdot \texttt{age} \tag{4.21}$$

to each group separately using the least-squares method at each voxel (Figure 1.1). The liner model fits show the dynamic pattern of different white matter density changes over time between groups. The pattern of growth in the corpus callosum is different. The autistic group shows lower white matter density compared to the control group at the lower age but gains white matter over time while the control group shows decreasing white matter density with age. There thus appears to be age differences for at least some regions of the corpus callosum and these should be accounted for.

One simple approach for removing the age effect would be to modulate the white matter density such that the age effect will not be present. First we estimate λ_1 and λ_2 for each group via the least squares method. Then adjust the white matter density $d(t)$ at time t via the transform

$$d(t) \to d(t) + \hat{\lambda}_2(\bar{t} - t),$$

where $\hat{\lambda}_2$ is the least-squres estimation of λ_2 and $\bar{t}$ is the mean age of both the controls and autistic combined together. This has an effect of modulating the densities measured at different age to the fixed reference age $\bar{t}$.

A more general statistical approach would be to use a general linear model (GLM). The general linear model (GLM) is a flexible framework that can be used in localizing the region of white matter concentration that are related to covariates such as age, IQ, brain size, gender and handness. We used the following GLM:

$$\texttt{density} = \lambda_1 + \lambda_2 \cdot \texttt{age} + \beta_1 \cdot \texttt{group}, \tag{4.22}$$

where the dummy variable $\texttt{group}$ is 1 for autism and 0 for control. In order to control the possible effect of the corpus callosum size differences, we also considered the following GLM sepeartely:

$$\texttt{density} = \lambda_1 + \lambda_2 \cdot \texttt{age} + \lambda_3 \cdot \texttt{area} + \beta_1 \cdot \texttt{group}, \tag{4.23}$$

where $\texttt{area}$ is the relative total corpus callosum area given in (4.17). In these formulations, we do not have separate linear equations as before but combine autism and control group data together and have a single linear equation. A similar linear model formulation in the VBM is used in localizing the region of the gray matter maturation in children (Paus *et al.*, 1999).

Once we obtained the statistical parametric maps from GLM, it is necessary to perform the multiple comparisons that account for spatially correlated error using the random field theory (Worsley, 1994; Worsley *et al.*, 1996b), the false discovery rates (Genovese *et al.*, 2002; Benjamini and Hochberg, 1995) or permutation tests (Nichols and Holmes, 2002).

4.3.4 *2D VBM Applied to Corpus Callosum*

In this section, we will show the detailed result of 2D VBM in localizing the regions of abnormal corpus callosum difference in autism. The detailed study results can be found in Chung *et al.* (2004).

Subjects. Gender and handedness usually affect the corpus callosum anatomy (Witelson, 1985, 1989) so all the 16 autistic and 12 control subjects used in this study are right-handed males except one subject who is ambidextrous. Sixteen autistic subjects were recruited for this study from a list of individuals with a diagnosis of high functioning autism in the Madison and Milwaukee area maintained for research purposes by the Waisman center at the University of Wisconsin-Madison. Diagnoses were confirmed with the Autism Diagnostic Interview - Revised (ADI-R) or clinical interview administered by a trained and certified psychologist at the Waisman center. All participants met DSM-IV criteria for autism or Asperger's pervasive developmental disorder. Twelve healthy, typically developing males with no current or past psychological diagnoses served as a control group. The average age for the control subject is 17.1 ± 2.8 and the autistic subjects is 16.1 ± 4.5. The age ranges for two groups are somewhat compatible; however, there might be still age effect on the white matter difference.

Image Acquisition. High resolution anatomical MRI scans were obtained using a 3-Tesla GE SIGNA (General Electric Medical Systems, Waukesha, WI) scanner with a quadrature head RF coil. A three-dimensional, spoiled gradient-echo (SPGR) pulse sequence was used to generate T1-weighted images. The imaging parameters were TR/TE 21/8 ms, flip angle $30°$, 240 mm field of view, 256x192 in-plane acquisition matrix (interpolated on the scanner to 256x256), and 128 axial slices (1.2 mm thick) covering the whole brain. Then the midsagittal cross-sections of the white matter segmented (Figures 4.8 and 4.9). Subsequently images are smoothed using 15 pixel wide FWHM 2D Gaussian kernel (Figure 4.8).

Age Effect on White Matter. The white matter density change over age was modeled using the linear growth model (4.21) to determine age effect. See Figure 1.1 for the resulting statistical parametric maps. The linear growth models were fitted for autism and control groups separately to show different pattern of white matter density change over time. Subjects with autism shows lower white matter concentration at the lower age range in almost all parts of the corpus callosum but the white matter density increases more rapidly over age to catch up with that of the control subjects.

The white matter increase of 2.5% per year in the genu of the autistic group is statistically significant (uncorrected p-value < 0.0014; corrected p-value < 0.16). Other regions of the corpus callosum do not show much age effect. The decrease of 2.5 per year in the midbody of the control group is not statistically significant (uncorrected p-value 0.1; corrected p-value $=$ 1). Since there is no age effect in the splenium, the white matter difference in the region should be largely due to the group difference while the white matter difference detected in the genu might be due to a possible age effect.

Removing the Effect of Age. Further to account for the possible global corpus callosum size difference among subjects, we have fitted GLM (4.23)

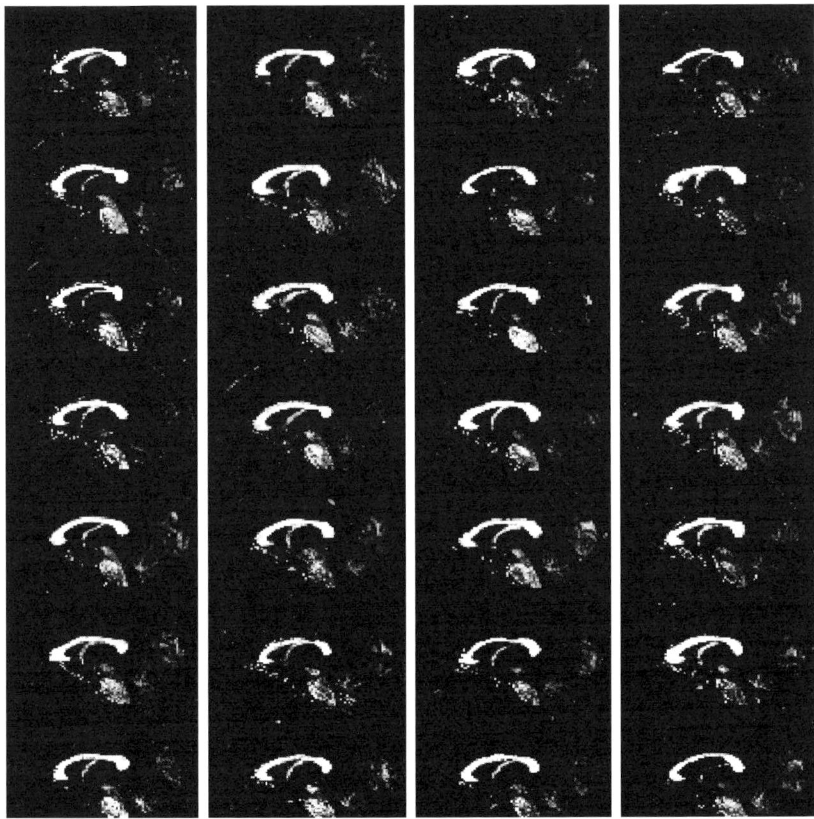

Fig. 4.9 The midsaggital cross-section images of segmented corpus callosum for 28 subjects. Starting from the first column, the first 16 subjects are autistics subjects while the next 12 subjects are control subjects. We are interested in localizing the white matter concentration difference between the two groups. All segmented images in the normalized MNI space.

controlling for both age and the total corpus callosum area. Statistically significant less white matter concentration in the splenium (corrected P-value 0.097, uncorrected p-value 0.0049, F-value 9.62), genu and rostrum regions (corrected p-value 0.16, uncorrected p-value 0.0086, F-value 8.18) were detected in the autistic subjects. This suggests impaired inter-hemispheric connectivity in frontal and particularly temporal and occipital regions.

Related Studies. It is interesting to note that Piven *et al.* (1996) found increased volume of the parietal, temporal and posterior lobes but not the frontal lobes in autism compared to normal control. Carper *et al.* (2002) did not find statistically significant frontal, temporal, parietal and occipital white matter volume differences between the groups in age range 7.5-11.5 years; however, their regression analysis showed the predicted white matter volume at age 12 is substantially lower in the autistic group. The orbital frontal cortex projects through the rostrum while occipital and inferior temporal cortex project through the splenium (Hardan *et al.*, 2000). So this findings indirectly suggest the impaired inter-hemispheric connectivity in those cortical regions.

The deficit in splenium white matter may be associated with the abnormalities in face processing and particularly in the identification of emotion in faces (Dalton *et al.*, 2003). In normal subjects, faces activate the right fusiform area and the verbal identification of the emotion in a face likely requires transfer of information between the hemispheres in the splenium region. The deficit found here in the autism group may at least in part underlie the abnormalities in emotional face processing observed in this group.

A similar result was also obtained using tensor-based morphometry where Vidal *et al.* (2003) compared 15 autistic subjects of age 9.9 ± 3.2 years to a group of 13 control subjects of age 10 ± 2.1 years. They found the most significant reduction of the corpus callosum size in the genu, splenium and midbody in decreasing order. The slight difference with our voxel-based morphometry result might be due to the different morphometric techniques plus manual segmentation used in Vidal *et al.* (2003) while no manual segmentation of any sort was applied in our VBM approach.

Using the white matter density as an index for neural connectivity (Hardan *et al.*, 2000), autism is shown to exhibit less white matter concentration in the region of the genu, rostrum and splenium while accounting for the anatomical variations due to age. Further it is shown that the less white matter concentration in the corpus callosum in autism is due to hypoplasia rather than atrophy.

Chapter 5

Geometry of Cortical Manifolds

Due to the geometric nature of convoluted cortical surfaces, differential geometric approaches have been often used in quantifying shape changes in the cortical surfaces. For an overview of differential geometry, see Boothby (1986), do Carmo (1992) and Kreyszig (1959). Given a cortical surface $\mathcal{M}$ which we assume to be a smooth twice-differentiable 2-dimensional manifold embedded in $\mathbb{R}^3$ (Joshi *et al.*, 1995), we have a parameterization of the surface $\mathcal{M}$:

$$X(u) = \{(x_1(u), x_2(u), x_3(u)) : u = (u^1, u^2) \in \mathcal{N}\}$$

where all partial derivatives of X up to the second order are continuous in a planar domain $\mathcal{N}$. It is a differential geometric convention to use the superscript to index the coordinates of the parameter space $\mathcal{N}$. The smooth map $X : \mathcal{N} \to \mathcal{M}$ is called a *parameterized surface* of $\mathcal{M}$ if the partial derivative vectors

$$X_1(u) = \left(\frac{\partial x_1}{\partial u^1}, \frac{\partial x_2}{\partial u^1}, \frac{\partial x_3}{\partial u^1}\right)'$$

and

$$X_2(u) = \left(\frac{\partial x_1}{\partial u^2}, \frac{\partial x_2}{\partial u^2}, \frac{\partial x_3}{\partial u^2}\right)'$$

form a basis for the tangent space $T_{\mathbf{p}}(\mathcal{M})$ at point $p \in \mathcal{M}$. For this to happen, we need $X_1(u) \times X_2(u) \neq 0$ for any $u \in \mathcal{N}$.

If X_1 and X_2 form a basis for the tangent space $T_{\mathbf{p}}(\mathcal{M})$, any vector $d\xi \in T_{\mathbf{p}}(\mathcal{M})$ can be written as a linear combination of the basis vectors X_1 and X_2, i.e.

$$d\xi = du^1 X_1 + du^2 X_2$$

for some constants du^1 and du^2. Then the length of the vector $d\xi$ in the Cartesian coordinate is given by

$$d\xi^2 \equiv \langle d\xi, d\xi \rangle = \sum_{i,j=1,2} \langle X_i, X_j \rangle du^i du^j. \tag{5.1}$$

The coefficients $g_{ij} = \langle X_i, X_j \rangle$ are called the *Riemannian metric tensor* and they measure the amount of deviation from the Cartesian coordinate system. If the basis are orthonormal, we have $g_{ij} = \delta_{ij}$, the Kroneker's delta. The bilinear form (5.1) is called the first fundamental form. The first fundamental form enables us to compute intrinsic properties of the surface such as lengths, angles and areas. If a curve on the surface $\mathcal{M}$ is given by $X(u(s))$, where the curvilinear coordinates $u(s) = (u^1(s), u^2(s))$ is parameterized by a parameter s, its length is given by

$$\int \left\| \frac{du}{ds} \right\| ds = \int \left(\sum_{i,j=1,2} g_{ij} \frac{du^i}{ds} \frac{du^j}{ds} \right)^{1/2} ds.$$

The angle θ between two vectors $\xi, \eta \in T_{\mathbf{p}}(\mathcal{M})$ can be computed in terms of the Riemannian metric tensor in the following way:

$$\cos\theta = \frac{\langle \xi, \eta \rangle}{\|\xi\| \|\eta\|} = \frac{\sum_{i,j} g_{ij} \xi^i \eta^j}{(\sum_{i,j} g_{ij} \xi^i \xi^j)^{1/2} (\sum_{i,j} g_{ij} \eta^i \eta^j)^{1/2}}.$$

The total surface area of a region $A \subset \mathcal{M}$ is

$$\int_{X^{-1}(A)} \sqrt{\det g} \, du^1 du^2,$$

where $\det g = g_{11} g_{22} - g_{12}^2$ and it is invariant under parameterization X (do Carmo, 1992). Note that $\sqrt{\det g}$ is the *local surface area element* and has been used in measuring the local surface area change at cortical mesh vertices (Chung *et al.*, 2003c).

Let us review few important surface parameterization methods. Surface parameterization is probably the most important procedure in mathematically modeling cortical and subcortical surfaces.

5.1 Surface Parameterization

Cortical surfaces are usually segmented and represented as high resolution unstructured triangular meshes. In order to compute differential geometric quantities, it is necessary to parameterize the coordinates of mesh vertices analytically using smooth functions. While parameterizing a curve can be done easily using arclength, it is not trivial to parameterize an arbitrary surface since there is no natural ordering of points on the surface (Staib and Duncan, 1996).

5.1.1 *B-Spline Parameterization*

One of the most widely used surface parameterization method is to extend the B-Spline curves to surfaces via tensor product. Let us start with Bézier curves which are special cases of B-spline curves (Guéziec, 1996; McLeod and Baart, 1998). It is originally developed by Bézier and De Casteljau in the 1970's for CAD/CAM operations for car manufacturing industry. Then it became the foundation of the entire Adobe Postscript drawing model.

The simplest Bézier curve is a line segment $\mathbf{p}_{0,1}(u)$ joining two points $\mathbf{p}_0$ and $\mathbf{p}_1$ and parameterized by $u \in (0,1)$ as

$$\mathbf{p}_{i,j}(u) = (1-u)\mathbf{p}_i + u\mathbf{p}_j, \ u \in (0,1).$$

For three points $\mathbf{p}_0, \mathbf{p}_1$ and $\mathbf{p}_2$, a quadratic Bézier curve is given by

$$\begin{aligned}\mathbf{p}_{0,2}(u) &= (1-u)\mathbf{p}_{0,1} + u\mathbf{p}_{1,2} \\ &= (1-u)^2\mathbf{p}_0 + 2(1-u)\mathbf{p}_1 + u^2\mathbf{p}_2.\end{aligned}$$

In general, m-th order Bézier curve is given by

$$\mathbf{p}_{0,m}(u) = \sum_{j=0}^{m} \phi_{j,m}(u)\mathbf{p}_j, \ u \in (0,1)$$

where the basis functions

$$\phi_{j,m}(u) = \binom{m}{j}(1-u)^{m-j}u^j, \ j = 0,\ldots,m$$

are Bernstein polynomials of degree m. Cubic Bézier curves are the most often used Bézier curve because cubics satisfy the minimum curvature property (Guéziec, 1996) or the strain energy property (McLeod and Baart, 1998), which make them a more suitable tool for a smooth curve approximation.

5.1.2 *B-Spline Curves*

To avoid increasing the degree of the Bézier curve, we need to connect cubic together Bézier curves in a piecewise fashion. If continuity conditions are satisfied for each Bézier curve segments, the result is a B-spline curve. In general, a B-spline curve of degree $K-1$ with $m+1$ vertices $\mathbf{p}_0, \cdots \mathbf{p}_m \in \mathbb{R}^d$ is defined as

$$X(u) = \sum_{j=0}^{m} B_{j,K}(u)\mathbf{p}_j,$$

where the B-spline functions $\{B_{j,K}(u), j = 0, \cdots, m\}$ are defined recursively with $m + K + 1$ knot values u_j such that

$$B_{j,1}(u) = \begin{cases} 1, & u_j \le u < u_{j+1} \\ 0, & \text{otherwise} \end{cases}$$

and

$$B_{j,k} = \frac{u - u_j}{u_{j+k-1} - u_j} B_{j,k-1}(u) + \frac{u_{j+k} - u}{u_{j+k} - u_{j+1}} B_{j+1,k-1}(u).$$

It is possible to generate surfaces using the tensor product on B-splines. Consider a rectangular mesh with vertices $\mathbf{p}_{ij}$. A B-spline surface parameterization X of degree $K - 1$ for points $\mathbf{p}_{ij} \in \mathbb{R}^3$ can be defined by the tensor product:

$$X(u^1, u^2) = \sum_{i,j} B_{i,K}(u^1) B_{j,K}(u^2)\mathbf{p}_{ij}. \tag{5.2}$$

The advantage for using B-spline to represent the surface is that it is easy to evaluate the curvature of a surface or other geometric characteristics of the surface because polynomial functions can be differentiated easily. The disadvantage of using the tensor B-spline is that it is not easy to modify the above formulation which works so well for a rectangular mesh to a irregular triangular mesh.

5.1.3 *Quadratic Parameterization*

Instead of using B-splines to form a parametric surface, there is a simpler method based on the polynomial regression. This is a smoothing technique to fit the given points $\mathbf{p}_0, \ldots, \mathbf{p}_m$ by the least-squares method to a polynomial function of the form

$$f(x, y) = \sum_{i+j \le p} \beta_{ij}\, x^i y^j. \tag{5.3}$$

Then for $\mathbf{p}_i = (x^i, y^i, z^i)$, $(p + 1)(p + 2)/2$ unknown coefficients β_{ij} are chosen to minimize the residual

$$\sum_{i=0}^{m} \left[z^i - f(x^i, y^i)\right]^2.$$

The drawback of the polynomial regression is that there is a tendency to weave the outer most vertices to find vertices in the center. Therefore this is not advisable to directly fit (5.3) when the z-coordinate values rapidly change. Polynomial regression is not recommended for global surface parameterization.

In estimating various differential geometric measures such as the Laplace-Beltrami operator or curvatures, it is not necessary to find such global parameterization of the surface $\mathcal{M}$. A local surface parameterization in the neighborhood of $\mathbf{p}$ can be obtained via the projection of the local surface onto the tangent plane $T_{\mathbf{p}}(\mathcal{M})$.

Let Q be an orthogonal matrix which rotates the normal vector $\mathbf{n} = (n_1, n_2, n_3)$ to align with the x_3-axis, i.e. $Q\mathbf{n} = (0, 0, 1)'$. Algebraic manipulation shows that

$$
Q = \begin{pmatrix} n_3 & 0 & -\sqrt{n_1^2 + n_2^2} \\ 0 & 1 & 0 \\ \sqrt{n_1^2 + n_2^2} & 0 & n_3 \end{pmatrix} \begin{pmatrix} \frac{n_1}{\sqrt{n_1^2+n_2^2}} & \frac{n_2}{\sqrt{n_1^2+n_2^2}} & 0 \\ -\frac{n_2}{\sqrt{n_1^2+n_2^2}} & \frac{n_1}{\sqrt{n_1^2+n_2^2}} & 0 \\ 0 & 0 & 1 \end{pmatrix}
$$

is such an orthogonal matrix assuming $n_1, n_2 \neq 0$. If $n_1 = n_2 = 0$, we can take Q to be an identify matrix.

Let $x \in \mathcal{M}$ be a point in the neighborhood of p. Under the transformation $(u^1, u^2, u^3)' : x \to Q(x - p)$, the local surface patch translates to the origin and then rotates by Q (Figure 5.1). With respect to the new coordinates (u^1, u^2, u^3), the local surface patch can be explicitly written as the standard explicit form $u_3 = f(u^1, u^2)$ for some function f assuming local smoothness of the surface. By identifying (u^1, u^2) as the parameter space $\mathcal{N}$, we have the following local parameterization in the neighborhood of p:

$$
X(u^1, u^2) = p + Q'\left(u^1, u^2, f(u^1, u^2)\right)'. \tag{5.4}
$$

Then the basis on the tangent plane $T_p(\mathcal{M})$ is

$$
X_1 = Q'\left(1, 0, \left.\frac{\partial f}{\partial u^1}\right|_{(0,0)}\right)'
$$

and

$$
X_2 = Q'\left(0, 1, \left.\frac{\partial f}{\partial u^2}\right|_{(0,0)}\right)'.
$$

Thus the Riemannian metric tensor is given by

$$
g_{ij} = \langle X_i, X_j \rangle = \delta_{ij} + \left.\frac{\partial f}{\partial u^i}\right|_{(0,0)} \cdot \left.\frac{\partial f}{\partial u^j}\right|_{(0,0)}. \tag{5.5}
$$

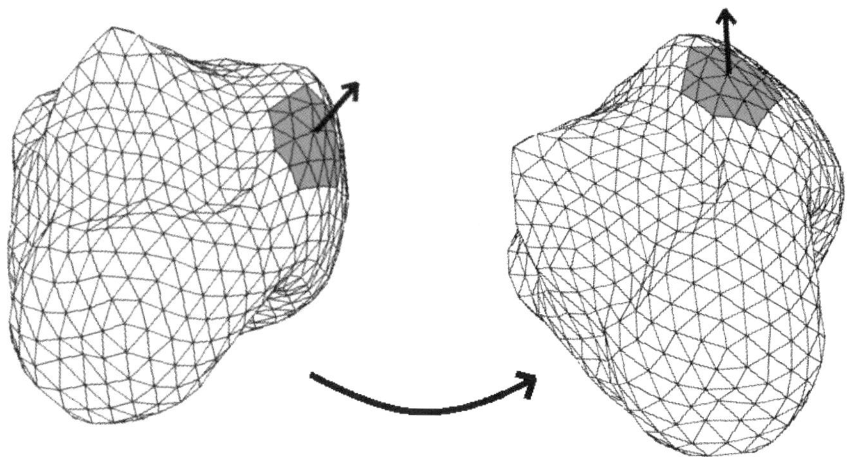

Fig. 5.1 A surface has been rotated by an orthogonal matrix Q so that the normal vector $\mathbf{n}$ is aligning with the x_3-axis.

Hence the metric tensor at p is completely determined by the derivatives of the function f evaluated at $(0,0)$ and it is independent of the rotation of the tangent plane by Q. Similarly, the coefficients of the second fundamental form are invariant under such a transformation.

In the neighborhood of $(0,0)$, we have the Taylor approximation of the function f:

$$f(u^1, u^2) = \beta_1 u^1 + \beta_2 u^2 + \beta_3 (u^1)^2 + \beta_4 u^1 u^2 + \beta_5 (u^2)^2 + \cdots . \quad (5.6)$$

Since we are forcing the function f to pass through the origin, there is no constant term in the Taylor expansion. The problem of estimating the parameters β_j can be formulated in terms of least-squares estimation. For m neighboring points $p_1, \cdots, p_m$, let

$$u_i = (u_i^1, u_i^2, u_i^3)' = Q(p_i - p).$$

Then the unknown parameters β_i are chosen to be the least-squares estimates of linear equations $Y = \mathbf{X}\beta$, where

$$\beta = (\beta_1, \cdots, \beta_5)',$$
$$Y = (u_1^3, \cdots, u_m^3)'$$

and the $m \times 5$ matrix $\mathbf{X}$ is given by

$$\mathbf{X} = \begin{pmatrix} u_1^1 & u_1^2 & (u_1^1)^2 & u_1^1 u_1^2 & (u_1^2)^2 \\ u_2^1 & u_2^2 & (u_2^1)^2 & u_2^1 u_2^2 & (u_2^2)^2 \\ \cdots\cdots\cdots\cdots\cdots\cdots\cdots \\ u_m^1 & u_m^2 & (u_m^1)^2 & u_m^1 u_m^2 & (u_m^2)^2 \end{pmatrix}.$$

The least-squares estimation is

$$\widehat{\beta} = (\mathbf{X}'\mathbf{X})^-\mathbf{X}'Y, \tag{5.7}$$

where $^-$ denotes a generalized inverse, which can be obtained through the singular value decomposition (Lawson and Hanson, 1974). Then from (5.5), the fundamental forms can be estimated and consequently the mean and the Gaussian curvatures as well. In practice, g_{ii} can be any number bigger than 1. The smoother the triangular mesh, the closer g_{11}, g_{22} are to the value 1. When $g_{ij} = \delta_{ij}$, we have locally Euclidean space, which is the smoothest possible space.

5.1.4 *Fourier Descriptors*

Beyond B-splines and quadratic surfaces, other surface representation technique such as Fourier descriptors (Staib and Duncan, 1996) spherical harmonic representation (Chung *et al.*, 2008a) are also available. In these approaches, we use sine or cosine basis or spherical harmonics in smoothly representing mesh vertices. For instance, we can have

$$f(x,y) = \sum_{i,j=0}^{k} a_{ij} \sin(i\omega_1 x)\sin(j\omega_2 y) + b_{ij}\sin(i\omega_1 x)\cos(j\omega_2 y)$$
$$+ c_{ij}\cos(i\omega_1 x)\sin(j\omega_2 y) + d_{ij}\cos(i\omega_1 x)\cos(j\omega_2 y).$$

Such a surface requires a large number of coefficients $a_{ij}, b_{ij}, c_{ij}, d_{ij}$ to fit. The fundamental frequencies ω_1, ω_2 has to be determined as well. In general, surface fitting based on finite Fourier series is computationally intensive although the fit is expected to be better than the polynomial fit. Fourier descriptors and spherical harmonic representation will be discussed in detail in the later chapters.

5.2 Surface Normals and Curvatures

Curvature of surfaces provide important knowledge in a number of applications such as structural bioinformatics (Koh *et al.*, 2006) and computer vision (Meyer *et al.*, 2002). To characterize the geometrical properties of surface folding pattern for instance, surface normal vectors need to be estimated first. Then curvatures can be computed from the normal vectors. In most applications including brain imaging, we do not have the smooth functional representation of surfaces to start with. Instead we need to deal with unstructured polygonal meshes.

5.2.1 *Surface Normals*

In order to compute the Riemannian metric tensors on a triangulated surface, we first estimate the tangent plane and its normal vector at each node then find a local parameterization in the neighborhood of each node. Normal vectors can be computed during the triangulation process. In the anatomic segmentation using proximities (ASP)method (MacDonald *et al.*, 2000), the outward unit normal vector $\mathbf{n}$ at each node p is computed as the weighted average of the unit normals of the incident triangles. If $\mathbf{p}_1, \ldots, \mathbf{p}_m$ are m neighboring points of $\mathbf{p} = \mathbf{p}_0$ in the counter-clockwise direction with respect to the tangent plane $T_{\mathbf{p}}(\mathcal{M})$ at $\mathbf{p}$ (Figure 5.2), the unit normal vector $\mathbf{n}$ is estimated as

$$\mathbf{n} = \frac{\sum_{i=1}^{m} \varphi_i \mathbf{n}_i}{\sum_{i=1}^{m} \varphi_i},$$

where the unit vectors $\mathbf{n}_i$ are normal to each triangle T_i.

$$\mathbf{n}_i = \frac{(\mathbf{p}_{i+1} - \mathbf{p}) \times (\mathbf{p}_i - \mathbf{p})}{\|(\mathbf{p}_{i+1} - \mathbf{p}) \times (\mathbf{p}_i - \mathbf{p})\|}$$

and the interior angles are

$$\varphi_i = \cos^{-1} \frac{\langle \mathbf{p}_{i+1} - \mathbf{p}, \mathbf{p}_i - \mathbf{p} \rangle}{\|\mathbf{p}_{i+1} - \mathbf{p}\| \|\mathbf{p}_i - \mathbf{p}\|}.$$

Alternatively, we may employ a method similar to principal components analysis (PCA) (Jolliffe, 2002). The equation of the plane with the unit normal vector $\mathbf{n}$ passing through the point p is $\langle \mathbf{n}, x \rangle = \langle \mathbf{n}, \mathbf{p} \rangle$. The distance from the point $\mathbf{p}_i$ to the plane is the length of the projection of $\mathbf{p}_i - \mathbf{p}$ onto the unit normal vector $\mathbf{n}$, i.e. $\langle \mathbf{n}, \mathbf{p}_i - \mathbf{p} \rangle$. Then we find the best fitting tangent plane in the sense of minimizing the sum of squared distance of the points $\mathbf{p}_1, \ldots, \mathbf{p}_m$ to the plane:

$$\min_{\mathbf{n}} \sum_{i=1}^{m} \langle \mathbf{n}, \mathbf{p}_i - \mathbf{p} \rangle^2 = \min_{\mathbf{n}} \mathbf{n}' \mathbf{C} \mathbf{n},$$

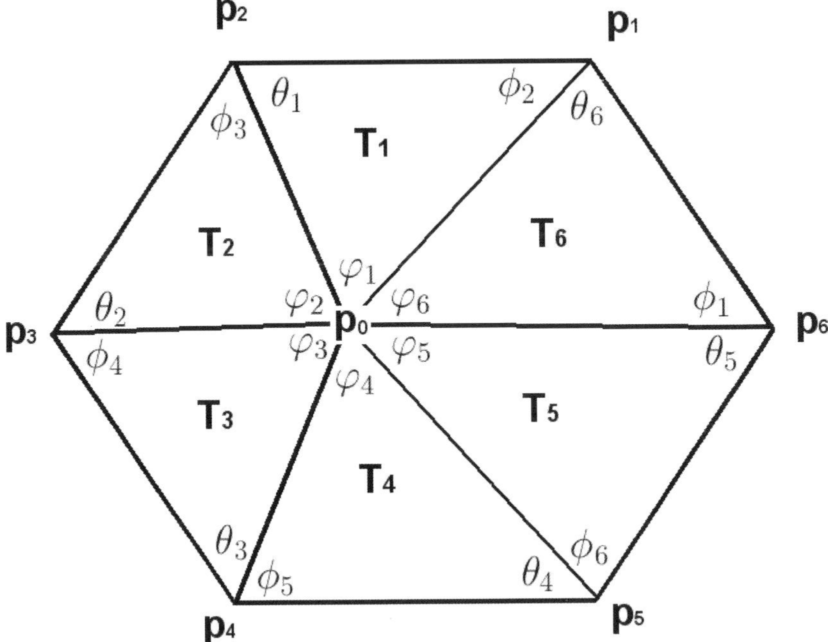

Fig. 5.2 A usual first order neighbors around the center vertex $\mathbf{p}_0$. Most of differential geometric quantities can be discretely approximated using the first order neighbors.

where

$$\mathbf{C} = \sum_{i=1}^{m} (\mathbf{p}_i - \mathbf{p})(\mathbf{p}_i - \mathbf{p})'.$$

If the fitting plane is not forced to pass through the point $\mathbf{p}$, $\mathbf{C}$ becomes the sample covariance matrix of $\mathbf{p}_1, \ldots, \mathbf{p}_m$ and the optimization problem is exactly the standard PCA. Since $\mathbf{n}'\mathbf{n} = 1$, using the Lagrange multiplier γ minimize

$$\mathbf{n}'\mathbf{C}\mathbf{n} - \gamma(\mathbf{n}'\mathbf{n} - 1).$$

Differentiating with respect to $\mathbf{n}$, $\mathbf{C}\mathbf{n} - \gamma\mathbf{n} = 0$. Thus, γ is an eigenvalue of $\mathbf{C}$. Note that we are minimizing $\mathbf{n}'\mathbf{C}\mathbf{n} = \mathbf{n}'\gamma\mathbf{n} = \gamma$. So the unit normal vector $\mathbf{n}$ of the best fitting tangent plane should be the eigenvector $\mathbf{n}$ that corresponds to the smallest eigenvalue.

If the interior angle of triangles joining the vertex $\mathbf{p}$ is acute, the best fitting plane passing through $\mathbf{p}$ might end up perpendicular to the tangent plane $T_{\mathbf{p}}(\mathcal{M})$. In this case, the unit normal vector $\mathbf{n}$ to $T_{\mathbf{p}}(\mathcal{M})$ should be the eigenvector that corresponds to the largest eigenvalue.

5.2.2   *Gaussian and Mean Curvatures*

The unit outward normal vector $\mathbf{n}$ to the surface is given by

$$\mathbf{n} = \frac{X_1 \times X_2}{\sqrt{\det g}}.$$

The vectors $(X_1, X_2, \mathbf{n})$ form an orthogonal basis in the 3D Euclidean space. So the partial derivative of the basis vectors X_1, X_2 and $\mathbf{n}$ can be again expressed in terms of the basis:

$$\frac{\partial X_i}{\partial u^j} = \Gamma^1_{ij} X_1 + \Gamma^2_{ij} X_2 + \Gamma^3_{ij} \mathbf{n},$$

$$\frac{\partial \mathbf{n}}{\partial u^j} = \Gamma^1_{3j} X_1 + \Gamma^2_{3j} X_2 + \Gamma^3_{3j} \mathbf{n},$$

where the coefficients Γ^k_{ij} are called the Christoffel symbols. The second fundamental form is then given by

$$-\langle d\xi, d\mathbf{n} \rangle = \sum_{i,j=1,2} l_{ij} du^i du^j, \tag{5.8}$$

where $l_{ij} = \langle X_{ij}, \mathbf{n} \rangle$ and

$$X_{ij} = \frac{\partial X_i}{\partial u^j} = \left(\frac{\partial^2 x_1}{\partial u^i \partial u^j}, \frac{\partial^2 x_2}{\partial u^i \partial u^j}, \frac{\partial^2 x_3}{\partial u^i \partial u^j} \right)'.$$

Let $g = (g_{ij})$ and $l = (l_{ij})$.

Principal Curvatures. The principal curvatures κ_1 and κ_2 are defined as the eigenvalues of $g^{-1}l$ and the mean curvature K_M and the Gaussian curvature K_G can be given in terms of the principal curvatures as

$$K_M = (\kappa_1 + \kappa_2)/2 = \operatorname{tr}(g^{-1}l)/2$$

and

$$K_G = \kappa_1 \kappa_2 = \det(l)/\det(g).$$

Figure 5.3 shows the mean and Gaussian curvatures of a brain surface.

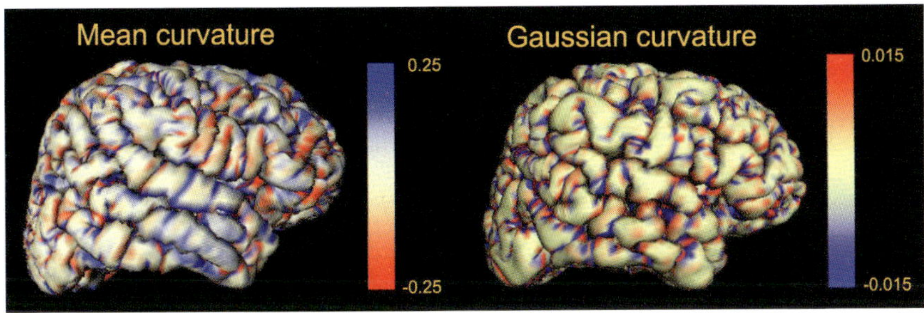

Fig. 5.3   The mean and Gaussian curvature maps of a cortical surface based on quadratic polynomial fit.

Estimating curvatures and surface normals on triangulated meshes is not an easy problem due to the possible inaccuracy and instability of estimation for noisy meshes. To solve these problems, various methods have been proposed. The covariance matrix of the surface normals has been used (Angelopoulou, 1999). There is also a finite element version of the mean curvature estimation using the cotan formulation (Desrun *et al.*, 1999; Meyer *et al.*, 2002; Ohtake *et al.*, 2000). Local quadratic surface fitting is also popular (Joshi *et al.*, 1995; Chung *et al.*, 2003c).

5.2.3   *Curvatures of Polynomial Surfaces*

Consider a polynomial surface of the form

$$f(x_1, x_2) = \beta_0 + \beta_1 x_1 + \beta_2 x_2 + \frac{1}{2}\beta_3 x_1^2 + \beta_4 x_1 x_2 + \frac{1}{2}\beta_5 x_2^2. \qquad (5.9)$$

The surface can be parameterized as

$$X(u^1, u^2) = \left(u^1, u^2, f(u^1, u^2)\right)$$

with $u^1 = x_1$ and $u^2 = x_2$. An algebraic manipulation will show that

$$X_1 = (1, 0, \beta_1), \ X_2 = (0, 1, \beta_2),$$

$$X_{11} = (0, 0, \beta_3), \ X_{12} = (0, 0, \beta_4), \ X_{22} = (0, 0, \beta_5)$$

at the origin $(u^1, u^2) = (0, 0)$. The normal vector $\mathbf{n}$ is

$$\mathbf{n} = \frac{(-\beta_1, -\beta_2, 1)}{(1 + \beta_1^2 + \beta_2^2)^{1/2}}.$$

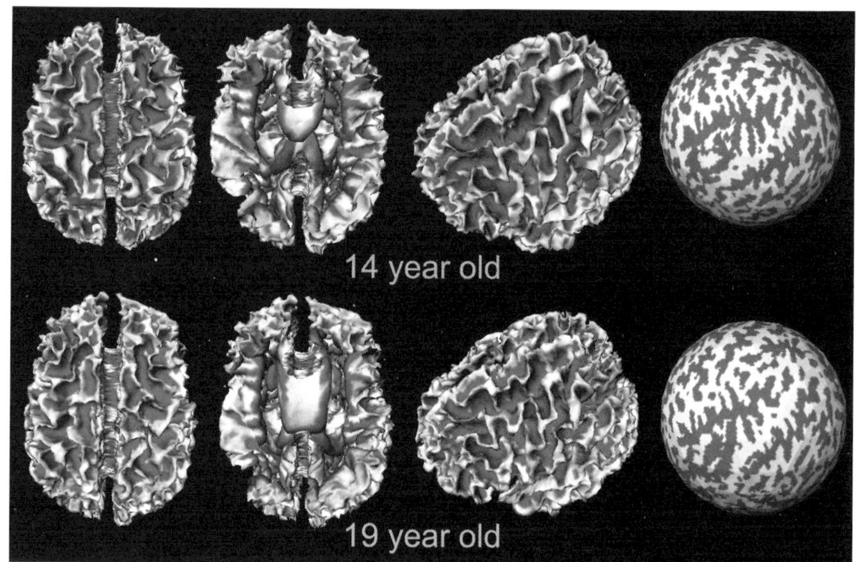

Fig. 5.4   Growth pattern of the inner cortical surface of a subject at age 14 and 19 (Chung *et al.*, 2003c). The enlarged ventricle is visible. Mean curvature was thresholded at 0.01 to visualize the sulcal patterns. The patterns at age 14 and 19 are globally similar although there are local variations. Surface-based morphometric techniques should be able to pick out such local pattern variations.

From (5.1) and (5.8), the coefficients of the fundamental forms at the origin are given by

$$g = \begin{pmatrix} 1 + \beta_1^2 & \beta_1\beta_2 \\ \beta_1\beta_2 & 1 + \beta_2^2 \end{pmatrix},$$

$$l = \frac{1}{(1 + \beta_1^2 + \beta_2^2)^{1/2}} \begin{pmatrix} \beta_3 & \beta_4 \\ \beta_4 & \beta_5 \end{pmatrix}.$$

Then the mean curvature is given by

$$K_M = \frac{\beta_3(1 + \beta_2^2) + \beta_5(1 + \beta_1^2) - 2\beta_1\beta_2\beta_4}{(1 + \beta_1^2 + \beta_2^2)^{3/2}}. \tag{5.10}$$

The parameters β_j in (5.9) can be estimated by projecting the local surface patch in the neighborhood of a vertex p onto the tangent plane $T_p(\mathcal{M})$. See (5.7) for the least squares estimation. Figure 5.3 illustrates the local polynomial fitting based curvature estimation of a cortical surface. Surface curvatures can be used in quantifying cortical shape variations (Figure 5.4).

When the local quadratic surface patch is used, it is easy to estimate geometric quantities such as local surface area, length and curvatures. Because of this simplicity, quadratic surface fitting has been often used in estimating curvatures on cortical surfaces. The drawback of the quadratic fit, and polynomial fit in general, is that there is tendency to wave the outer most data so it usually breaks down near boundary.

5.3   Laplace-Beltrami Operator

The gradient ∇_X of F on the tangent plane $T_{\mathbf{p}}(\mathcal{M})$ is defined as

$$\nabla_X F = \sum_{i,j} g^{ij} \frac{\partial F}{\partial u^j} X_i, \tag{5.11}$$

where $(g^{ij}) = g^{-1}$. The generalized Laplacian called the *Laplace-Beltrami operator* Δ_X corresponding to the surface parameterization X is defined as the divergence of the gradient operator such that

$$\Delta_X F = \nabla_X \cdot (\nabla_X F) = \frac{1}{|g|^{1/2}} \sum_{i,j} \frac{\partial}{\partial u^i} \left(|g|^{1/2} g^{ij} \frac{\partial F}{\partial u^j} \right), \tag{5.12}$$

where $|g|$ is the determinant of g (Kreyszig, 1959; Marsden and Hughes, 1983). For the derivation of the Laplace-Beltrami operator without using differential geometry, one may approach the problem in terms of a curvilinear coordinate transform (Courant and Hilbert, 1953). The most important intrinsic property of the Laplace-Beltrami operator is that it is independent of the parameterization of $\mathcal{M}$. If $\widetilde{X} = X \circ \Phi$ is another parameterization, we have

$$\Delta_{\widetilde{X}} \widetilde{F} = \widetilde{\Delta_X F}.$$

However, one should be careful in choosing a proper parameterization which stabilizes the numerical computation and minimizes the variances of errors in estimating the Laplace-Beltrami operator.

The Laplace-Beltrami operator is *self-adjoint* so if F and G are twice differentiable functions in $\mathcal{M}$,

$$\int_{\mathcal{M}} G\Delta F \, d\mu = \int_{\mathcal{M}} F\Delta G \, d\mu$$

$$= -\int_{\mathcal{M}} \langle \nabla F, \nabla G \rangle \, d\mu,$$

where the inner product is defined as

$$\langle \nabla F, \nabla G \rangle = \sum_{ij} g^{ij} \frac{\partial}{\partial u^i} F \frac{\partial}{\partial v^i} G$$

and the surface area element $d\mu = \sqrt{\det g}\, du^1 du^2$ (Grigoryan, 1999).

The *conformal coordinates* are defined as a coordinate system $u = (u^1, u^2)$ whose metric is given by

$$d\xi^2 = \lambda(du^1)^2 + \lambda(du^2)^2$$

for some function $\lambda = \lambda(u)$. With respect to the conformal coordinates, the Laplace-Beltrami operator is simplified to

$$\Delta_X = \frac{1}{\lambda}\left(\frac{\partial}{\partial u^1} + \frac{\partial}{\partial u^2} \right).$$

For an arbitrary smooth surface and a fixed point p, we can always find conformal coordinates such that $p = X(u)$ and $\lambda(u) = 1$ (do Carmo, 1992). Therefore, if we find a conformal coordinate system at each $p \in \mathcal{M}$, the computation of the Laplace-Beltrami operator at $p = X(u)$ can be simplified to the planar Laplacian at u.

5.3.1 *Eigenfunctions of Laplace-Beltrami Operator*

The eigenfunctions and the eigenvalues of the Laplace-Beltrami operator has been used in many different contexts in image analysis (Lévy and Inria-Alice, 2006; Zhang *et al.*, 2010). Qiu *et al.* (2006) constructed splines on a cortical surface with boundary using the eigenfunctions. Seo *et al.* (2010) constructed the heat kernel as a series expansion of eigenfunctions and formulated diffusion as heat kernel smoothing. Vallet and Lévy (2008) used the eigenfunctions to analytically formulate geometric filtering problems. Dong *et al.* (2006) proposed a quadrangular remeshing of surfaces using the evenly distributed extrema of eigenfunctions. The eigenvalues and eigenfunctions used in shape analysis (Reuter *et al.*, 2009) and shape segmentation and registration (Reuter, 2010). In this study, we mainly use the eigenfunctions and eigenvalues to be used in smoothing out mesh noises. Further the second eigenfunction is used as a way to extract the centerline of the mandible.

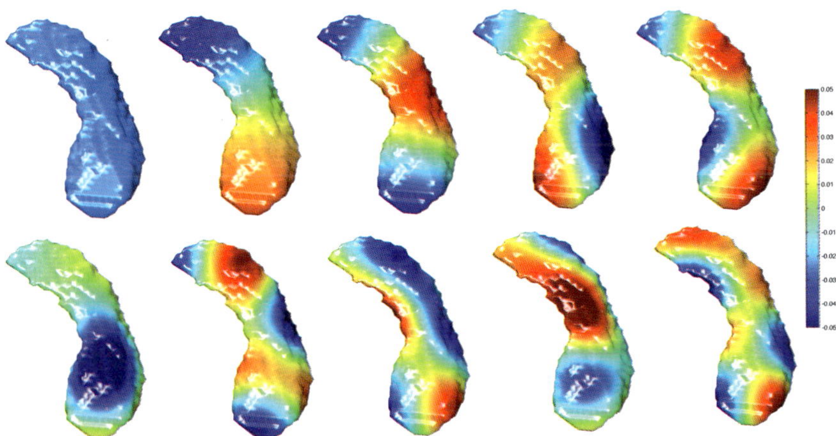

Fig. 5.5   The first ten eigenfunctions of the Laplace-Beltrami operator on a left hippocampus surface.

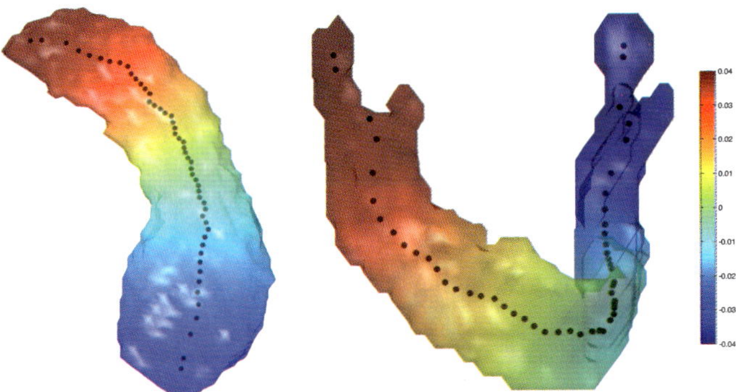

Fig. 5.6   The second eigenfunction ψ_1 of the Laplace-Beltrami operator for an elongated object obtains its maximum and minimum at two extremes. This is related to the hotspots conjecture (Banuelos and Burdzy, 1999). Here we have a left hippocampus surface and a mandible surface. Since ψ_1 is monotonically increasing from one end to the other end, the centerline of the elongated object can be obtained by connecting the centroids of the successive level contours of ψ_1.

Since the Laplace-Beltrami operator is self-adjoint and elliptic, we have discrete eigenvalues

$$0 = \lambda_0 \leq \lambda_1 \leq \lambda_2 \leq \cdots$$

and the corresponding eigenfunctions ψ_j satisfying

$$\Delta\psi_j = \lambda_j\psi_j. \tag{5.13}$$

The eigenfunctions ψ_j form orthonormal basis in $L^2(\mathcal{M})$, the space of square integrable functions in $\mathcal{M}$. Numerically, eigenfunctions can be made into orthonormal by scaling the eigenvalues. The first eigenfunction is trivially given as $\psi_0 = 1/\sqrt{\mu(\mathcal{M})}$ and $\lambda_0 = 0$ for a closed compact surface. However, other eigenfunctions are not known analytically unless the manifold $\mathcal{M}$ is algebraically given. The spherical harmonics Y_{lm} are a well known example of eigenfuctions on a unit sphere (Wahba, 1990). For arbitrary manifolds such as cortical and hippcampus surfaces, the eigenfunctions has to be numerically computed using finite element method, which is discussed in a later section. Figures 5.5 and 5.6 show the eigenfunctions on a left hippocampus and human mandible surfaces.

5.3.2   *Multiplicity of Eigenfunctions*

It is possible to have multiple eigenfunctions corresponding to a single eigenvalue. For instance, $2l + 1$ spherical harmonics $Y_{l,-l}, \cdots, Y_{l,l}$ correspond to a single eigenvalue $l(l+1)$. The exact number of multiplicity is unknown for arbitrary manifolds (Hoffmann-Ostenhof *et al.*, 1999). For smooth genus zero surfaces, the multiplicity m is bounded by

$$m(\lambda_k) \leq 2k - 3 \text{ for } k \geq 2.$$

Suppose $\psi_{k1}, \cdots \psi_{kk_i}$ are k_i eigenfunctions corresponding to eigenvalue λ_k, i.e.

$$\Delta\psi_{kj} = \lambda_k\psi_{kj}.$$

Then any linear combination of basis $\sum_j w_j\psi_{kj}$ satisfy

$$\Delta\left(\sum_j w_j\psi_{kj}\right) = \lambda_k \sum_j w_j\psi_{kj}$$

as well. Hence, within the same degree, the space of eigenfunctions form a vector space. For instance, spherical harmonics of degree l span the vector space so any linear combination of spherical harmonics of the same degree is again are eigenfunctions. The eigenfunctions form a complete orthonormal basis in the space of square integrable functions, $L^2(\mathcal{M})$, so all other possible orthonormal basis is a linear combination of eigenfunctions.

Note that since ψ_{kj} are orthonormal, we have

$$\int_{\mathcal{M}} \left(\sum_j w_j \psi_{kj} \right)^2 d\mu = \sum_j w_j^2.$$

If we normalize the linear combination in such a way that $\sum_j w_j^2 = 1$, $\sum_j w_j \psi_{kj}$ is also orthonormal with respect to other eigenfunctions.

5.3.3 *Laplace-Beltrami Shape Descriptors*

The eigenvalues can be used as a global geometric descriptors . They have been used in caudate shape discriminant (Niethammer *et al.*, 2007). Unfortunately eigenvalues do not completely characterize the shape of surface as explained in M. Kac's seminal paper *Can One hear the Shape of a Drum?* (Kac, 1966). From the Weyl's formula (Chavel, 1984), for compact 2D Riemannaian manifolds, eigenvalues are asymptotically given as

$$\lambda_k \to \frac{4\pi k}{\mu(\mathcal{M})}$$

as $k \to \infty$.

Figure 5.7 shows the plot of eigenvalues up to degree 1000 for control (gray) and autistic (black) subjects. The two sample t-test performed at each degree separately does not detect statistically significant group difference at 0.01 level. This is somewhat expected since the global amygdala shapes are not very distinguishable between autistic and control subjects

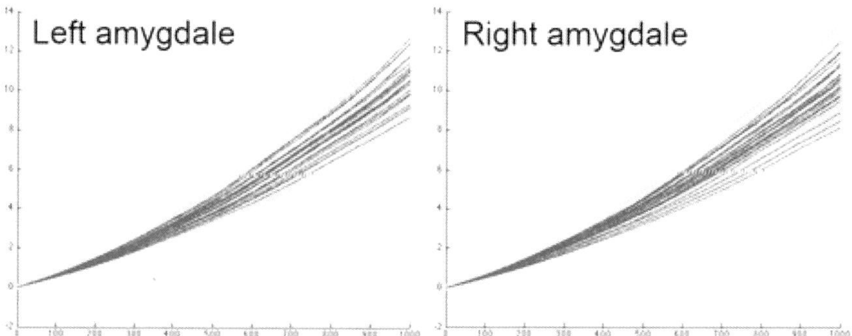

Fig. 5.7 The plot of eigenvalues λ_k for control (gray) and autistic (black) subjects for degree $0 \leq k \leq 1000$. The eigenvalues for the two groups overlap and do not show statistically significant group separation at 0.01 level.

(Chung *et al.*, 2008c). A lack of significant difference in eigenvalues does not imply there is no local shape difference. It may be that the eigenvalues themselves might be inefficient discriminant measures. Therefore, a better intrinsic framework is needed for the Laplace-Beltrami spectrum approaches to work in discriminating similarly shaped objects. One promising new framework is a data embedding techniques (Belkin and Niyogi, 2002; Jones *et al.*, 2008). Belkin and Niyogi (Belkin and Niyogi, 2002) developed an embedding framework for mapping graphs into $\mathbb{R}^m$ and clustering subsequently. The eigenvaules of the Laplace-Beltrami operator depends on the size of anatomy. The larger the size of anatomy, larger the eigenvalues. If the metric g changes to cg, the eigenvalues scale to λ_j/c while the eigenfunctions scale to $\psi_j/\sqrt{c}$. So we need to come up with a representation that is invariant of scale. One way of doing this is the global point signature (GPS) embedding of a manifold (Rustamov, 2007) which basically expand signal with respect to the basis $\psi_j/\sqrt{\lambda_j}$ rather than ψ_j.

5.3.4 *Second Eigenfunctions*

Other than the first eigenfunction, which is trivially given as $\psi_0 = 1/\sqrt{\mu(\mathcal{M})}$, all other eigenfunctions are unknown for an arbitrary manifold. However, the second eigenfunction ψ_1 exhibits a very interesting characteristic that deserves a special attention. The second eigenfunction can be used to establish the intrinsic coordinate system for elongated tubular structures like mandible, hippocampus or the bundle of white matter fiber tracts. Basically the second eigenfunction follows the shape of elongated objects (Lévy and Inria-Alice, 2006). The maximum and the minimum of ψ_1 usually occurs at the two extremes of an elongated object (Figure 5.6). So the gradient of the second eigenfunction follows the shape of elongated objects. In computer vision and medical imaging literature, this *monotonicity property* was observed by many researchers but without any mathematical justification (Gebal *et al.*, 2009; Lévy and Inria-Alice, 2006; Shi *et al.*, 2008b; Zhang *et al.*, 2007b). Many treated it as a well known mathematical fact although the general statement was not proved yet. This seems so obvious and trivial but the general statement is extremely difficult to prove and still a challenging open problem related to the hot spots conjecture of J. Rauch in differential geometry (Banuelos and Burdzy, 1999), which states that the second eigenfunction corresponding to the Laplace-Beltrami operator on a domain with Neumann boundary conditions attains its maximum and minimum on the boundary. Although we will not attempt to prove the general statement, we will discuss the hot spots conjecture in detail.

5.3.5 *Dirichlet Energy*

Let $\mathcal{E}(f)$ be the Dirichlet energy functional of f:

$$\mathcal{E}(f) = \int_{\mathcal{M}} \langle \nabla f, \nabla f \rangle \, d\mu(p).$$

The second eigenfunction is then given by the minimizer of Dirichlet energy as

$$\psi_1 = \arg \min_{\|f\|=1} \mathcal{E}(f) \tag{5.14}$$

$$\lambda_1 = \min_{\|f\|=1} \mathcal{E}(f) \tag{5.15}$$

The Dirichlet energy measures the smoothness of the function f so the second eigenfunction should be the smoothest possible map among all possible functions. This is the reason why ψ_1 needs to be as smooth as possible. Further since ψ_0 and ψ_1 are orthonormal, we must have

$$\langle \psi_0, \psi_1 \rangle = \frac{1}{\sqrt{\mu(\mathcal{M})}} \int_{\mathcal{M}} \psi_1(p) \, d\mu(p) = 0. \tag{5.16}$$

Therefore, ψ_1 is positive on half of the surface and negative on the other half. However, (5.14) still does not explicitly tell us such the smooth function has to be monotonically changing from one end to the other end. This phenomenon is also observed in Zhang *et al.* (2007b) but without explanation.

Let us introduce Rauch's *hot spots conjecture*, which has not been proved for a general statement other than few specific examples mostly on a planar shape (Athreya, 2000; Banuelos and Burdzy, 1999; Kawohl, 1985). The hot spots conjecture basically says that the second eigenfunction corresponding to the Laplace-Beltrami operator on a domain with Neumann boundary conditions attains its maximum and minimum on the boundary.

Conjecture 5.1. *Let $\mathcal{M}$ be an open connected bounded subset. Let $f(t,p)$ be the solution of heat equation*

$$\frac{\partial f}{\partial \sigma} = \Delta f \tag{5.17}$$

with the initial condition $f(0,p) = g(p)$ and the Neumann boundary condition $\frac{\partial f}{\partial n}(\sigma, p) = 0$ on the boundary $\partial \mathcal{M}$. n is the unit normal vector on $\partial \mathcal{M}$. Then for most initial conditions g, if p_{hot} is a point at which the function $f(\cdot, p)$ attains its maximum (hot spots), then the distance from p_0 to $\partial \mathcal{M}$ tends to zero as $\sigma \to \infty$ (Banuelos and Burdzy, 1999).

We can also claim similar statement for minimum (cold spots) as well. We may wonder how the second eigenfunction is related to the hot spots conjecture. The solution to heat equation (5.17) is given by heat kernel expansion (Chung *et al.*, 2007, 2008b; Rosenberg, 1997):

$$K_\sigma * g(p) = \sum_{j=0}^{\infty} e^{-\lambda_j \sigma} \beta_j \psi_j(p), \qquad (5.18)$$

where $\beta_j = \langle \psi_j, g \rangle$ are Fourier coefficients. The bandwidth σ is interpreted as a diffusion time. Since $\lambda_0 = 0$ and $\psi_0 = 1/\sqrt{\mu(\mathcal{M})}$, we have

$$K_\sigma * g(p) = \frac{\int_{\mathcal{M}} g(p)\, d\mu(p)}{\mu(\mathcal{M})} + \beta_1 e^{-\lambda_1 \sigma} \psi_1(p) + R(\sigma, p), \qquad (5.19)$$

where the first term is the average signal and R goes to faster to zero than $e^{-\lambda_1 \sigma}$ as $\sigma \to \infty$ (Banuelos and Burdzy, 1999). Due to the expansion (5.19), the behavior of diffusion is basically governed by the eigenfunction ψ_1. The pattern of the second eigenfunction shoud be similar to a harmonic map obtained by solving a Laplace equation with the Dirichlet boundary condition on its surface, an approach used in establishing surface parametrization (Brechbuhler *et al.*, 1995; Zhu and Jiang, 2004). The harmonic map is the equilibrium solution when $\sigma \to \infty$ so it is expected that the patterns of the harmonic map and the second eigenfunction behave almost identically. However, the second eigenfunction approach avoids the pole selection step which is required in constructing the harmonic map. There are few variations on the hot spots conjecture but the most relevant and intuitive statement related to our study is the following.

Conjecture 5.2. *For every $q \in \mathcal{M}$, we have*

$$\inf_{p \in \partial \mathcal{M}} \psi_1(p) \leq \psi_1(q) \leq \sup_{p \in \partial \mathcal{M}} \psi_1(p).$$

The conjecture has been proved for specific shapes such as parallelepipeds, balls and annuli (Banuelos and Burdzy, 1999; Kawohl, 1985). Conjecture 5.2 basically asserts that the hot and cold spots of eigenfunctions occurs at the boundary. Since the second eigenfunction has to be smooth as possible, the heat gradient of ψ_1 has to follow very closely to the geodesic path from the hot spots to the cold spots. Obviously not every objects have a boundary. So what will happen if there is no boundary? In the case of closed manifold with no boundary, the Neumann boundary condition simply disappears so the direct application of the hot spots conjecture is not valid.

For a closed surface with no boundary, the hot and cold spots have to move away from each other as far as possible to make ψ_1 as smooth as possible. So here is the conjecture for closed surfaces.

Conjecture 5.3. *Consider a close and sufficiently smooth simply connected surface $\mathcal{M}$ with no boundary. If there exist points p_1 and p_2 such that the geodesic distance d between p_1 and p_2 is maximum among all possible points, i.e.*

$$d(p, q) \leq d(p_1, p_2) \ \text{for all } p, q \in \mathcal{M}.$$

Then we claim that the hot and cold spots occur exactly at p_1 and p_2, and the ψ_1 basically forms heat gradient from the hot to cold spots.

Figure 5.8 and 5.9 illustrate Conjecture 5.3. For very complicated branching tree structures like Figure 5.9, the hot and cold spots occur at the two extreme points along the longest geodesic path. The hot spots conjecture basically dictates that it is possible to find the maximum possible geodesic path by simply finding the maximum and the minimum in the second eigenfunction and connecting them. It is possible to prove the statement for algebraic surfaces such as an ellipsoid but obviously there is no general statement available yet. We will not pursue the problem any further.

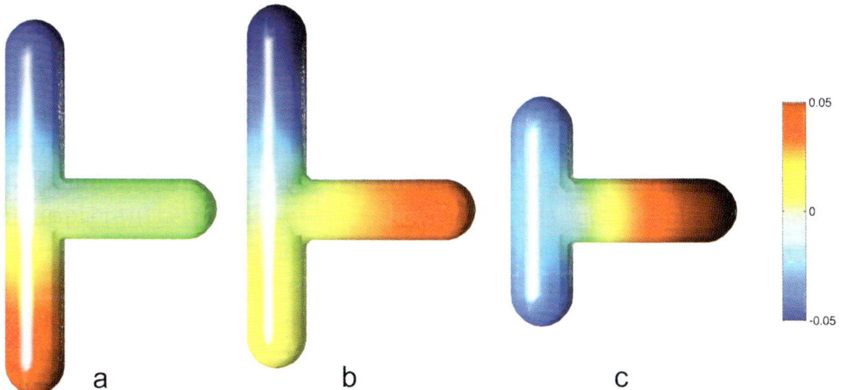

Fig. 5.8 The second eigenfunction for various T-shaped tubular structure with symmetry (a,c) and without symmetry (b). The hot and cold spots occur at the extreme points that gives the maximum geodesic distance along the surface. Even they are similarly shaped, the gradient pattern drastically changes depending on where the hot spots occur.

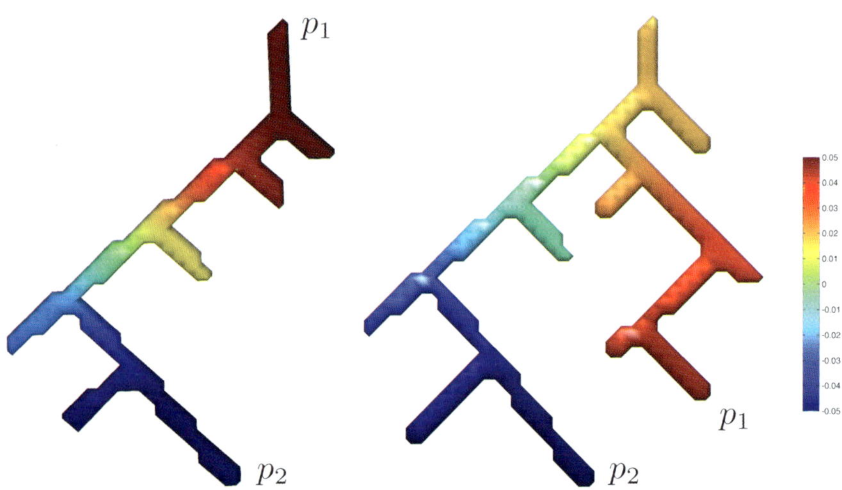

Fig. 5.9   The second eigenfunction ψ_1 of branching tubular structures. The maximum and the minimum of ψ_1 always occur at the points of maximum geodesic distance.

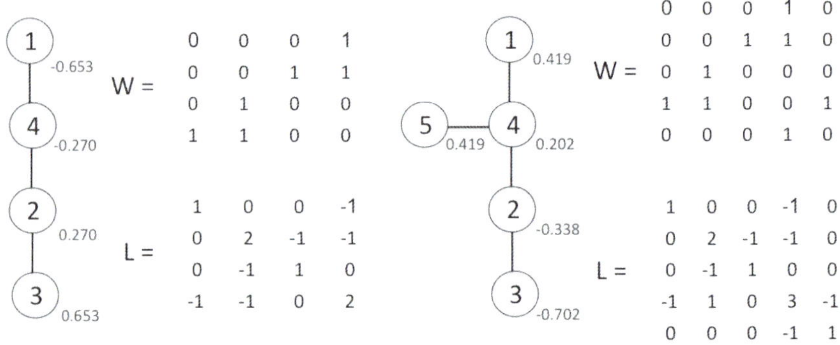

Fig. 5.10   A graph, the weights W and the graph Laplacian L. The weights are simply the adjacency matrix. The second eigenfunction ψ_1 value is displayed in blue. (a) This example is given in Hall (1970). The maximum geodesic distance is obtained between the nodes 1 and 3, which are also hot and cold spots. (b) In this example, there are two hot spots 1 and 5 which corresponds to two maximal geodesic paths 1-4-2-3 and 5-4-2-3.

5.3.6 *Fiedler's Vector*

Surface meshes can be considered as graphs. The connection between the eigenfunctions of continuous and discrete Laplacians have been well established by many authors (Gladwell and Zhu, 2002; Tlusty, 2007). Many properties of eigenfunctions of Laplace-Beltrami operator discrete analogues. The second eigenfunction of the discrete graph Laplacian is called the Fiedler vector and it has been studied in connection to the graph and mesh manipulation, manifold learning and the minimum linear arrangement problem (Fiedler, 1973; Ham *et al.*, 2005; Lévy and Inria-Alice, 2006; Ham *et al.*, 2004, 2005).

Let $G = \{V, E\}$ be the graph with the vertex set V and the edge set E. G is the discrete approximation of the underlying continuous manifold $\mathcal{M}$. We will simply index the node set as $V = \{1, 2, \cdots, n\}$. If two nodes i and j form an edge, we denote it as $i \sim j$. Various forms of graph Laplacian have been proposed but almost all proposed graph Laplacian $L = (l_{ij})$ is a real symmetric matrix of the form

$$l_{ij} = \begin{cases} -w_{ij}, & i \sim j \\ \sum_{i \neq j} w_{ij}, & i = j \\ 0, & \text{otherwise} \end{cases}$$

for some edge weight w_{ij}. The graph Laplacian L can be decomposed as $L = D - W$ where $D = (d_{ij})$ is the diagonal matrix with $d_{ii} = \sum_{j=1}^{n} w_{ij}$ and $W = (w_{ij})$. For a vector $\mathbf{f} = (f_1, \cdots, f_n)'$ observed at the n nodes, the discrete analogue of the Dirichlet energy (5.14) is given by

$$\mathcal{E}(\mathbf{f}) = \mathbf{f}'L\mathbf{f} = \sum_{i,j=1}^{n} w_{ij}(f_i - f_j)^2 = \sum_{i \sim j} w_{ij}(f_i - f_j)^2. \tag{5.20}$$

The discrete Dirichlet energy (5.20) is also called the linear placement cost in the minimum linear arrangement problem (Koren and Harel, 2002). The Fiedler vector $\mathbf{f}$ evaluated at n nodes is obtained as the minimizer of the quadratic polynomial:

$$\min_{\boldsymbol{f}} \mathcal{E}(f)$$

subject to the quadratic constraint

$$\|\mathbf{f}\|^2 = \mathbf{f}'\mathbf{f} = \sum_i f_i^2 = 1. \tag{5.21}$$

The solution can be interpreted as the kernel principal components of a Gram matrix given by the generalized inverse of L (Ham *et al.*, 2004, 2005).

Since ψ_1 is required to be orthonormal with ψ_0, which is constant, we also have an additional constraint on $\boldsymbol{f}$:

$$\sum_i f_i = 0. \tag{5.22}$$

This optimization problem was first introduced for the minimum linear arrangement problem in 1970's (Hall, 1970; Koren and Harel, 2002). The optimization can be solved using the Lagrange multiplier (Holzrichter and Oliveira, 1999).

Let g be the constraint (5.21) so that

$$g(\mathbf{f}) = \mathbf{f}'\mathbf{f} - 1 = 0.$$

Then the constraint minimum should satisfy

$$\nabla \mathcal{E} - \mu \nabla g = 0, \tag{5.23}$$

where μ is the Lagrange multiplier. (5.23) can be written as

$$2L\mathbf{f} - \mu \mathbf{f} = 0 \tag{5.24}$$

Hence, $\mathbf{f}$ must be the eigenvector of L and $\mu/2$ is the corresponding eigenvalue. But which eigenvector and eigenvalue? By multiplying $\mathbf{f}'$ on the both sides of (5.24), we have

$$2\mathbf{f}'L\mathbf{f} = \mu \mathbf{f}'\mathbf{f} = \mu.$$

Since we are minimizing $\mathbf{f}'L\mathbf{f}$, $\mu/2$ should be the second eigenvalue λ_1.

In most literature (Holzrichter and Oliveira, 1999), the condition $\sum_i f_i = 0$ is incorrectly stated as a necessary constraint for the Fiedler's vector. However, the constraint $\sum_i f_i = 0$ is not really needed in minimizing the Dirichlet energy. This can be further seen from introducing a new constraint

$$h(\mathbf{f}) = \mathbf{e}'\mathbf{f} = \sum_i f_i = 0,$$

where $\mathbf{e} = (1, \cdots, 1)'$.

So far the optimization problem tells us that ψ_1 embeds the the graph into 1-dimension but it still does not tell us much about the monotonicity property of ψ_1 mathematically. The constraint (5.21) and (5.22) forces ψ_1 to have at least two differing *sign domains* in which ψ_1 has one sign. But it is unclear how many differing sign domains ψ_1 can possibly have. The upper bound is given by Courant's nodal line theorem (Courant and Hilbert, 1953; Gladwell and Zhu, 2002; Tlusty, 2007). The *nodal set* of eigenfunctions ψ_i is defined as the zero level set $\psi_i(p) = 0$. Courant's nodal line theorem states

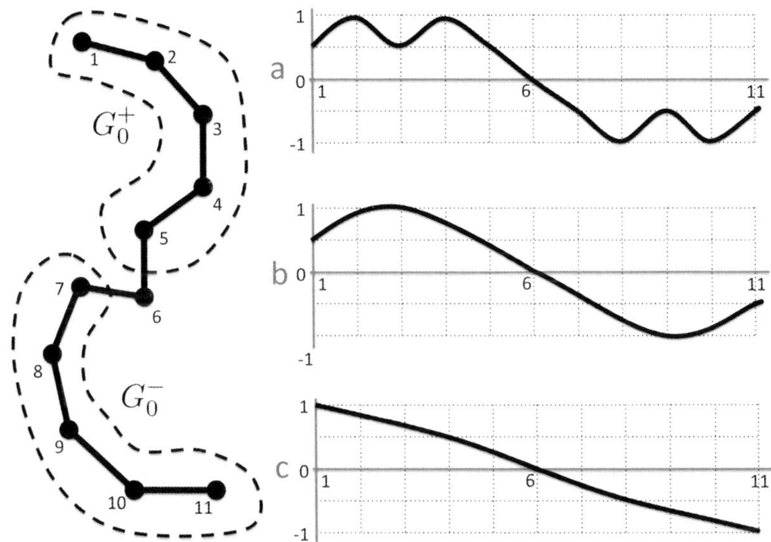

Fig. 5.11 A path with with positive (G_0^+) and negative (G_0^-) sign domains. Due to symmetry, the possible eigenfunction ψ_1 has to be an odd function.

that the nodal set of the i-th eigenfunction ψ_{i-1} divide the manifold into no more than i sign domains. Hence, the second eigenfunction has exactly 2 disjoint sign domains. At the positive sign domain, we have the global maximum and at the negative sign domain, we have the global minimum. This property is illustrated in the T-shaped tubular structure in Figure 5.8.

The hot spot conjecture can be proved for specific cases. Although it is difficult to prove in general cases. Here we provide a heuristic proof for a path, which is a graph with maximal degree 2 and without a cycle.

Definition 5.1. For a function **f** defined on the vertex set V, let G_s^- be the subgraph induced by the vertex set $V_s^- = \{i \in V | f_i < s\}$. Similarly, let G_s^+ be the subgraph induced by the vertex set $V_s^+ = \{i \subset V | f_i > s\}$. For any s, if G_s^- and G_s^+ are either connected or empty, then **f** is tight (Tlusty, 2007).

The concept of tightness is crucial in proving the statement. When $s = 0$, G_0^+ and G_0^- are sign graphs. If we relax the condition so that G_s^+ contains nodes satisfying $f_i \geq s$, we have weak sign graphs. It can be shown that the second eigenfunction on a graph with maximal degree 2 (cycle or path) is tight (Tlusty, 2007). Figure 5.11 shows an example of a path with

11 nodes. Among three candidates for the second eigenfunction, (a) and (b) are not tight while (c) is. Note that the candidate function (a) have two disjoint components for $G_{0.5}^+$ so it can not be tight. In order to be tight, the second eigenfunction cannot have a positive minimum or a negative maximum at the interior vertex in the graph (Gladwell and Zhu, 2002). This implies that the second eigenfunction must decrease monotonically from the positive to negative sign domains as shown in (c). Therefore, the hot and cold spots must occur at the two end points 1 and 11, which gives the maximum geodesic distance of 11.

5.4 Finite Element Methods

Since the closed form expression for the eigenfunctions of the Laplace-Beltrami operator on an arbitrary surface is unknown, the eigenfunctions are numerically computed by discretizing the Laplace-Beltrami operator. To solve the eigensystem (5.13) numerically, we need to discretize it on a triangular mesh using the Cotan formulation, which was first introduced in Chung *et al.* (2001b) and then subsequently in Chung and Taylor (2004) and Qiu *et al.* (2006). The eigenfunctions are used as basis for performing smoothing on an arbitrary triangulated mesh. Qiu *et al.* (2006) presented a similar Cotan discretization of the eigensystem and used to construct splines on a manifold. Seo *et al.* (2010) constructed heat kernel using the eigenfunctions to isotropically diffuse signal along the surface.

5.4.1 *Pieacewise Linear Functions*

Let N_T be the number of triangles in the mesh that approximates the underlying manifold $\mathcal{M}$. We seek a piecewise differentiable solution f_i in the i-th triangle T_i such that the solution $f_i(x)$ is continuous across neighboring triangles. A slightly different formulation of FEM for the surface flattening problem is given in (Angenent *et al.*, 1999). The solution f for the whole mesh is then

$$f(x) = \sum_{i=1}^{N_T} f_i(x).$$

Let $p_{i_1}, p_{i_2}, p_{i_3}$ be the vertices of element T_i. In T_i, we estimate f_i linearly as

$$f_i(x) = \sum_{k=1}^{3} \xi_{i_k} f(p_{i_k}),$$

where nonnegative ξ_{i_k} are given by the *barycentric coordinates* (Chung, 2001; Sadiku, 1989, 1992; Tang *et al.*, 1999). In the barycentric coordinates, any point $x \in T_i$ is uniquely determined by two conditions:

$$x = \sum_{k=1}^{3} \xi_{i_k}(x) p_{i_k}, \quad \sum_{k=1}^{3} \xi_{i_k}(x) = 1.$$

Similarly, an arbitrary piecewise linear function g can be written as

$$g(x) = \sum_{i=1}^{N_T} \sum_{k=1}^{3} \xi_{i_k}(x) g_{i_k}, \tag{5.25}$$

where $g_{i_k} = g(p_{i_k})$ are the values of function g evaluated at vertices p_{i_k} of T_i. For the function f, we can represent similarly as $f_{i_k} = f(p_{i_k})$. Since the Laplace-Beltrami operator is *self-adjoint*, we have

$$\int g \Delta f \, d\mu = -\int \langle \nabla f, \nabla g \rangle \, d\mu = \int f \Delta g \, d\mu.$$

Then the integral version of the eigensystem $\Delta f = -\lambda f$ in the triangle T_i can be written as

$$\int_{T_i} g \lambda f \, d\mu = \int_{T_i} \langle \nabla f, \nabla g \rangle \, d\mu. \tag{5.26}$$

5.4.2 *Mass and Stiffness Matrices*

The left-hand term in (5.26) can be written further as

$$\int_{T_i} g \lambda f \, d\mu = \sum_{k,l=1}^{3} g_{i_k} \lambda f_{i_l} \int_{T_i} \xi_{i_k} \xi_{i_l} \, d\mu \tag{5.27}$$

$$= \lambda \mathbf{G}_i' \mathbf{A}^i \mathbf{F}_i, \tag{5.28}$$

where $\mathbf{G}_i = (g_{i_1}, g_{i_2}, g_{i_3})'$, $\mathbf{F}_i = (f_{i_1}, f_{i_2}, f_{i_3})'$ and 3×3 *mass matrix*

$$\mathbf{A}^i = (A_{kl}^i), \quad A_{kl}^i = \int_{T_i} \xi_{i_k} \xi_{i_l} \, d\mu.$$

It can be shown that

$$\mathbf{A}^i = \frac{|T_i|}{12} \begin{pmatrix} 2 & 1 & 1 \\ 1 & 2 & 1 \\ 1 & 1 & 2 \end{pmatrix}, \tag{5.29}$$

where $|T_i|$ is the area of the triangle T_i (Sadiku, 1989, 1992). Similarly, the right-hand term in (5.26) is

$$\int_{T_i} \langle \nabla f, \nabla g \rangle \, d\mu = \sum_{k,l=1}^{3} g_{i_k} f_{i_l} \int_{T_i} \langle \nabla \xi_{i_k}, \nabla \xi_{i_l} \rangle \, d\mu \tag{5.30}$$

$$= \mathbf{G}_i' \mathbf{C}^i \mathbf{F}_i, \tag{5.31}$$

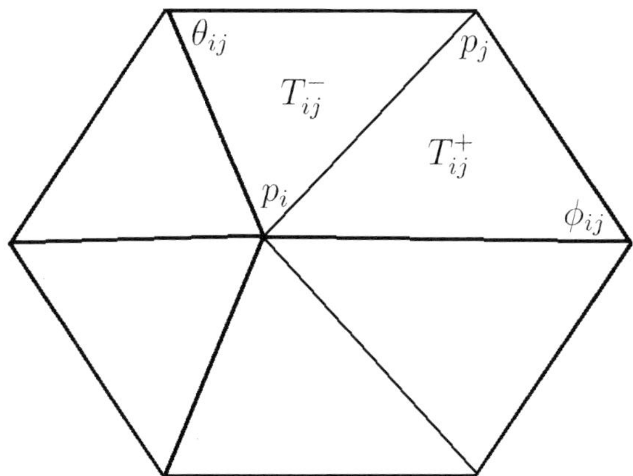

Fig. 5.12 A typical first order neighbor of vertex p_i. θ_{ij} and ϕ_{ij} are the angles opposite to the edge $p_i p_j$. T_{ij}^- and T_{ij}^+ are triangles sharing the edge $p_i p_j$.

where 3×3 *stiffness matrix* $\mathbf{C}^i$ is given by

$$\mathbf{C}^i = (c_{kl}^i), \quad c_{kl}^i = \int_{T_i} \langle \nabla \xi_{i_k}, \nabla \xi_{i_l} \rangle \, d\mu. \tag{5.32}$$

Since T_i is planar, the gradient $\nabla \xi_{i_k}$ is the standard planar gradient. The matrix $\mathbf{C}^i$ can be further written as

$$\frac{1}{2} \begin{pmatrix} \cot \theta_{i_2} + \cot \theta_{i_3} & -\cot \theta_{i_3} & -\cot \theta_{i_2} \\ -\cot \theta_{i_3} & \cot \theta_{i_1} + \cot \theta_{i_3} & -\cot \theta_{i_1} \\ -\cot \theta_{i_2} & -\cot \theta_{i_1} & \cot \theta_{i_1} + \cot \theta_{i_2} \end{pmatrix},$$

where θ_{i_k} is the incident angle of vertex p_{i_k} in triangle T_i (Sadiku, 1989, 1992; Silvester and Ferrari, 1983). See Figure 5.2 for notations. By equating (5.28) and (5.31), we obtain

$$\mathbf{A}^i \lambda \mathbf{F}_i = \mathbf{C}^i \mathbf{F}_i. \tag{5.33}$$

We solve (5.33) by assembling all triangles. To simply the indexing, we will use slightly different notations from now on. Let $N(p_i)$ be the set of neighboring vertices around p_i, and let T_{ij}^- and T_{ij}^+ denote two triangles sharing vertices p_i, and p_j. Let two angles opposite to the edge containing p_i and p_j be ϕ_{ij} and θ_{ij} respectively for T_{ij}^+ and T_{ij}^- (Figure 5.12). Then, the assembled sparse matrices $\mathbf{A} = (A_{ij})$ is computed as follows. The diagonal entries are

$$A_{ii} = \frac{1}{12} \sum_{p_j \in N(p_i)} (|T_{ij}^|| + +|T_{ij}^-|), \tag{5.34}$$

and the off-diagonal entries are

$$A_{ij} = \frac{1}{12}\left(|T_{ij}^+| + |T_{ij}^-|\right),\tag{5.35}$$

if p_i and p_j are adjacent, and $A_{ij} = 0$ otherwise. When we construct A matrix numerically, we compute the off-diagonal elements first and the diagonal elements next by summing the off-diagonal terms in the first ring neighbors.

The global coefficient matrix $\mathbf{C} = (c_{ij})$, which is the assemblage of individual element coefficients is given similarly using the cotan formulation. The contribution to c_{ij} comes from all elements containing vertices i and j. The diagonal entries are

$$c_{ii} = \frac{1}{2} \sum_{p_j \in N(p_i)} (\cot\theta_{ij} + \cot\phi_{ij}),\tag{5.36}$$

and the off diagonal entries are

$$c_{ij} = -\frac{1}{2}(\cot\theta_{ij} + \cot\phi_{ij}),\tag{5.37}$$

if p_i and p_j are adjacent, and $c_{ij} = 0$ otherwise. For example, in the case of a hexagonal triangulation in Figure 5.2, $\mathbf{C}$ is given by

$$\begin{pmatrix}
c_{00}^1 + \cdots + c_{00}^6 & c_{01}^1 + c_{01}^6 & c_{02}^1 + c_{02}^2 & c_{03}^2 + c_{03}^3 & c_{04}^3 + c_{04}^4 & c_{05}^4 + c_{05}^5 & c_{06}^5 + c_{06}^6 \\
c_{01}^1 + c_{01}^6 & c_{11}^1 + c_{11}^6 & c_{12}^1 & 0 & 0 & 0 & c_{16}^6 \\
c_{02}^1 + c_{02}^2 & c_{12}^1 & c_{22}^1 + c_{22}^2 & c_{23}^2 & 0 & 0 & 0 \\
c_{03}^2 + c_{03}^3 & 0 & c_{23}^2 & c_{33}^2 + c_{33}^3 & c_{34}^3 & 0 & 0 \\
c_{04}^3 + c_{04}^4 & 0 & 0 & c_{34}^3 & c_{44}^3 + c_{44}^4 & c_{45}^4 & 0 \\
c_{05}^4 + c_{05}^5 & 0 & 0 & 0 & c_{45}^4 & c_{55}^4 + c_{55}^5 & c_{56}^5 \\
c_{06}^5 + c_{06}^6 & c_{16}^6 & 0 & 0 & 0 & c_{56}^5 & c_{66}^5 + c_{66}^6
\end{pmatrix},$$

where c_{kl}^i is the cotan entry for the i-th element (5.32). Note that the matrix $\mathbf{A}$ has similar structure as $\mathbf{C}$ so we write $a_{01} = a_{01}^1 + a_{01}^6$ instead of $c_{01} = c_{01}^1 + c_{01}^6$ for instance.

When we construct $\mathbf{A}$ and $\mathbf{C}$ matrices, we compute the off diagonal elements first and the diagonal elements next by summing the off-diagonal terms in the first ring neighbors. Finally, we can obtain the following generalized eigenvalue problem:

$$\mathbf{C}\psi = \lambda \mathbf{A}\psi,\tag{5.38}$$

For large sparse matrices $\mathbf{C}$ and $\mathbf{A}$, (5.38) can be solved using the Implicitly Restarted Arnoldi Method (Hernandez *et al.*, 2006; Lehoucq *et al.*, 1998) without consuming large amount of memory and time for sparse entries

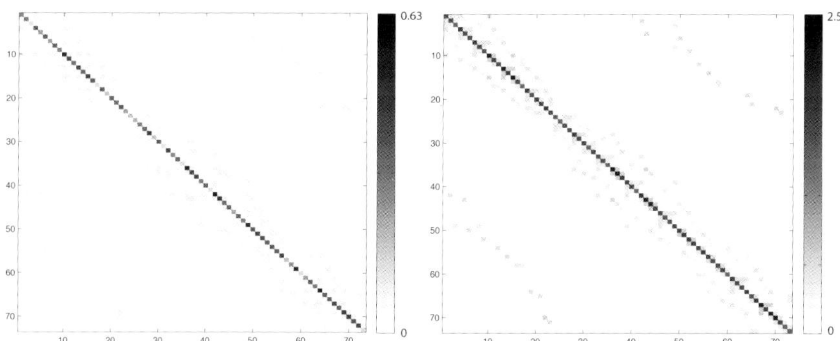

Fig. 5.13   The absolute values of matrices **A** (left) and **C** (right) show the sparse structures. The generalized eigenvalue problem can be solved more efficiently incorporating
the sparsity of matrices.

using `LAPACK` (Anderson *et al.*, 1999). Figure 5.13 shows the usual sparse
structure of matrices **A** and **C**. Figure 5.5 shows the first 10 eigenfunctions
on a left hippocampus surface.   The `MATLAB` implementation for solving
(5.38) is given at `http://brainimaging.waisman.wisc.edu/~chung/lb` .

Chapter 6

Smoothing on Cortical Manifolds

In brain imaging, cortical and subcortical surfaces obtained from MRI are often represented as triangular meshes. Image acquisition, segmentation and surface extraction process themselves are likely to introduce noise. Further processing such as thickness computation, surface registration and parameterization on the meshes are expected to introduce more noise in cortical measures. It is thus imperative to reduce noise measurements on the meshes. For instance, in order to increase the signal-to-noise ratio (SNR) and smoothness of data required for the subsequent random field theory based inference, some type of surface-based smoothing is necessary (Kiebel *et al.*, 1999). The SNR is usually defined as the ratio:

$$\text{SNR} = \frac{\text{Variance of signal}}{\text{Variance of noise}}.$$

An alternate definition is also available:

$$\text{SNR} = \frac{\text{Mean of signal}}{\text{Variance of noise}}.$$

The precise definition of SNR using the spectral density can be found in Dougherty (1999) and Worsley (1996). Among many image smoothing methods, *Gaussian kernel smoothing* has emerged as a de facto smoothing technique among brain imaging researchers due to its simplicity in numerical implementation (Kovačič and Bajcsy, 1999; Perona and Malik, 1990). Gaussin kernel smoothing also increases statistical sensitivity and statistical power as well as Gausianess. Gaussian kernel smoothing can be viewed as weighted averaging of voxel values. Then from the central limit theorem, the weighted average should be more Gaussian.

The Gaussian kernel weights an observation according to its Euclidean distance. However, data residing on the convoluted brain surface fails to be isotropic in the Euclidean sense. On the curved surface, a straight line

127

between two points is not the shortest distance so one may incorrectly assign less weights to closer observations. So when the observations lie on the cortical surface, it is more natural to assign the weights based on the geodesic distance along the surface. For this purpose *diffusion smoothing* has been developed for smoothing data along the cortex (Andrade *et al.*, 2001; Chung *et al.*, 2001b, 2003c). By solving a diffusion equation on a manifold, Gaussian kernel smoothing can be indirectly generalized.

Diffusion equations have been widely used in image processing as a form of noise reduction starting with Perona and Malik in 1990 (Perona and Malik, 1990). Motivated by Perona and Malik's work, numerous image smoothing methods have been devised in computer vision for surface fairing, mesh regularization (Desrun *et al.*, 1999; Sochen *et al.*, 1998; Malladi and Ravve, 2002; Tang *et al.*, 1999; Taubin, 1995, 2000) and anisotropic smoothing of intensity images, where the image intensities are taken as surfaces to be smoothed (Sochen *et al.*, 1998). On the other hand, in brain imaging, the explosion of various functional data such as MEG, EEG or fMRI on cortical surfaces, and multitude of surface geometric measures such as cortical bending, cortical thickness from MRI provide a tremendous motivation for smoothing surface data using diffusion (Andrade *et al.*, 2001; Chung *et al.*, 2001b; Cachia *et al.*, 2003a,b; Chung *et al.*, 2003c; Joshi *et al.*, 2009). Andrade *et al.* (2001) and Chung *et al.* (2001b) were the first few that tried to smooth out measurements defined on surface for the subsequent data analysis. Andrade *et al.* (2001) was the first paper, although not correctly formulated, to use isotropic diffusion on smoothing signal cortical surfaces. It is followed by the more accurate Cotan approach (Chung *et al.*, 2001b; Chung, 2001) in estimating the Laplace-Beltrami operator.

When solving a diffusion equation on a curved surface, the Laplacian somehow has to incorporate the geometry of the curved surface. The extension of the Euclidean Laplacian to an arbitrary Riemannian manifold is called the *Laplace-Beltrami operator* (Kreyszig, 1959) and was discussed extensively in Section 5.3. In this section, we will start with how to represent the Laplace-Beltrami operator explicitly for an arbitrary triangular surface mesh using the finite element method (FEM). Afterwards the explicit representation of the Laplacian is used in the finite difference method (FDM) for solving a diffusion equation iteratively on the human brain surface for the cortical thickness and curvature measurements (Chung, 2001). There are extensive literature on the Cotan formulation for estimating the Laplace-Beltrami operator and solving related problems including the eigenfunctions of the operator (Chung *et al.*, 2003c; Desrun *et al.*, 1999; Qiu *et al.*, 2006; Shi *et al.*, 2008a).

6.1 Gaussian Kernel Smoothing

We will review Gaussian kernel smoothing, which is the basis of more advanced surface-based smoothing. Consider the integral transform

$$Y(t) = \int K(t, s) X(s) \, ds, \tag{6.1}$$

where K is the *kernel* of the integral. Given the input signal X, Y represents the output signal. The smoothness of the output depends on the smoothness of the kernel. We assume the kernel to be unimodal and isotropic. When the kernel is isotropic, it has radial symmetry and should be invariant under rotation. So it has the form

$$K(t, s) = f(\|t - s\|)$$

for some function f. Since the kernel only depends on the difference of the arguments, with the abuse of notation, we can simply write K as

$$K(t, s) = K(t - s).$$

We may further assume the kernel is normalized such that

$$\int K(t) \, dt = 1.$$

Then (6.1) can be written as

$$Y(t) = K * X(t) = \int K(t - s) X(s) \, ds$$

and it is called *kernel smoothing*. We may further assume K to be dependent on some parameter σ such that

$$\lim_{\sigma \to 0} K(t, s; \sigma) \to \delta(t - s),$$

where δ is the Dirac-delta function (Berline *et al.*, 1991; Dirac, 1981). The Dirac-delta function is a special case of *generalized functions* or *distributions* (Gel'fand *et al.*, 1964; Stakgold, 2000). It is usually defined as $\delta(t) = 0$ if $t \neq 0$ and $\int \delta(t) \, dt = 1$. This is also referred to as the *impulse function* in engineering literature. Figure 6.1 illustrates Gaussian kernel smoothing in 2D image.

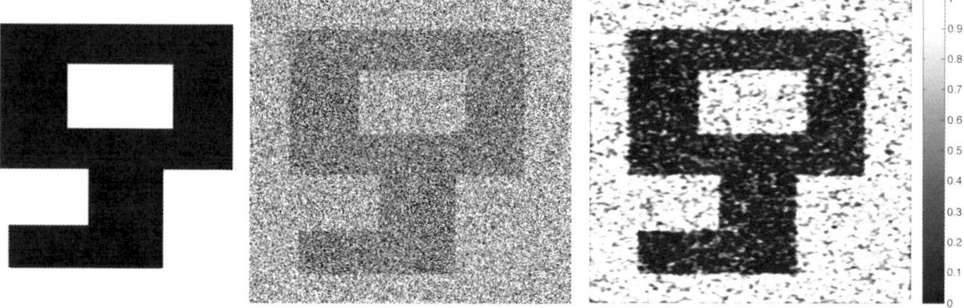

Fig. 6.1   Illustration of Gaussian kernel smoothing as a form of signal detection. Gaussian white noise $N(0, 2^2)$ is added to the binary image. Kernel smoothing with Gaussian kernel K_2 is applied to the noise image to recover the original shape.

6.1.1   *Isotropic Gaussian Kernel*

Gaussian kernel smoothing is probably the most widely used image smoothing technique in brain imaging. An isotropic Gaussian kernel in 1D is defined as

$$K(t) = \frac{1}{\sqrt{2\pi}} e^{t^2/2}.$$

Let's scale the kernel by the parameter σ:

$$K_\sigma(t) = \frac{1}{\sigma} K\left(\frac{t}{\sigma}\right).$$

This is the density function of the normal distribution with mean 0 and variance σ^2. The *bandwidth* σ defines the spread of kernel. In brain imaging, the spread of kernel is usually measured in terms of the *full width at the half maximum* (FWHM) of Gaussian kernel K_σ, which is given by $2\sqrt{2\ln 2}\,\sigma$.

The n-dimensional isotropic Gaussian kernel is defined as the product of n 1D kernel. Let $x = (x_1, \cdots, x_n)' \in \mathbb{R}^n$. Then the n-dimensional kernel is given by

$$\begin{aligned} K_\sigma(x) &= K_\sigma(x_1) K_\sigma(x_2) \cdots K_\sigma(x_n) \\ &= \frac{1}{(2\pi)^{n/2}\sigma^n} \exp\left(\frac{x_1^2 + x_2^2 + \cdots + x_n^2}{2\sigma^2}\right). \end{aligned}$$

Subsequently, n-dimensional isotropic Gaussian kernel smoothing can be done by applying 1-dimensional smoothing n times in each direction by factorizing the kernel as

$$\int K_\sigma(x-y)X(y)\,dy$$

$$= \int K_\sigma(x_1-y_1)K_\sigma(x_2-y_2)\cdots K_\sigma(x_n-y_n)X(y)\,dy$$

$$= \int K_\sigma(x_1-y_1)\cdots K_\sigma(x_{n-1}-y_{n-1})\,dy_1\cdots dy_{n-1}\int K_\sigma(x_n-y_n)X(y)\,dy_n$$

6.1.2 *Anisotropic Gaussian Kernel*

Assume $H = H'$. The isotropic kernel under linear transform $x \to H^{1/2}x$ changes the shape of the kernel to an *anisotropic kernel*

$$K_H(x) = \frac{1}{(2\pi)^{n/2}\det H^{1/2}}K(x'H^{-1}x/2). \tag{6.2}$$

$\det H^{1/2}$ is the Jacobian determinant of the transformation that normalize the kernel. Note that this is the density of n-dimensional multivariate normal with the covariance matrix HH', i.e. $N(0, HH')$. The matrix H is called the *bandwidth matrix* and it measures the amount of smoothing. It can be shown that K_H is the Dirac-delta function when all the eigenvalues $\lambda_1, \cdots, \lambda_n$ of H go to zero, i.e.

$$\lim_{\lambda_1,\cdots,\lambda_n \to 0} K_H(x) = \delta(x).$$

From now on we will denote $H \to 0$ if all $\lambda_i \to 0$ and $H \to \infty$ if all $\lambda_i \to \infty$.

Given noise observation

$$X(t) = \mu(t) + \epsilon(t),$$

where ϵ is a mean zero random field and μ is unknown signal, the kernel smoothing estimator of μ is given by

$$\widehat{\mu}(t) = K_H * X(t) = \int K_H(t-s)X(s)\,ds$$

The important properties of the estimator are

(1) $\lim_{H\to 0}\widehat{\mu}(t) = \int \delta(t-s)X(s)\,ds = X(t)$.

(2) $\lim_{H\to\infty}\widehat{\mu}(t) = 0$.

(3) $\mathbb{E}\widehat{\mu}(t) = K_H*\mu(t) \to \mu(t)$ as $H \to 0$. The kernel estimator becomes more unbiased as $H \to 0$.

(4) Assuming the mean signal is bounded, i.e. $|\mu| < \infty$,

$$\mathbb{E}\widehat{\mu}(t) \leq \int K_H(t) \sup \mu(t) \, dt \leq \sup_t \mu(t).$$

Similarly we can bound from below so that

$$\inf_t \mu(t) \leq \mathbb{E}\widehat{\mu}(t) \leq \sup \mu(t).$$

(5) Another interesting property is

$$\int K_H * X(t) \, dt = \int_t \int_s K_H(t-s)X(s) \, ds \, dt$$

$$= \int X(s) \, ds.$$

This implies that the integral mean signal is preserved after kernel smoothing.

Truncated Kernel. In general, it is cumbersome to manipulate kernels with infinite support numerically. We usually truncate kernel K_H in outside some compact subset $\mathcal{M}$. We define a truncated and normalized kernel

$$\widetilde{K}_H(x) = \frac{K_H(x)\mathbf{1}_{\mathcal{M}}(x)}{\int_{\mathcal{M}} K_H(x) \, dx},$$

where $\mathbf{1}_{\mathcal{M}}$ is an indicator function that is zero everywhere except $\mathcal{M}$ where it is one. The kernel smoothing estimator is then given by

$$\widehat{\mu}(x) = \widetilde{K}_H * X(x).$$

Even though functional signal X is continues, it will be observed at n discrete points x_i so the signal can be written as

$$X(x) = \sum_{i=1}^{n} X(x_i)\delta(x - x_i).$$

From the property of the Dirac-delta function, we have

$$\widehat{\mu}(\mathbf{x}) = \sum_{i=1}^{n} \widetilde{K}_H(\mathbf{x} - \mathbf{x}_i)X(\mathbf{x}_i)$$

where $\widetilde{K}_H$ is now a discrete normalized kernel

$$\widetilde{K}_H(x - x_i) = \frac{K_H(x - x_i)}{\sum_{x_j \in \mathcal{M}} K_H(x - x_j)}.$$

The discrete normalized kernel estimator in the nonparametric regression setting is usually called *Nadaraya-Watson kernel estimator* (Nadaraya, 1964; Watson, 1964).

6.2 Diffusion Smoothing

Gaussian kernel smoothing $K_\sigma * X$ is the unique solution to a diffusion equation

$$\frac{\partial f}{\partial t} = \Delta f, \ f(x, t = 0) = X(x) \tag{6.3}$$

with $t = \sigma^2/2$. This relationship was exploited in developing diffusion smoothing on cortical manifolds (Chung *et al.*, 2001b, 2003c).

6.2.1 *Diffusion in Euclidean Space*

With respect to the spherical coordinates, the n-dimensional Gaussian kernel is given by

$$K_\sigma(r) = \frac{1}{(2\pi)^{n/2}\sigma^n} \exp\left[-\frac{r^2}{2\sigma^2}\right],$$

where $r = \sum_{i=1}^n x_i^2$. Since the Gaussian kernel is isotropic, it is the function or radius r only. The Laplacian Δ in both the Cartesian and spherical coordinates for isotropic functions like K_σ is given by

$$\Delta = \sum_{i=1}^n \frac{\partial^2}{\partial x_i^2}$$
$$= \frac{\partial^2}{\partial r^2} + \frac{n-1}{r}\frac{\partial}{\partial r}.$$

The algebraic manipulation can show that

$$\frac{1}{\sigma}\frac{\partial K_\sigma}{\partial \sigma} = \Delta K_\sigma. \tag{6.4}$$

Although (6.4) does not look like a diffusion equation, actually it is in a different time scale $t = \sigma^2/2$. Using the differential $dt = \sigma d\sigma$, (6.4) transforms to

$$\frac{\partial K_\sigma}{\partial t} = \Delta K_\sigma.$$

Since the both sides are linear, we can convolve the both sides with observation X.

$$\frac{\partial K_\sigma * X}{\partial t} = \Delta\big[K_\sigma * X\big].$$

Hence $K_\sigma * X$ is a unique solution of (6.3).

Note that

$$\lim_{\sigma \to 0} K_\sigma * X(x) = X(x)$$

so the solution satisfies the initial condition. If we diffuse observation X for the duration $t = \sigma^2/2$, it should be equivalent to kernel smoothing with bandwidth σ. This is a remarkable result that has been used in many imaging applications. The solution to (6.3) is identical to Gaussian kernel smoothing estimate so diffusion smoothing estimator should inherit all the statistical properties of kernel smoothing estimator and vice versa.

The drawback of Gaussian kernel smoothing is that it does not respect the natural boundaries of objects. We would like to encourage smoothing within a region rather than smoothing across the boundaries. This could be achieved by solving the diffusion equation with the condition $X(x,t) = 0$ on the boundaries. Solving a partial differential equation with such boundary condition is called the boundary value problem (BVP) and such smoothing method is usually referred as *diffusion smoothing* or diffusion filtering. J.O. Ramsay has solved the BVP to smooth data constrained within a region (Ramsay, 2000). Extending the work of A. Witkin (Witkin, 1983), P. Pernona and J. Malik (Perona and Malik, 1990) first introduced the concept of anisotropic diffusion in the problem of edge enhancement and detection by running the diffusion equation backwards in time. Diffusion smoothing has been also used in the analysis of functional magnetic resonance imaging (fMRI) data on the brain surface (Andrade *et al.*, 2001) and detecting the regions of surface area change in brain development (Chung *et al.*, 2001b).

Despite the simplicity of Gaussian kernel smoothing, it has the problem of shrinkage toward the mean near the data boundary and the shrinkage worsens as the bandwidth gets larger. However, it is possible to correct such boundary bias of Gaussian kernel smoothing by using *boundary kernels* (Ramsay and Silverman, 1997).

6.2.2 *Diffusion in 1D*

Consider 1-dimensional diffusion equation

$$\frac{\partial f}{\partial t} = \frac{\partial^2 f}{\partial^2 x}, \ f(x,0) = g(x). \tag{6.5}$$

The diffusion equation (8.48) can be solved iteratively by the finite difference method:

$$f(x^i, t_{j+1}) = f(x^i, t_j) + (t_{j+1} - t_j)\frac{\widehat{\partial f}}{\partial x}(x^i, t_j), \tag{6.6}$$

where $\frac{\widehat{\partial f}}{\partial x}(x^i, t_j)$ is an estimator of $\frac{\partial f}{\partial x}(x^i, t_j)$. To simplify the problem, take the same iteration step size $\Delta t = t_{j+1} - t_j$ and iterate until t_j hits $\sigma^2/2$

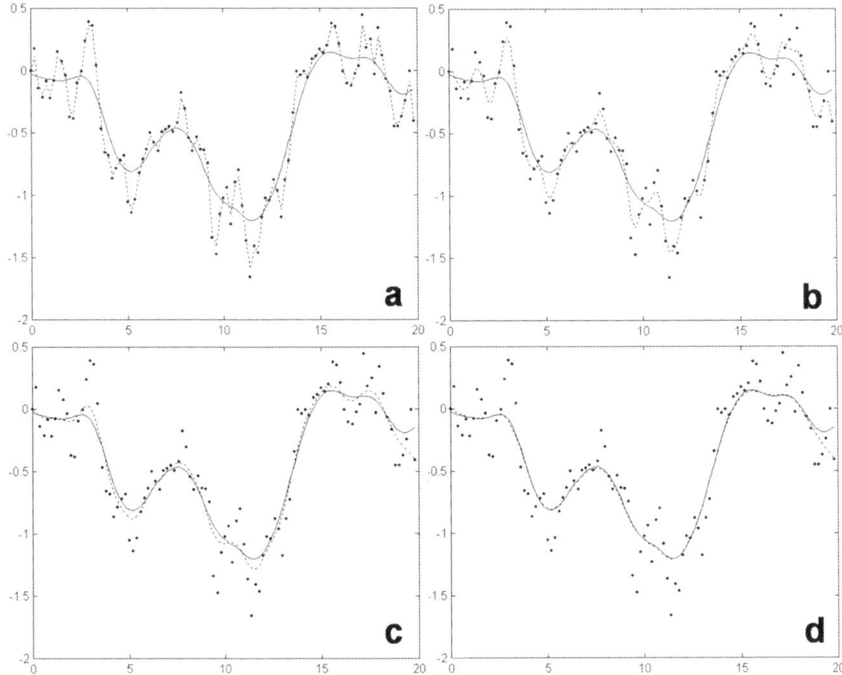

Fig. 6.2   Comparison between Gaussian kernel smoothing with $\sigma = 1$ (solid line) and diffusion smoothing (dotted line). The diffusion smoothing is done iteratively. (a) before the iteration. (b) after 5th iterations. (c) after 25th iterations. (d) after 50th iteration.

(Figure 6.3). Estimating the second derivative of a function requires at least three data points. One way of estimating $\frac{\partial f(x^i)}{\partial x}$ is to differentiate a quadratic function that passes through three points

$$\left(x^{i-1}, f(x^{i-1})\right), \left(x^i, f(x^i)\right), \left(x^{i+1}, f(x^{i+1})\right).$$

It can be shown that the estimation based on the quadratic interpolation is

$$\widehat{\frac{\partial^2 f}{\partial x^2}}(x^i) = \frac{\frac{f(x^{i+1})-f(x^i)}{x^{i+1}-x^i} - \frac{f(x^i)-f(x^{i-1})}{x^i-x^{i-1}}}{\frac{x^{i+1}-x^{i-1}}{2}}.$$

We can not interpolate at the end points x^1 and x^N so we are forced to set up boundary conditions $F(x^1, t_j) = f(x^1), F(x^N, t_j) = f(x^N)$ for all t_j in our iteration scheme. With these boundary conditions, we are numerically solving a BVP of PDE and this is why diffusion smoothing will outperform Gaussian kernel smoothing near boundary. Figures 6.2

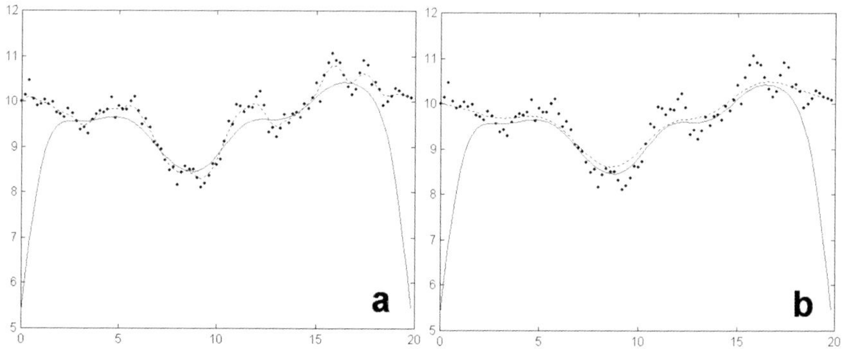

Fig. 6.3   Breakdown of Gaussian kernel smoothing with $\sigma = 1$ at the boundary (solid line). Diffusion smoothing solved with the boundary condition (dotted line). (a) after 0.25 seconds (25th. iteration). (b) after 0.5 seconds equivalent to $\sigma = 1$ (50th. iteration).

and 6.3 show the comparison between Gaussian kernel smoothing in and the equivalent diffusion smoothing. Note that there are slight discrepancies near the edges due to the fact that the diffusion equation was solved with the boundary conditions while Gaussian kernel smoothing is not.

6.2.3   *Diffusion on Triangular Mesh*

We present the FEM scheme for performing diffusion smoothing. We will follow the notations given in Section 5.4 in discretizing the diffusion equation

$$\frac{\partial f}{\partial t} = \Delta f. \tag{6.7}$$

The only difference between solving eigenfunctions of the Laplace-Beltrami operator in Section 5.4 is the discretization of the temporal derivative. Let g and $f(x, t)$ be arbitrary piecewise linear functions. We discretize (6.7) in each triangle element T_i. Following the discretization of the eigenequation of the Laplace-Beltrami operator in (5.26), we discretize (6.7) as

$$\int_{T_i} g \frac{\partial f}{\partial t} \, d\mu = -\int_{T_i} \langle \nabla f, \nabla g \rangle \, d\mu. \tag{6.8}$$

The left-hand term of (6.8) is

$$\int_{T_i} g \frac{\partial f}{\partial t} \, d\mu = \sum_{k,l=1}^{3} g_{i_k} \frac{\partial f(p_{i_l}, t)}{\partial t} \int_{T_i} \xi_{i_k} \xi_{i_l} \, d\mu$$

$$= \mathbf{G}'_i \mathbf{A}^i \frac{d}{dt} \mathbf{F}_i,$$

where $\mathbf{G}_i = (g_{i_1}, g_{i_2}, g_{i_3})'$, $\mathbf{F}_i = (f_{i_1}, f_{i_2}, f_{i_3})'$ and $\mathbf{A}^i$ is given in (5.29). The right-hand term of (6.8) is given in (5.31). Then equating the left and right hand sides, we get

$$\mathbf{G}_i' \mathbf{A}^i \frac{d}{dt} \mathbf{F}_i = -\mathbf{G}_i' \mathbf{G}^i \mathbf{F}_i. \tag{6.9}$$

Since the equation (6.9) should be satisfied for an arbitrary vector $\mathbf{G}_i$, we have a system of ordinary differential equations (ODE) given by

$$\frac{d\mathbf{F}_i}{dt} = -(\mathbf{A}^i)^{-1} \mathbf{C}^i \mathbf{F}_i \text{ for all } i. \tag{6.10}$$

(6.10) discretizes the diffusion equation in a triangle element T_i. Having discretized an element, the next step is to assemble all such elements in m incident triangles around vertex p. Let $p_1, \cdots, p_m$ be the m neighboring vertices around $p = p_0$ in the counter-clockwise direction. Let p, p_i, p_{i+1} be the vertices of the element T_i (Figure 5.2). By combining all elements, we have

$$\int_{T_1 \cup \cdots \cup T_m} \langle \nabla f, \nabla g \rangle \, d\mu = \sum_{i=1}^{m} \int_{T_i} \langle \nabla f, \nabla g \rangle \, d\mu$$
$$= \mathbf{G}' \mathbf{C} \mathbf{F},$$

where

$$\mathbf{F} = [f(p, t), f(p_1, t), \cdots, f(p_m, t)]',$$
$$\mathbf{G} = [g(p), g(p_1), \cdots, g(p_m)]'.$$

The matrix $\mathbf{C} = (C_{ij})$ is the global coefficient matrix given in (5.36) and (5.37). Similarly

$$\int_{T_1 \cup \cdots \cup T_m} G \frac{\partial F}{\partial t} \, d\mu = \mathbf{G}' \mathbf{A} \frac{d\mathbf{F}}{dt},$$

where $\mathbf{A} = (A_{ij})$ are given in (5.34) and (5.35).

Equating the above equations, we have

$$\mathbf{G}' \mathbf{A} \frac{d\mathbf{F}}{dt} = -\mathbf{G}' \mathbf{C} \mathbf{F}. \tag{6.11}$$

Since equation (6.11) should be satisfied for an arbitrary G, we have

$$\frac{d\mathbf{F}}{dt} = -\mathbf{A}^{-1} \mathbf{C} \mathbf{F}. \tag{6.12}$$

At first glance, it seems like we need to solve a system of large linear equations iteratively. Note that the first row of the simultaneous ODE (6.12) gives the discrete diffusion equation at the vertex $p = p_0$:

$$\frac{dF(p, t)}{dt} = -\sum_{i,k=0}^{m} A_{0k}^{-1} C_{ki} F(p_i, t), \tag{6.13}$$

where A_{0k}^{-1} is the $0k$-th element of A^{-1}. Comparing this with the diffusion equation $\frac{\partial f(p,t)}{\partial t} = \Delta f(p,t)$, we can see that the right-hand side of equation (6.13) should be the discrete estimation of Laplacian of function F evaluated at vertex p. Simplifying the matrix inversion using the computational algebraic system MAPLE, we have the cotan estimation of the Laplace-Beltrami operator given by

$$\widehat{\Delta} f(p) = \sum_{i=1}^{m} w_i \left[f(p_i) - f(p) \right] \tag{6.14}$$

with the weights

$$w_i = \frac{\cot \theta_i + \cot \phi_i}{\sum_{i=1}^{m} |T_i|},$$

where θ_i and ϕ_i are the two angles opposite to the edge $p_i - p$ (Figure 5.2). This is an improved formulation from (Andrade *et al.*, 2001), where the Laplace-Beltrami operator is simply estimated as the planar Laplacian after locally flattening the triangular mesh consisting of nodes $p_0, \cdots, p_m$ onto a flat plane. In the numerical implementation, we can use the relationship

$$\cot \theta_i = \frac{\langle p_{i+1} - p, p_{i+1} - p_i \rangle}{\|(p_{i+1} - p) \times (p_i - p)\|},$$

$$\cot \phi_i = \frac{\langle p_{i-1} - p, p_{i-1} - p_i \rangle}{\|(p_{i+1} - p) \times (p_i - p)\|}.$$

Computing the weights w_i for the Laplace-Beltrami operator takes a fair amount of time in MATLAB but once the weights are computed once, it is applied through the subsequent finite scheme repeatedly.

6.2.4   *Finite Difference Scheme*

The diffusion equation is then solved by the finite difference scheme:

$$f(p, t_{n+1}) = f(p, t_n) + (t_{n+1} - t_n)\widehat{\Delta} f(p, t_n) \tag{6.15}$$

where $\widehat{\Delta} f(p, t_n)$ is estimated by (6.14). We can fix the iteration step size $t_{n+1} - t_n = \delta t$. We need to choose δt sufficiently small that the finite difference converges. For the convergence of the finite difference scheme, δt is chosen to satisfy the following harmonic condition (Chung *et al.*, 2003b)

$$\min_i f(p_i, t_n) \leq f(p, t_n + \delta t) \leq \max_i f(p_i, t_n). \tag{6.16}$$

The inequality (6.16) states that the diffused heat must be anywhere between the highest and the lowest heat. The minimum case follows similarly.

The inequality (6.16) may break down if δt is large. From (6.15) and (6.16), the iteration step size must satisfy

$$\delta t \leq \left| \frac{\max_i f(p_i, t_n) - f(p, t_n)}{\widehat{\Delta} f(p, t_n)} \right|, \left| \frac{\min_i f(p_i, t_n) - f(p, t_n)}{\widehat{\Delta} f(p, t_n)} \right|. \qquad (6.17)$$

The denominator $\widehat{\Delta} f$ behaves like the sample covariance of F at $p, p_1, \cdots, p_m$. The smoother the function F is, the smaller the Laplace-Beltrami operator of f is. In such a case, the iteration step size δt can be large. By changing the iteration step size δt with respect to the inequality at each node p, we can have *spatially adaptive smoothing*, which depends on the smoothness of f. In order to determine the critical iteration step size for the isotropic diffusion (with respect to the local conformal coordinates) with the spatially fixed δt, it is best to measure the smoothness of the function f first and then estimate the δt accordingly. The signal $f(p, t_n)$ tends to become smoother as n increases, in which case, the ratio between the numerator and the denominator in (6.17) gets larger. Therefore, if δt satisfies the inequality (6.17) at every nodes in the first iteration $n = 1$, the inequality (6.16) will likely to be satisfied for the later iteration $n \geq 1$. Note that the iteration time step should be in the order of

$$\delta t < \text{nodal distance} \times \left| \frac{\text{the first derivative of F}}{\text{the second derivatives of F}} \right|$$

to guarantee the convergence and the stability of the finite difference scheme. The relation between the critical iteration step size and the nodal distance has also been briefly pointed out in Andrade *et al.* (2001).

If the iteration step size is bigger than the desired inequality (6.16), the finite difference scheme diverges as illustrated in Figure 6.4, where the large iteration step size $\delta t = 1.5$ causes the numerical singularity in iteration. Ideally, the finite difference scheme should converge to the stationary solution of the diffusion equation, i.e. the Laplace equation given by $\Delta f = 0$ as the number of iterations increases. After N iterations, the finite difference scheme gives an approximate solution of the diffusion of the initial heat after time $N\delta t$. Figure 6.5 shows another example of diffusion smoothing applied to the noisy mean curvature estimation of the outer cortical surface.

The Laplace-Beltrami operator in the conformal coordinate system (Kreyszig, 1959) (u^1, u^2) can be written as

$$\Delta = \frac{\partial^2}{\partial (u^1)^2} + \frac{\partial^2}{\partial (u^2)^2}.$$

So locally the Laplace-Beltrami operator is viewed as the Laplacian in $\mathbb{R}^2$. We can represent the FWHM of diffusion smoothing locally as the FWHM

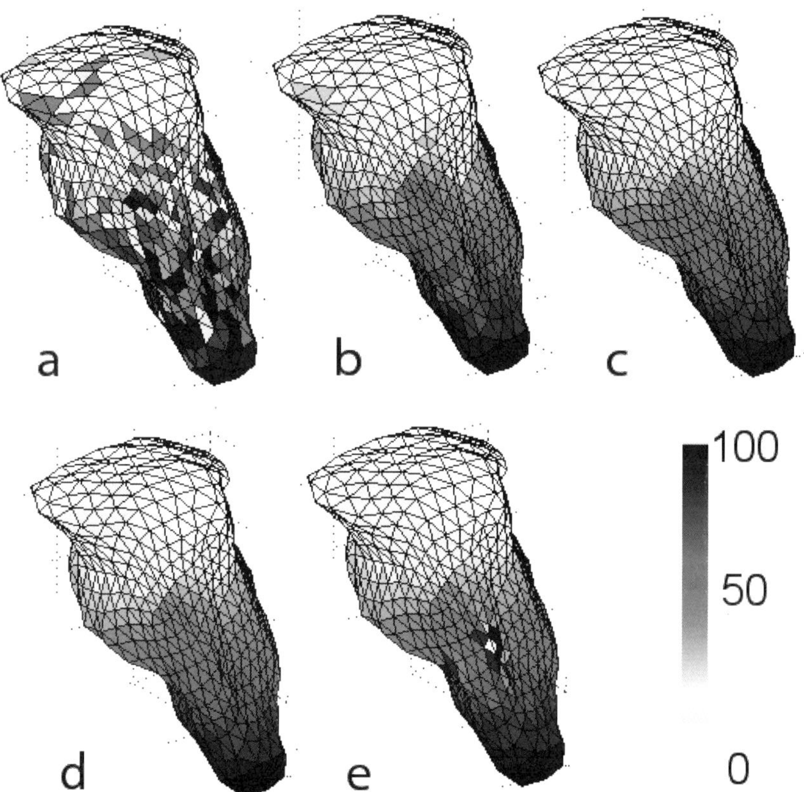

Fig. 6.4   Diffusion smoothing of simulated signal on the brain stem consisting of 1280 triangles. (a) The initial signal, (b) After 10 iterations with $\delta t = 0.5$, (c) After 20 iterations with $\delta t = 0.5$, (d) After 50 iterations with $\delta t = 0.2$. (e) After 10 iterations with $\delta t = 1.5$. Because the iteration step size is large, the iteration breaks down. This shows the step size should be smaller than 1.5.

of the corresponding Gaussian kernel in the conformal coordinate system. Then diffusion smoothing with N iterations and the step size δt in $\mathbb{R}^2$ would be equivalent to Gaussian kernel smoothing with

$$\text{FWHM} = 4\sqrt{\ln 2 \cdot N\delta t}. \tag{6.18}$$

For instance, in order to have 10mm FWHM Gaussian kernel smoothing in Euclidean space, we should have $N\delta t = 4.33$. If the iteration step size is taken at $\delta t = 0.2$, then $N = 22$ iterations are sufficient to get the 10mm FWHM smoothing assuming the iterations are stable. Equivalently $\delta t = 0.1$ with $N = 44$ will give the identical result. So the number of iterations that

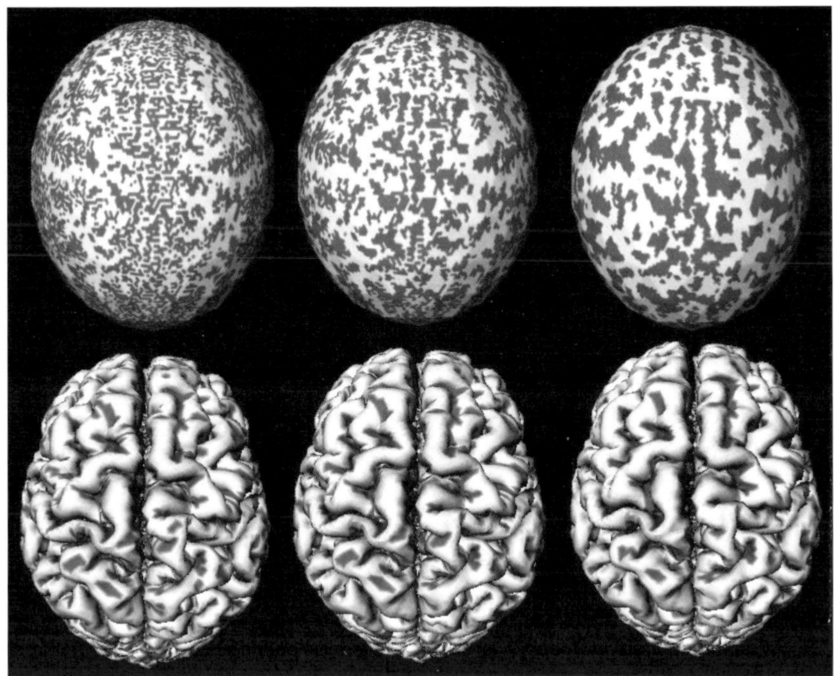

Fig. 6.5 Diffusion smoothing is applied to smooth out the mean curvature of the brain cortex and projected onto a sphere to show how the hidden sulcal pattern. From the left to right: initial mean curvature, after 20 iterations with $\delta t = 0.2$, and after 100 iterations.

is required is inversely proportional to the iteration step size δt. The smaller the iteration step size, the longer it takes to achieve the same result. This has been illustrated in Figure 6.4 (c) and (d), which show almost identical results. It should be noted that the above argument about 10mm FWHM Gaussian kernel smoothing is only an analogy applied to the curved surface and should not be taken exactly. In fact, FWHM of heat kernel on a sphere is different from that of Gaussian kernel in $\mathbb{R}^2$ (Figure 6.6) (Chung *et al.*, 2007).

6.3 Heat Kernel Smoothing

Diffusion smoothing requires using the finite element or finite difference methods which are known to suffer numerical instability if the forward Euler scheme is used. So instead of trying to solve diffusion equations directly,

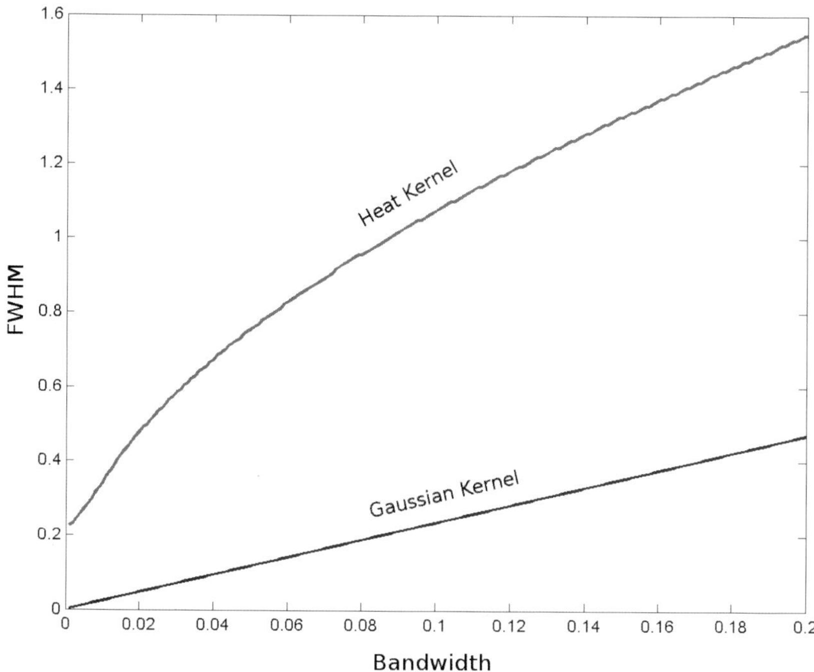

Fig. 6.6 Plot of FWHM over smoothing bandwidth for both 2D heat and 2D Gaussian kernels. FWHM of heat kernel does not proportionally increase as the bandwidth increases. This causes sever underestimation of FWHM in iterated Gaussian kernel smoothing which approximates heat kernel smoothing. The FWHM has to be numerically estimated in the case of the heat kernel. The estimated FWHM can be used in the random field theory as a measure of smoothness.

approximate but more stable kernel smoothing has been proposed. Gaussian kernels are only defined in the Euclidean space. The generalization of the Gaussian kernel to arbitrary manifolds is a heat kernel. By convolving signal given in an manifold with the corresponding heat kernel, we perform *heat kernel smoothing*. There are many different numerical implementations for Gaussian kernel smoothing depending on how we approximate Gaussian kernel. For instance, one can do weighted averaging only using 6-neighbors in 3D voxel space while others may use 14-neighbors. Similar to Gaussian kernel smoothing, we can have various numerical implementations for heat kernel smoothing. Heat kernel smoothing and its variants have been the most widely used framework for smoothing data along the cortical surface. It has been used in smoothing various cortical data: cortical curvatures (Luders *et al.*, 2006b; Gaser *et al.*, 2006), cortical thickness

(Luders *et al.*, 2006a; Bernal-Rusiel *et al.*, 2008), hippocampus (Shen *et al.*, 2006; Zhu *et al.*, 2007), magnetoencephalography (MEG) (Han *et al.*, 2007) and functional-MRI (Hagler Jr., 2006; Jo *et al.*, 2007).

6.3.1 *Heat Kernel*

If we want to perform Gaussian kernel smoothing on cortical surfaces, we need to reshape the kernel to adapt the geometric structure of surfaces. Let ψ_j be eigenfunctions of the Laplace-Beltrami operator Δ satisfying

$$\Delta \psi_j = -\lambda_j \psi_j, \tag{6.19}$$

where λ_j are ordered eigenvalues such that

$$0 = \lambda_0 < \lambda_1 \leq \lambda_2 \leq \cdots .$$

Then the *heat kernel* K_σ is a positive definite function defined on a manifold $\mathcal{M}$ as

$$K_\sigma(p, q) = \sum_{j=0}^{\infty} e^{-\lambda_j \sigma} \psi_j(p)\psi_j(q). \tag{6.20}$$

On a two-sphere, the heat kernel is analytically given in terms of the spherical harmonics Y_{lm} as

$$K_\sigma(p, q) = \sum_{l=0}^{\infty} \sum_{m=-l}^{l} e^{-l(l+1)\sigma} Y_{lm}(p)Y_{lm}(q). \tag{6.21}$$

Figure 6.7 shows the shape of heat kernels for different bandwidths. The detailed mathematical exposition of heat kernel is given in Berline *et al.* (1991) and Rosenberg (1997).

Although the exact analytic form of heat kernel is unknown when the underlying manifold is not algebraically given, using the parametrix expansion, we can at least approximate the heat kernel using the Gaussian kernel as

$$K_\sigma(p, q) = \frac{1}{(4\pi\sigma)^{1/2}} e^{-\frac{d^2(p,q)}{4\sigma}} \left[1 + O(\sigma^2)\right] \tag{6.22}$$

for small geodesic distance $d(p, q)$ (Rosenberg, 1997; Wang, 1997). When the Riemannian metric tensors are identity, i.e. $g_{ij} = \delta_{ij}$, $\mathcal{M}$ becomes flat and the the geodesic distance becomes the usual Euclidean distance $\| \cdot \|$. Then the heat kernel (6.22) collapses to the usual Gaussian kernel

$$K_\sigma(p, q) = \frac{1}{(4\pi\sigma)^{1/2}} \exp\left[-\frac{\|p - q\|^2}{4\sigma} \right].$$

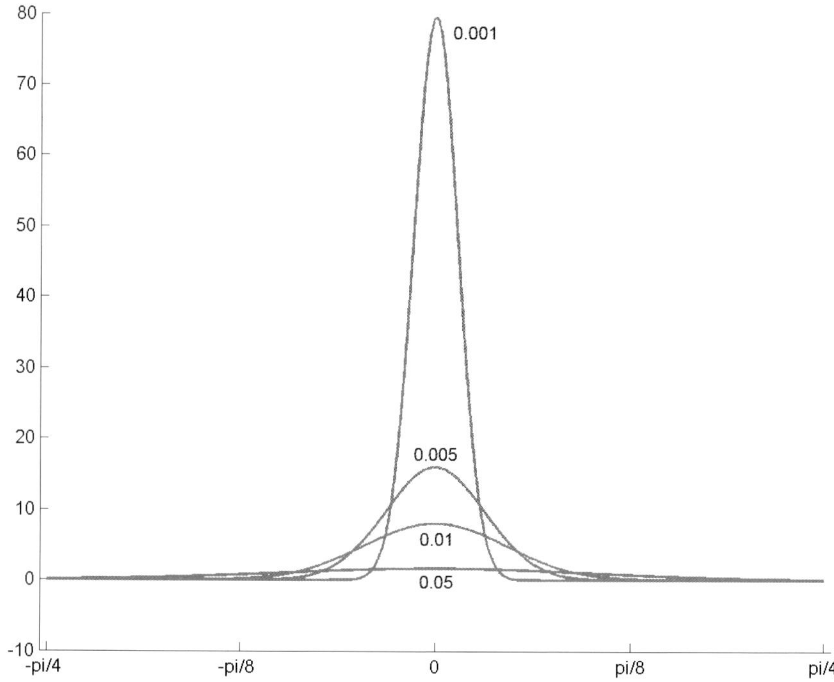

Fig. 6.7 The shape of the heat kernel $K_\sigma(p, q)$ for various bandwidths σ in S^2. The shape is computed from the harmonic addition theorem. The point p is fixed to be the north pole and the horizontal axis is the angle $\cos^{-1}(p \cdot q)$.

Hence, heat kernel is a natural extension of the Gaussian kernel. If we rescale the bandwidth to $2\sigma = \tau^2$, we obtain the Gaussian probability density

$$K_\tau(p, q) = \frac{1}{\sqrt{2\pi}\tau} \exp\left[-\frac{\|p - q\|^2}{2\tau^2} \right]. \tag{6.23}$$

Care should be taken in which scale we are formulating heat kernel smoothing. Note that (6.23) is the probability density for Gaussian random variable with variance τ^2 so it provides a more straightforward statistical interpretation. The heat kernel can be also interpreted as the transition probability density for an isotropic diffusion process with respect to the surface area element (Wang, 1997).

The kernel is symmetric, i.e. $K_\sigma(p, q) = K_\sigma(q, p)$ and isotropic with respect to the geodesic distance d defined along the manifold. The property of a kernel being isotropic needs some explanation. A function f is *isotropic* in a manifold $\mathcal{M}$ if $f(p) = $ constant for all point p on the geodesic circle $d(0,p) = $ constant. Since $K_\sigma(p,q)$ has two arguments while symmetric, the isotropic property should holds for either one of the arguments.

6.3.2 *Heat Kernel Smoothing*

Heat kernel smoothing of functional data f is defined as the convolution:

$$K_\sigma * f(p) = \int_{\mathcal{M}} K_\sigma(p,q) f(q) \, d\mu(q), \tag{6.24}$$

where μ is the Lebegue measure in $\mathcal{M}$. Figure 6.8 demonstrates heat kernel smoothing applied to cortical thickness along the outer cortical surface.

By substituting (6.20) into (6.24), we can write heat kernel smoothing as a series expansion:

$$K_\sigma * f(p) = \sum_{j=0}^{\infty} e^{-\lambda_j \sigma} f_j \psi_j(p), \tag{6.25}$$

where

$$f_j = \int_{\mathcal{M}} f(q) \psi_j(q) \, d\mu(q)$$

is the Fourier coefficient of signal f with respect to the basis ψ_j. This is the *weighted Fourier series representation* (Chung et al., 2007). The special case of the representation using spherical harmonics will be discussed in detail in a later chapter. Here we list few additional properties of heat kernel smoothing:

(1) Since $\psi_0 = 1/\sqrt{\mu(\mathcal{M})}$, we have

$$K_\sigma * f(p) = \frac{\int_{\mathcal{M}} f(p) \, d\mu(p)}{\mu(\mathcal{M})} + f_1 e^{-\lambda_1 \sigma} \psi_1(p) + R(\sigma, p), \tag{6.26}$$

where the first term is the average signal, f_1 is a constant and R goes to 0 faster than $e^{-\lambda_1 \sigma}$ as $\sigma \to \infty$ (Banuelos and Burdzy, 1999). Due to expansion (6.26), the behavior of diffusion is basically governed by the second eigenfunction ψ_1.

(2) As $\sigma \to 0$, $K_\sigma(p,q)$ becomes the Dirac-delta function $\delta(p,q)$ so heat kernel smoothing becomes unbiased as $\sigma \to 0$, i.e.

$$\lim_{\sigma \to 0} K_\sigma * f(p) = f(p).$$

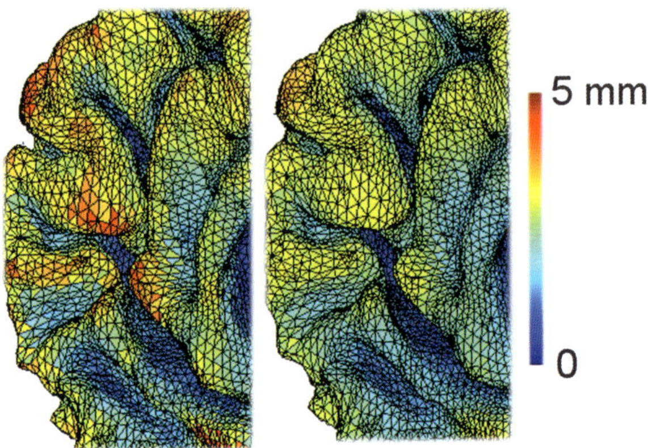

Fig. 6.8 Cortical thickness obtained from FreeSurfer package is smoothed using heat kernel smoothing with $\sigma = 1$ and $m = 100$ iterations.

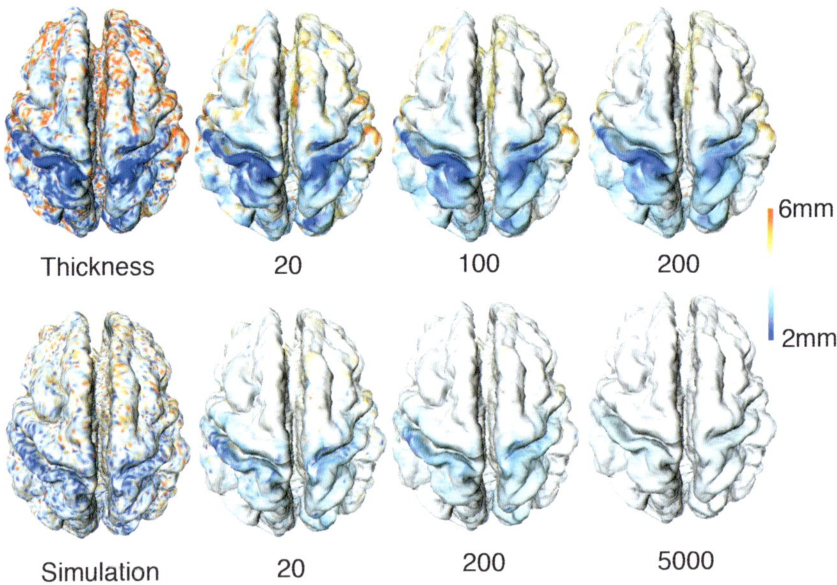

Fig. 6.9 Iterated kernel smoothing of cortical thickness with bandwidth $\tau = 1$ and different number of iterations . Iterated kernel smoothing on real (top) and simulated (bottom) cortical thickness data.

(3) As σ gets larger, the bias increases. However, the total bias over $\mathcal{M}$ is always zero, i.e.

$$\int_{\mathcal{M}} \left[K_\sigma * f(p) - f(p) \right] d\mu(p) = 0.$$

This can be seen from taking one more integral on (6.24) and realizing

$$\int_{\mathcal{M}} f(q) \int_{\mathcal{M}} K_\sigma(p, q) \, d\mu(p) \, d\mu(q) = \int_{\mathcal{M}} f(p) \, d\mu(p)$$

since K integrate to 1.

(4) $K_\sigma * f$ is the unique solution of the following isotropic diffusion:

$$\frac{\partial g}{\partial \sigma} = \Delta g, \ f(p, 0) = f(p). \tag{6.27}$$

The bandwidth σ is interpreted as diffusion time. If we use the different scale $2\sigma = \tau^2$, (6.27) is written as

$$\frac{1}{\tau} \frac{\partial g}{\partial \tau} = \Delta g.$$

This is a well known result given in Chung *et al.* (2005a) and Rosenberg (1997). By definition, a Green's function or a fundamental solution $G(p, q)$ of the Cauchy problem (6.27) is given by

$$\frac{\partial g}{\partial \sigma} = \Delta g, \ f(p, 0) = \delta(p), \tag{6.28}$$

where δ is the Dirac delta function. It can be shown that the heat kernel K_σ is a Green's function of (6.28) (Evans, 1998). Since all the operators are linear in (6.28), we can further convolve all the terms with initial functional data f so that we have

$$\frac{\partial}{\partial \sigma} (K_\sigma * f) = \Delta (K_\sigma * f), \ K_\sigma * f = f(p).$$

Hence $K_\sigma * f$ is a solution of (6.27).

(5) As $\sigma \to \infty$, heat kernel smoothing converges to the mean signal over $\mathcal{M}$, i.e.

$$\lim_{\sigma \to \infty} K_\sigma * f = \frac{1}{\mu(\mathcal{M})} \int_{\mathcal{M}} f(p) \, d\mu(p),$$

where $\mu(\mathcal{M})$ is the total surface area. Figure 6.9 shows the convergence of heat kernel smoothing to the within-subject mean thickness 4mm as the bandwidth increases.

The problem with the heat kernel smoothing (6.24) is that the explicit analytic form of the heat kernel is unknown. Therefore, iterative kernel smoothing has been developed, where the weights are spatially adapted to follow the shape of heat kernel in discrete fashion along a surface mesh (Chung *et al.*, 2005a). The algorithm has been implemented in MAT-LAB and it is freely available in `http://www.stat.wisc.edu/~mchung/softwares/hk/hk.html`. We decompose the kernel with large bandwidth to k-iterated kernels with smaller bandwidth. Then approximate the kernel with the smaller bandwidth with (6.22).

In iterated kernel smoothing, kernel weights are spatially adapted to follow the shape of the heat kernel in a discrete fashion along a manifold. In the tangent space of the manifold, the heat kernel can be approximated linearly using the Gaussian kernel for small bandwidth. A kernel with large bandwidth is then constructed iteratively applying the kernel with small bandwidth. However, this process compounds the linearization error at each iteration as we will demonstrate in the paper.

Smoothing implemented in FreeSurfer package is based on the similar iterative averaging of nearest neighbors (Han *et al.*, 2006; Kuperberg *et al.*, 2003). At each iteration, data at a surface vertex is updated by the average of the values at the 1st order neighbors and at its own location (Kuperberg *et al.*, 2003). Although this approximates a heat kernel linearly, the FWHM estimation of the kernel can be severely biased (Figure 6.6). Instead of simple averaging, heat kernel can be approximated using a Gaussian kernel with the 1st order neighbors (Chung *et al.*, 2005a). As in Gaussian kernel which has an infinite support, the support of heat kernel spans whole surface. As the bandwidth increases, heat kernel converges to the inverse of surface area. So it has the effect of averaging all measurements on the cortical surface. On the other hand, wavelets have finite supports so it should perform better for rapidly changing signals. For instance, Bernal-Rusiel *et al.* (2008) used spherical wavelet based smoothing to improve sensitivity and specificity compared to heat kernel smoothing.

6.3.3 *Iterated Kernel Smoothing*

Denote the k-fold iterated kernel as

$$K_\sigma^{(k)} = \underbrace{K_\sigma * \cdots * K_\sigma}_{k \text{ times}}.$$

We can show that

$$K_{k\sigma} * f = K_{\sigma}^{(k)} * f. \tag{6.29}$$

This can be seen as a scale space property of diffusion. $K_{\sigma}^{(2)} * f$ is equivalent to the diffusion of signal f after time 2σ. Hence we have

$$K_{\sigma}^{(2)} f = K_{2\sigma} * f.$$

Arguing inductively we see that the general statement holds. The relationship (6.29) is the basis of iterated heat kernel smoothing used to smooth data in irregular grids such as cortical surfaces (Chung *et al.*, 2005a,b). Heat kernel with a large bandwidth is equivalently performed by applying heat kernel smoothing with a smaller bandwidth multiple times.

An alternate proof can be obtained by noting that $K_{\sigma}^{(k)}$ is the density of the sum of k independent and identically distributed Gaussian random variables. Heat kernel with a large bandwidth is decomposed into heat kernels with smaller bandwidth. For instance, iterated heat kernel smoothing with $\tau = 1$ and $k = 200$ will generate heat kernel smoothing with the effective bandwidth of 200. Figure 6.9 shows the process of iterated heat kernel smoothing. If we change the scale to $2\sigma = \tau^2$, (6.29) takes a slightly different form:

$$K_{\tau}^{(k)} * f = K_{\sqrt{k}\tau} * f.$$

The original paper Chung *et al.* (2005a) formulates heat kernel smoothing in τ-scale while Chung *et al.* (2008b) formulates it in σ-scale. So the care should be taken in what scale smoothing and modeling are done.

For small bandwidth, all the kernel weights are concentrated near the center of kernel, so can truncate the kernel in the first order neighbors of a given vertex in a mesh. Let $p_1, \cdots, p_m$ be m neighboring vertices of the center vertex $p = p_0$. The geodesic distance between p and its adjacent vertex p_i is the length of edge between these two vertices in the mesh. So the discretized and truncated version of heat kernel is given by

$$W_{\sigma}(p, p_i) = \frac{\exp\left(-\frac{\|p - p_i\|^2}{4\sigma}\right)}{\sum_{j=0}^{m} \exp\left(-\frac{\|p - p_i\|^2}{4\sigma}\right)}.$$

Note that $\sum_{i=0}^{m} K_{\sigma}(p, p_i) = 1$. Then we define the discrete version of heat kernel smoothing as

$$W_{\sigma} * f(p) = \sum_{i=0}^{m} W_{\sigma}(p, p_i) f(p_i).$$

This is repeatedly applied to obtain the desired effective smoothing bandwidth. The discrete version should converges to heat kernel smoothing (6.24) as the mesh resolution increases. This is the form of the Nadaraya-Watson kernel estimator applied to surface data (Chaudhuri and Marron, 2000). Figures 6.8 and 6.9 illustrate how heat kernel smoothing can enhance the thickness pattern by increasing the signal-to-noise ratio.

6.3.4   *Smoothing via Laplace-Beltrami Eigenfunctions*

In iterated kernel smoothing, kernel weights are spatially adapted to follow the shape of the heat kernel in a discrete fashion along a manifold. In the tangent space of the manifold, the heat kernel can be approximated linearly using the Gaussian kernel for small bandwidth. A kernel with large bandwidth is then constructed iteratively applying the kernel with small bandwidth. However, this process compounds the linearization error at each iteration. To remedy this problem, a new analytic framework has been developed (Seo *et al.*, 2010), where the heat kernel is analytically constructed using the eigenfunctions of the Laplace-Beltrami operator, avoiding the need for the linear approximation (Chung *et al.*, 2005a,b; Han *et al.*, 2006). Although solving for the eigenfunctions of the Laplace-Beltrami operator requires the finite element method, heat kernel is constructed analytically in a sense that it is represented as a series expansion explicitly. Obviously the whole framework can not be analytic which is theoretically impossible when we deal with real data. The proposed method represents isotropic heat diffusion analytically as a series expansion so it avoids the numerical instability associated with solving the diffusion equations numerically using the forward Euler scheme (Andrade *et al.*, 2001; Chung *et al.*, 2003c; Cachia *et al.*, 2003a). This radically different framework can bypass various numerical problems associated with previous approaches: numerical instability, slow convergence, and accumulated linearization error. Although there are many papers on solving diffusion equations on arbitrary triangular meshes (Andrade *et al.*, 2001; Joshi *et al.*, 2009; Tasdizen *et al.*, 2006), Seo *et al.* (2010) was the first paper that explicitly and correctly constructs heat kernel for an arbitrary surface and solved heat diffusion using the eigenfunctions of Laplace-Beltrami operator.

Section 5.4 discussed the finite element method for numerically computing the eigenfunction of the Laplace-Beltrami operator. Once we obtain the eigenfunctions, we construct the subspace $\mathcal{H}_k$, which is spanned by up to k-th degree basis. Then we approximate the functional data Y in $\mathcal{H}_k$ by minimizing the sum of squared residual:

$$\arg\min_{f\in\mathcal{H}_k}\|f-Y\|^2=\sum_{j=0}^{k}\beta_j\psi_j(p),\qquad(6.30)$$

where

$$\beta_j=\langle Y,\psi_j\rangle\qquad(6.31)$$

are Fourier coefficients to be estimated.

Using the FEM discretization (5.25), we can write two functions Y and ψ_j as piecewise linear functions

$$Y(x)=\sum_{i=1}^{N_T}\sum_{k=1}^{3}\xi_{i_k}(x)Y_{i_k}\qquad(6.32)$$

and

$$\psi_j(x)=\sum_{i=1}^{N_T}\sum_{k=1}^{3}\xi_{i_k}(x)\psi_{j_{i_k}},\qquad(6.33)$$

where $Y_{i_k}=Y(p_{i_k})$ and $\psi_{j_{i_k}}$ are function values evaluated at vertices p_{i_k} of the triangle element T_i. Then the inner product (6.31) can be written as

$$\beta_j=\sum_{i=1}^{N_T}\sum_{k,l=1}^{3}Y_{i_k}\psi_{j_{i_l}}\int_{T_i}\xi_{i_k}\xi_{i_l}\,d\mu.\qquad(6.34)$$

Following the argument similar to deriving the generalized eigenvalue problem, (6.34) can be rewritten into a matrix form

$$\beta_j=\mathbf{Y}'\mathbf{A}\boldsymbol{\psi}_j,\qquad(6.35)$$

where $\mathbf{Y}=(Y(p_1),\cdots,Y(p_n))'$ and $\boldsymbol{\psi}_j=(\psi_j(p_1),\cdots,\psi_j(p_n))'$ (Zhang *et al.*, 2007b).

The FEM discretization (6.35) is one way of computing the Fourier coefficients. For the spherical harmonic representation, the least squares method has been most widely used (Chung *et al.*, 2008b; Shen *et al.*, 2004; Styner *et al.*, 2006). The advantage of the least squares method is that it does not require knowing the mass matrix $\mathbf{A}$ but at the expense of inverting a matrix involving the basis functions. So the least squares method has been the more often used in the case where the basis functions are already known. On a unit sphere, the eigenfunctions of the Laplace-Beltrami operator is explicitly given so there is no need to compute the mass matrix $\mathbf{A}$. Note that the relation

$$\boldsymbol{\psi}_i\mathbf{A}\boldsymbol{\psi}_j=\delta_{ij}$$

is numerically exact if the basis functions are computed via FEM. However, if the basis functions are already given or computed in other ways, this relationship is approximate. For this reason, it would be better to use the least squares method in validation against spherical harmonics.

Consider the triangular mesh for $\mathcal{M}$ consisting of n nodes $p_1, \cdots, p_n$. Then we solve for

$$\underbrace{\begin{pmatrix} Y(p_1) \\ Y(p_2) \\ \vdots \\ Y(p_n) \end{pmatrix}}_{\mathbf{Y}} = \underbrace{\begin{pmatrix} \psi_0(p_1) & \psi_1(p_1) & \cdots & \psi_k(p_1) \\ \psi_0(p_2) & \psi_1(p_2) & \cdots & \psi_k(p_2) \\ \vdots & \vdots & \ddots & \vdots \\ \psi_0(p_n) & \psi_1(p_n) & \cdots & \psi_k(p_n) \end{pmatrix}}_{\mathbf{\Psi}} \underbrace{\begin{pmatrix} \beta_0 \\ \beta_1 \\ \vdots \\ \beta_k \end{pmatrix}}_{\boldsymbol{\beta}}. \tag{6.36}$$

Then the least squares estimation for $\boldsymbol{\beta}$ is given by

$$\widehat{\boldsymbol{\beta}} = (\mathbf{\Psi}'\mathbf{\Psi})^{-1}\mathbf{\Psi}'\mathbf{Y}. \tag{6.37}$$

Since the size of matrix $\mathbf{\Psi}'\mathbf{\Psi}$, i.e. $k \times k$, can become fairly large for large number of basis, it may be difficult to directly invert it when there is a need to obtain large number of basis. This is evident when the spherical harmonic basis are used. The problem with inverting extremely large matrix can be overcome by decomposing the subspace $\mathcal{H}_k$ into smaller subspaces and iteratively estimating the parameters in the smaller subspaces using the *iterative residual fitting (IRF) algorithm* (Chung et al., 2007, 2008b). The IRF-algorithm starts decomposing the subspace $\mathcal{H}_k$ into smaller subspaces as the direct sum

$$\mathcal{H}_k = \mathcal{I}_0 \oplus \mathcal{I}_1 \cdots \oplus \mathcal{I}_k,$$

where each subspace $\mathcal{I}_j$ is the projection of $\mathcal{H}_k$ along the j-th eigenfunction. Instead of directly solving the normal equation (6.36), we project the normal equations into a smaller subspace $\mathcal{I}_j$ and find the corresponding coefficient β_j in an iterative fashion from increasing the degree from 0 to k. The details of the IRF-algorithm is given in a later section and we will not discuss it here. Once we obtain the Fourier coefficients, the analytic version of heat kernel smoothing (6.25) is performed (Figure 6.10). Figure 6.11 shows an example of heat kernel smoothing using the Laplace-Beltrami eigenfunctions on a hippocampus surface.

6.4   Smoothness of Random Fields

Many brain imaging studies assume images to be stationary Gaussian fields and a general linear model (GLM) is often used in determining the effect

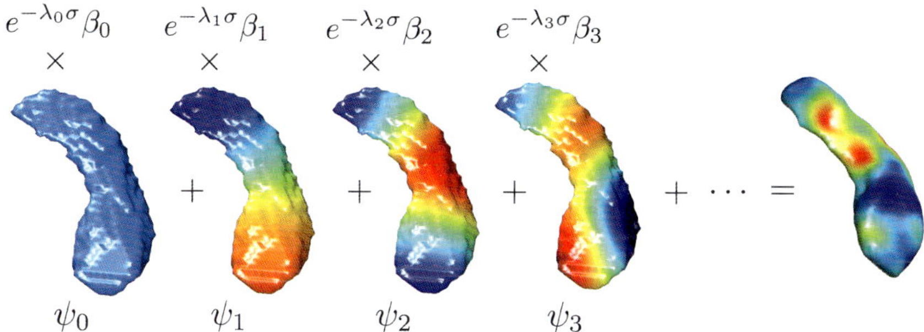

Fig. 6.10 Schematic of heat kernel smoothing using the eigenfunctions of the Laplace-Beltrami operator. Once we obtained the eigenfunctions, we multiply with the weighted Fourier coefficients $e^{-\lambda_j\sigma}\beta_j$ and sum them up.

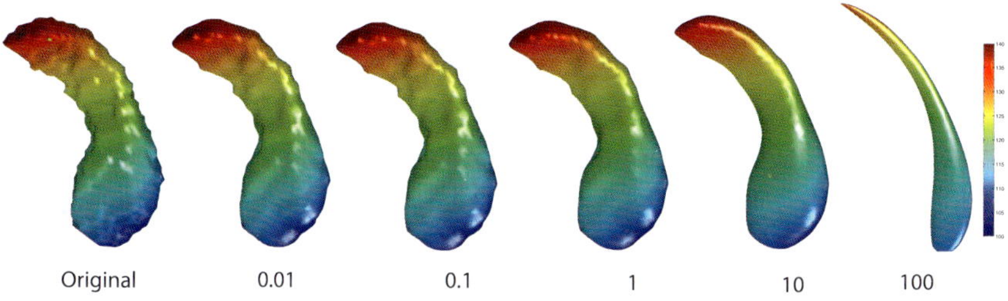

Fig. 6.11 Heat kernel smoothing with different bandwidths on a left hippocampus surface. The heat kernel is constructed using the Laplace-Beltrami eigenfunctions.

of explanatory variables. In order to determine the statistical significance associated with the GLM, it is necessary to estimate the roughness of such fields as the covariance matrix of the derivative of the fields. In earlier implementation of statistical parametric mapping (SPM) package, the roughness of images was assessed using the Gaussianized t-field but the estimation is not stable and biased (Kiebel *et al.*, 1999). Worsley proposed an unbiased way of estimating roughness more rigorously (Worsley *et al.*, 2004, 1996b; Worsley, 1994).

The covariance matrix of the spatial derivatives of the smoothed image is used in determining the statistical significance. For the t random field T, the probability that the maximum of the field exceeds h is approximately

$$P\left[\sup_{x\in\mathcal{M}} T(x) > h\right] \approx \mu(\mathcal{M})|\Lambda|^{1/2}(2\pi)^{-2}(h^2 - 1)e^{-\frac{1}{2}h^2} \qquad (6.38)$$

for high threshold h. Here, $\mu(\mathcal{M})$ is the volume of the search region $\mathcal{M}$ (Adler and Hasofer, 1976; Worsley *et al.*, 1992) and Λ is the covariance matrix of the partial derivative of the underlying Guassian error field η that is used in constructing the field T.

6.4.1 *Resels of Field*

The covariance matrix Λ can be given analytically if we assume the error field η is given as Gaussian kernel smoothing of white noise. Let $\eta = K_{\sigma'} * \epsilon$, where ϵ is Gaussian white noise. The smoothness of field η is then defined in terms of the covariance of the derivative field as

$$\Lambda = \mathrm{Cov}\left(\frac{\partial \eta}{\partial t}\right). \tag{6.39}$$

To simplify the computation in (6.39), we may assume a zero mean unit variance field for η. Instead of smoothing with the isotropic kernel K_σ, we will consider a more general setting with the anisotropic kernel K_H (6.2). The kernel K_H is given by

$$K_H(x) = \frac{1}{(2\pi)^{n/2}|H|} \exp\left[\frac{-x'(HH')^{-1}x}{2}\right].$$

Then it can be shown that Λ is given by (Adler, 1981; Worsley *et al.*, 1992)

$$\Lambda = \int \frac{\partial K_H(t)}{\partial t} \frac{\partial K_H(t)}{\partial t'} \, dt \Big/ \int K_H^2(t) \, dt.$$

An algebraic manipulation can show that $\Lambda = (HH')^{-1}/2$. If the principal axes of HH' are along the x, y and z axis direction then the offdiagonal elements of Λ are zero. If $\mathrm{FWHM}_x, \mathrm{FWHM}_y, \mathrm{FWHM}_z$ denote the full widths at half maximum along each axes, we can show that

$$\Lambda = 4\ln 2 \begin{pmatrix} 1/\mathrm{FWHM}_x^2 & 0 & 0 \\ 0 & 1/\mathrm{FWHM}_y^2 & 0 \\ 0 & 0 & 1/\mathrm{FWHM}_z^2 \end{pmatrix}.$$

Hence

$$|\Lambda|^{1/2} = (4\ln 2)^{3/2}(\mathrm{FWHM}_x\mathrm{FWHM}_y\mathrm{FWHM}_z)^{-1}.$$

Since it is cumbersome to express (6.38) using FWHMs, we define *resels*

$$R = \frac{\mu(\mathcal{M})}{\mathrm{FWHM}_x\mathrm{FWHM}_y\mathrm{FWHM}_z},$$

which is a measure of the number of resolution elements (Worsley *et al.*, 1992). If we are using an isotropic kernel, we have

$$\mathrm{FWHM} = \mathrm{FWHM}_x = \mathrm{FWHM}_y = \mathrm{FWHM}_z$$

and the resels is simply given as

$$R = \frac{\mu(\mathcal{M})}{\text{FWHM}^3}.$$ (6.40)

Then (6.38) is written as

$$P\left[\sup_{x \in \mathcal{M}} T(x) > h\right] \approx R(4\ln 2)^{3/2}(2\pi)^{-2}(h^2 - 1)e^{-\frac{1}{2}h^2}.$$ (6.41)

6.4.2 *Effective Bandwidth*

The problem with (6.41) is that the noise component needs to be exactly of the form $\eta = K_{\sigma'} * \epsilon$, which is unrealistic. To see this, consider the following GLM:

$$Y(t) = X\beta(t) + \epsilon(t),$$

where $\beta(t) = (\beta_1, \cdots, \beta_p)'$ is spatially varying parameters of the linear model and ϵ is the Gaussian white noise. The parameters of the model are usually estimated after smoothing with kernel K_σ to reduce noise. Unfortunately, the actual smoothing bandwidth σ is not going to be the observed amount of smoothing in the smoothed images due to the inhomogeneity of the field and numerical discrepancy. This relationship can be written as

$$K_\sigma * Y(t) = X\beta(t) + K_{\sigma'} * \epsilon(t),$$

where σ' is the observed amount of smoothing. The observed bandwidth σ' is often called the effective bandwdith. In terms of the full width at the half maximum (FWHM), it is called the effective-FWHM or eFWHM. Once we estimate eFWHM in smoothed image, we replace it with FWHM in (6.40).

6.4.3 *Unbiased Estimator of eFWHM*

The unbiased estimator of eFWHM is given first in Worsley *et al.* (1999), where it is estimated along edges in the lattice. Label the two voxels at the end of an edge by 1 and 2. Let the length of edge be Δx. Suppose there are n images in a group. Let r_{ij} denote the residual for the i-th image at voxel j. The normalized residuals at the two ends are

$$u_{ij} = \frac{r_{ij}}{\sqrt{\sum_{i=1}^n r_{ij}^2}}.$$

The roughness of the noise is defined as the standard deviation of the derivative of the noise divided by the standard deviation of the noise itself. Let

$$\Delta u = \sqrt{\sum_{i=1}^n (u_{i1} - u_{i2})^2}.$$

Then an unbiased estimator of the roughness is given by

$$\lambda = \frac{\Delta u}{\Delta x}.$$

Then the eFWHM along the edge is given by

$$e\text{FWHM} = \frac{\sqrt{4ln2}}{\lambda}.$$

6.5 Gaussianness of Random Fields

Smoothing not only increases the smoothness of underlying random fields, but it also increases the normality of data. Here we explain how to check the normality of imaging data. Checking the normality of imaging data is fairly important when the underlying statistical model assumes the normality of data. But how do we know the data will follow normality? This is easily checked using the *quantile-quantile (QQ) plot* first introduced by Wilk and Gnanadesikan (Wilk and Gnanadesikan, 1968). The QQ-plot displays quantiles from an empirical distribution on the vertical axis versus theoretical quantiles from a Gaussian distribution on the horizontal axis. It is used to check graphically if the empirical distribution follows the theoretical Gaussian distribution. If the data comes from a Gaussian field, then the QQ-plot should be close to a straight line.

6.5.1 *Quantiles*

The quantile point q for random variable X is a point that satisfies

$$P(X \leq q) = F_X(q) = p,$$

where F_X is the cumulative distribution function (CDF) of X. Assuming we can find the inverse of CDF, the quantile is given by

$$q = F_X^{-1}(p).$$

This function is mainly referred to as a quantile function. The quantile-quantile (QQ) plot of two random variables X and Y is then defined to be a parametric curve $\mathcal{C}(p)$ parameterized by $p \in [0, 1]$:

$$\mathcal{C}(p) = \left(F_X^{-1}(p), F_Y^{-1}(p) \right).$$

6.5.2 *Empirical Distribution*

The CDF $F_X(q)$ measures the proportion of random variable X less than given value q. So by counting the number of measurements less than q, we can empirically estimate the CDF. Let $X_1, \cdots, X_n$ be a random sample of size n. Then order them in increasing order

$$\min(X_1, \cdots, X_n) \le X_{(2)} \le \cdots \le X_{(n)} = X_{(1)} = \max(X_1, \cdots, X_n).$$

Suppose $X_{(j)} \le q < X_{(j+1)}$. This implies that there are j samples that are smaller than q. So we approximate the CDF as

$$\widehat{F_X}(q) = \frac{j}{n}.$$

The j/n-th *sample quantile* is $X_{(j)}$. Some authors define this as the $(j - 0.5)/n$-th sample quantile. The factor 0.5 is introduced to account for the descritization error.

In computer implementation, it is easier to implement the empirical distribution using the *step function* $\mathcal{I}_q(x)$ which is implemented as $\mathcal{I}_q(x) = 1$ if $x \le q$ and $\mathcal{I}_q(x) = 0$ if $x > q$. Then the CDF is estimated as

$$\widehat{F_X}(q) = \frac{1}{n} \sum_{i=1}^{n} \mathcal{I}_q(X_i),$$

where $\mathcal{I}_q(X_i)$ counts if X_i is less than q. A different possibly more sophisticated estimation can be found in Frigge *et al.* (1989).

6.5.3 *Quantile Quantile Plots*

The QQ-plot for two normal distributions is called the *normal probability plot* and it is a straight line. Suppose

$$X \sim N(\mu_1, \sigma_1^2) \text{ and } Y \sim N(\mu_2, \sigma_2^2).$$

Let $Z \sim N(0, 1)$ and $\Phi(z) = P(Z \le z)$, the CDF of the standard normal distribution. If we denote q_1 and q_2 to be the p-th quantiles for X and Y respectively, we have

$$p = P(X \le q_1) = P\left(\frac{X - \mu_1}{\sigma_1} \le \frac{q_1 - \mu_1}{\sigma_1}\right) = \Phi\left(\frac{q - \mu_1}{\sigma_1}\right).$$

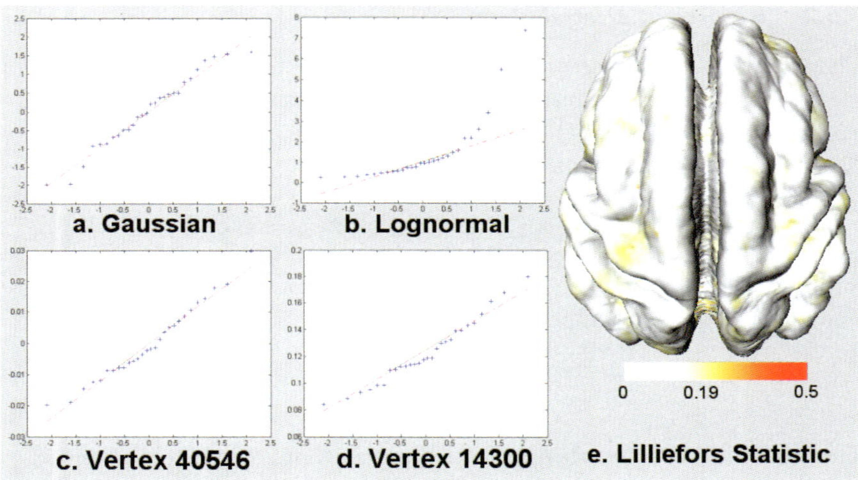

Fig. 6.12   QQ-plots of a Gaussian (a) and lognormal (b) distributions from simulation. (c), (d) QQ-plots of two vertices on the cortical surface. (e) Lilliefors statistic measures the maximum difference between the empirical and a theoretical Gaussian distributions. Most of cortex shows value less than the cutoff value 0.19 indicating that the Gaussian random field assumption is valid. See Chung *et al.* (2003c) for details.

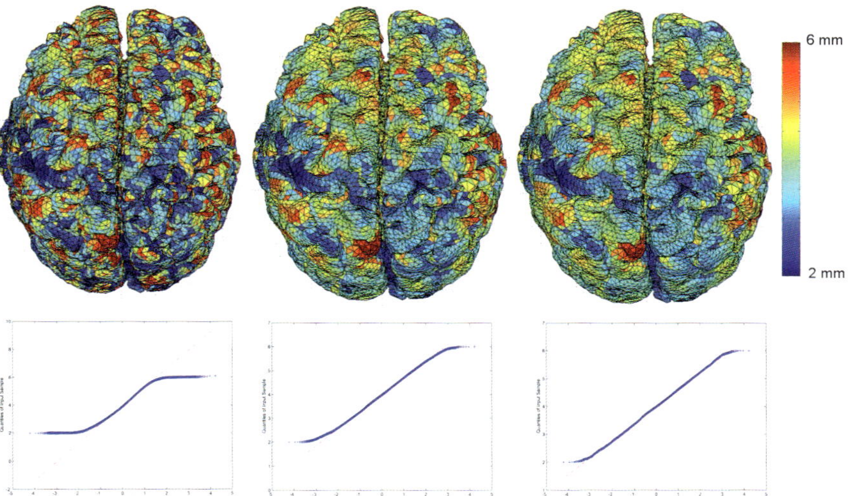

Fig. 6.13   Iterated heat kernel smoothing applied to cortical thickness with 0, 50 and 100 iterations with the bandwidth $\sigma = 1$. As the amount of smoothing increases, Gaussianness increases as shown in the normal probability plots.

Hence the parameterized QQ-plot is given by

$$q_1(p) = \mu_1 + \sigma_1 \Phi^{-1}(p),$$
$$q_2(p) = \mu_2 + \sigma_2 \Phi^{-1}(p).$$

The QQ-plot without the parameter p is given by

$$\frac{q_1 - \mu_1}{\sigma_1} = \frac{q_2 - \mu_2}{\sigma_2},$$

the equation for a line. This shows the QQ-plot of two normal distributions is a straight line. This idea can be used to determine the normality of a given sample. We can check how closely the sample quantiles corresponds to the normal distribution by plotting the QQ-plot of the sample quantiles vs. the corresponding quantiles of a normal distribution. In normal probability plot, we plot the QQ-plot of the sample against the standard normal distribution $N(0,1)$. Figure 6.12 demonstrates the normality of cortical thickness measures (Chung *et al.*, 2003c).

6.5.4 *Checking Gaussianness in Cortical Thickness*

In the usual random field theory, all cortical surface measures Λ such as surface area, cortical thickness, curvature dilatation rates are modeled as Gaussian random fields on the cortical surface, i.e.

$$\Lambda(\mathbf{x}) = \lambda(\mathbf{x}) + \epsilon(\mathbf{x}), \mathbf{x} \in \mathcal{M}, \tag{6.42}$$

where the deterministic part λ is the mean of the metric Λ and ϵ is a mean zero Gaussian random field. This theoretical model assumption can be checked using both Lilliefors test and quantile-quantile plots (qqplots) (Chung *et al.*, 2003c; Conover, 1980). If the data comes from a normal distribution, QQ-plot should shows a straight line (Figure 6.12 a). If the data comes from a lognormal distribution, it may not form a straight line (Figure 6.12 b). Because it is not possible to view QQ-plots for every vertices on the cortex, we measured the correlation coefficients γ of the vertical and horizontal coordinates in the QQ-plots. If the empirical distribution comes from Gaussian, γ should asymptotically converge to 1. For Gaussian simulation, $\gamma = 0.98 \pm 0.01$ and for lognormal simulation $\gamma = 0.84 \pm 0.08$ on the cortex. For the cortical thickness data, which has been filtered with the diffusion smoothing, $\gamma = 0.96 \pm 0.03$. So it does seems that the smoothed cortical thickness metric can be modeled as a Gaussian random field. Using Lilliefors statistic, we can statistically tested the Gaussian assumption as well. The Lilliefors test, which is a special case of the Komogorov-Smirnov test, looks at the maximum difference between the empirical and a theoretical Gaussian distribution when the mean and the variance of the distribution are not known. Since the Lilliefors statistics of the cortical thickness metric are mostly smaller than the cutoff value of 0.19 at 1% level (0.16 at 5% level), there is no reason to reject model (6.42). (Figure 6.12 e).

Figure 6.13 shows how the iterated kernel smoothing will increase Gaussianness as the amount of smoothing increases (Chung *et al.*, 2005a).

Chapter 7

Surface-Based Morphometry

The human cerebral cortex has the topology of a 2D highly convoluted gray matter shell of average thickness of 3mm. The interface between the gray matter and the cerebrospinal fluid (CSF) is the *outer cortical surface* while the interface between the gray and white matters is the *inner cortical surface* (Figures 7.1 and 7.2). The whole gray matter shell is folded outwardly to form *gyri* and inwardly to form *sulci*. The thickness of the gray matter shell is usually referred as the *cortical thickness*. Surface metrics out of these structures were found to be important biomarkers for the progression of various diseases. For cortical and subcortical structures, surface-based morphometric techniques that utilize the distance between surfaces, curvature of surfaces have been extensively used for surface-specific shape characterization.

In the surface-based morphometric framework, MRI intensity nonuniformity is usually corrected using the nonparametric nonuniform intensity normalization method (Sled *et al.*, 1988) and then the images are spatially normalized into the Montreal neurological institute (MNI) stereotaxic space using a global affine transformation (Collins *et al.*, 1994). Afterwards, an automatic tissue-segmentation algorithm based on a supervised artificial neural network classifier is used to classify each voxel as cerebrospinal fluid (CSF), gray matter, or white matter (Kollakian, 1996). Subsequently various ious surface segmentation and extraction algorithms are used to generate the outer and the inner cortical meshes. The standard method for triangulating the surface is the marching cubes algorithm (Lorensen and Cline, 1987). Alternative methods such as the level set method (Sethian, 2002) or deformable surfaces method (Davatzikos and Bryan, 1995; MacDonald *et al.*, 2000) are available but most methods for extracting cortical surfaces follows this framework.

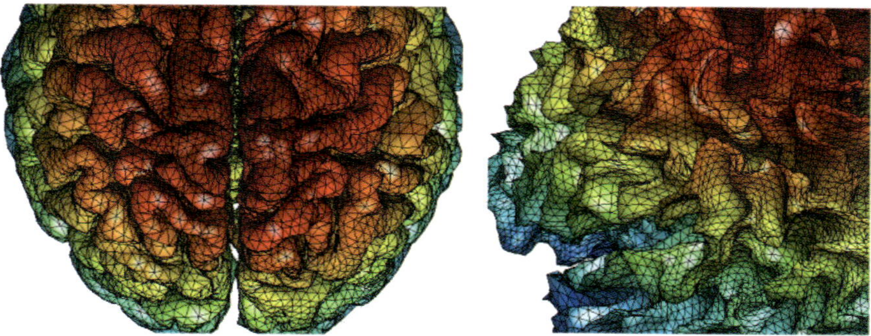

Fig. 7.1   The outer (left) and inner (middle) cortical meshes obtained from a deformable surface algorithm. The outer surface is more smooth compared to the inner surface.

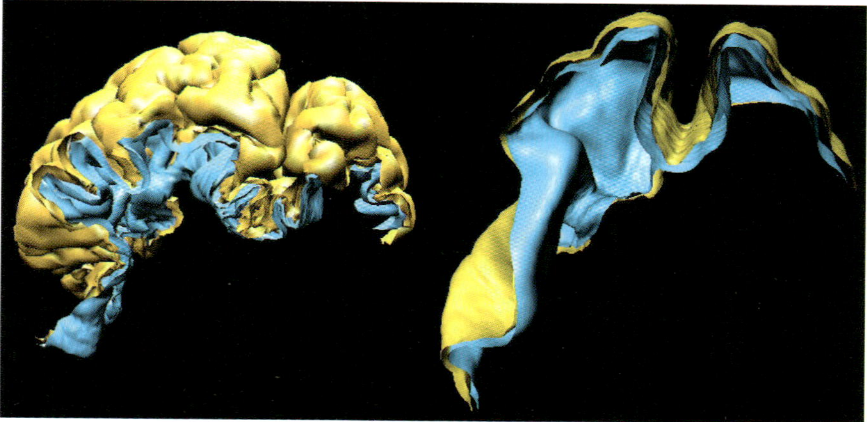

Fig. 7.2   Part of the cortex showing the outer (yellow) and inner (blue) surfaces that bound gray matter. The distance between the two surfaces is cortical thickness.

The main difficulty of obtaining cortical surfaces is the *partial volume effect* which is caused by a voxel having more than one tissue type. Due to the severe partial volume effect in sulcal regions, the outer cortical surface is mainly deformed from the inner cortical surface, which is easier to obtain. The deformable surface modeling has been probably the most widely used framework for extracting cortical surfaces. In particular, in the anatomic segmentation using proximities (ASP) method (MacDonald *et al.*, 2000), a variant of deformable surface algorithms, represent a hemisphere or the whole brain surface as 81,920 triangles. At this surface sampling rate, the average intervertex distance is about 3mm for whole brain (Figure 7.1). Constrained Laplacian-based Anatomic Segmentation with Proximities (CLASP) algorithm, which improves ASP, takes the advantage of partial volume information to improve the tissue segmentation and surface extraction (Kim *et al.*, 2005). The algorithms usually start with a spherical mesh to fit the interface between white matter and gray matter. Since image contrast is fairly high between white and gray matters, it is easier to extract the inner surface compared to the outer surface. The obtained inner surface is then expanded outward to the gray matter and CSF interface to obtain the outer surface.

7.1 Surface Flattening

Parameterizing cortical and subcortical surfaces to a simpler algebraic surface such as a sphere and plane is necessary to establish a standard coordinate system. One of the simplest way to parameterize cortical and subcortical surfaces smoothly is to find a smooth map from anatomical surfaces to a sphere. Deformable surface models usually provides a one-to-one mapping from the cortical surface to a sphere since the algorithm initially starts with a spherical mesh and deform it to match the tissue boundaries (MacDonald *et al.*, 2000). For example, ASP algorithm starts with the second level of triangular subdivision of icosahedron as the initial surface (Figure 7.3). After several iterations of deformation and triangular subdivision, the resulting cortical surface contains 40962 vertices and 81920 faces. In general, it is necessary to develop a surface flattening technique for an arbitrary given mesh. There are many surface flattening techniques such as conformal mappings (Angenent *et al.*, 1999; Gu *et al.*, 2004; Hurdal and Stephenson, 2004) quasi-isometric mappings (Timsari and Leahy, 2000) and area preserving mappings (Brechbuhler *et al.*, 1995), Laplace equation method (Chung *et al.*, 2008c).

Here we present a new and very fast surface flattening technique based on the propagation of heat diffusion using the Laplace equation (Chung *et al.*, 2008c). By tracing the integral curve of heat gradient from a heat source (anatomical surface) to a heat sink (sphere), we can obtain the flattening map. Since solving an isotropic heat equation in a 3D image volume is fairly straightforward, our proposed method offers a much simpler numerical implementation than previously available surface flattening methods.

The established spherical mapping can be used to parameterize an anatomical surface using two angles associated with the unit sphere. The

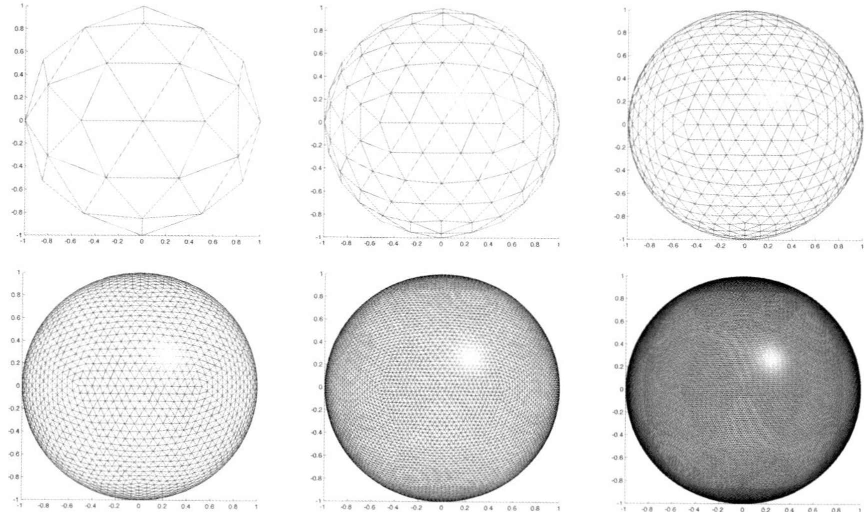

Fig. 7.3   Icosahedron (top left) has 20 triangles, 30 edges and 12 vertices. The trianglur subdivision of the icosahedron increases the number of triangles by a factor of 4. At each subdivision, the vertices are projected onto the sphere. At the subsequent level of refinement, we have (42, 80), (162, 320), (642, 1280), (2562, 5120), (10242, 20480), (40962, 81920) vertices and faces.

angles serve as coordinates for representing anatomical surfaces further possibly using, for instance, spherical harmonics. The streamlined tools containing the spherical harmonic representation and the flattening algorithm can be found in `http://www.stat.wisc.edu/~mchung/research/` `amygdala`. It should be pointed out that our representation and paramterization techniques are general enough to be applied to various brain structures such as hippocampus, caudate and cortical surfaces that are topologically equivalent to a sphere.

Once the binary segmentation $\mathcal{M}_a$ of an object is obtained either manually or automatically, the marching cubes algorithm (Lorensen and Cline, 1987) can beapplied to obtain a triangle surface mesh $\partial \mathcal{M}_a$. We start with putting a larger sphere $\mathcal{M}_s$ that encloses the binary object $\mathcal{M}_a$. The center of the sphere $\mathcal{M}_s$ is taken as the average of the mesh coordinates of $\partial \mathcal{M}_a$, which forms the surface mass center. The radius of the sphere $\mathcal{M}_s$ is taken in such a way that the shortest distance between the sphere to the binary object $\mathcal{M}_a$ is some specific distance. We found 5mm is sufficient for amygdale for instance. The final flattening map is definitely affected by the

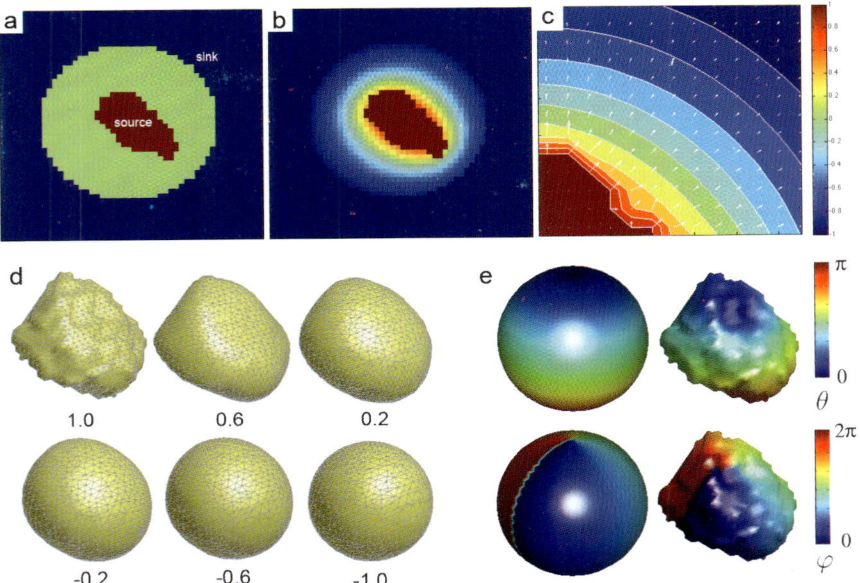

Fig. 7.4   (a) The heat source (amygdala) is assigned value 1 while the heat sink (outer sphere) is assigned the value -1. The diffusion equation is solved with these boundary condition. (b) After a sufficient number of iterations, the equilibrium state $f(x, \infty)$ is reached. (c) The gradient field $\nabla f(x, \infty)$ shows the direction of heat propagation from the source to the sink. The integral curve of the gradient field is computed by connecting one level set to the next level set of $f(x, \infty)$. (d) Amygala surface flattening is done by tracing the integral curve at each mesh vertex. The numbers $c = 1.0, 0.6, \cdots, -1.0$ correspond to the level sets $f(x, \infty) = c$. (e) The surface flattening to a sphere produces surface parameterization based on the spherical angles (θ, φ). The point $\theta = 0$ corresponds to the north pole of a unit sphere.

perturbation of the position of the sphere but since we are fixing it to be the mass center of surface for all amygdale, we do not need to worry about the perturbation effect.

The binary object $\mathcal{M}_a$ is assigned the value 1 while the enclosing sphere is assigned the value -1, i.e.

$$f(\mathcal{M}_a, \sigma) = 1 \text{ and } f(\mathcal{M}_s, \sigma) = -1 \tag{7.1}$$

for all $\sigma \in [0, \infty)$ (Figure 7.4). The parameter σ is the diffusion time. $\mathcal{M}_a$ and $\mathcal{M}_s$ serve as a heat source and a heat sink respectively. Then we solve isotropic diffusion

$$\frac{\partial f}{\partial \sigma} = \Delta f \tag{7.2}$$

with the given boundary condition (7.1). Δ is the 3D Laplacian. As $\sigma \to \infty$, the solution reaches the heat equilibrium state where the additional diffusion does not make any change in heat distribution. The heat equilibrium state is also obtained by letting $\frac{\partial f}{\partial \sigma} = 0$ and solving for the Laplace equation

$$\Delta f = 0 \tag{7.3}$$

with the same boundary condition. This will results in the equilibrium state denoted by $f(x, \sigma = \infty)$. Once we obtained the equilibrium state, we trace the path from the heat source to the heat sink for every mesh vertices on the isosurface of $\mathcal{M}_a$ using the gradient of the heat equilibrium $\nabla f(x, \infty)$.

A similar formulation has been used in estimating cortical thickness bounded by outer and inner cortical surfaces by establishing correspondence between two surfaces by tracing the gradient of the equilibrium state (Yezzi and Prince, 2001; Jones *et al.*, 2006; Lerch and Evans, 2005).

Iterative update scheme is needed to solve (7.3). Each iteration increases the numerical accuracy to the solution. Instead of solving (7.3) directly, we can solve (7.2) for sufficiently large σ. For the sufficiently large σ, we expect the heat diffusion to be close to the equilibrium state within some error bound. To solve (7.2), we can use iterative heat kernel smoothing (Chung *et al.*, 2005a).

The heat gradients form vector fields originating at the heat source and ending at the heat sink (Figure 7.4). The integral curve of the gradient field at a mesh vertex $p \in \partial \mathcal{M}_a$ establishes a smooth mapping from the mesh vertex to the sphere. The integral curve τ is obtained by solving a system of differential equations

$$\frac{d\tau}{dt}(t) = \nabla f(\tau(t), \infty)$$

with $\tau(t = 0) = p$. The integral curve approach is a widely used formulation in tracking white matter fibers using diffusion tensors (Basser *et al.*, 2000; Lazar *et al.*, 2003). These methods rely on discretizing the differential equations using the Runge-Kutta method; however, the such computation intensive approach is not needed here. Instead of directly computing the gradient field $\nabla f(x, \infty)$, we computed the level sets $f(x, \infty) = c$ of the equilibrium state corresponding to for varying c between -1 and 1. The integral curve is then obtained by finding the shortest path from one level set to the next level set and connecting them together in a piecewise fashion. This is done in an iterative fashion as shown in Figure 7.4, where five level sets corresponding to the values $c = 0.6, 0.2, -0.2, -0.6, -1.0$ are used to flatten the amygdala surface. Once we obtained the spherical mapping, we can then project the angles (θ, φ) onto $\partial \mathcal{M}_a$ and the two angles serve as the underlying parameterization.

For the proposed flattening method to work, the binary object has to be close to star-shape or convex. For shapes with a more complex structure, the gradient lines that correspond to neighboring nodes on the surface will fall within one voxel in the volume, creating singularities in mapping to the sphere. Other more complex mapping methods such as conformal mapping use the complexity to avoid this problem but more numerically demanding (Angenent *et al.*, 1999; Gu *et al.*, 2004; Hurdal and Stephenson, 2004). On the other hands, our approach is simpler and more computationally efficient because it works for a limited class of shapes.

7.2 Cortical Thickness

Once we obtain the both outer and inner cortical surfaces of a subject, *cortical thickness*, which is the distance between the outer and inner surfaces, is computed at each vertex of the outer surface (MacDonald *et al.*, 2000) (Figure 7.2). Since different clinical populations are expected to show different patterns of cortical thickness variations, cortical thickness has been used as a quantitative index for characterizing a clinical population (Chung *et al.*, 2005a). Cortical thickness varies locally by region and is likely to be influenced by aging, development and disease (Barta *et al.*, 2005). By analyzing how cortical thickness differs locally in a clinical population with respect to a normal population, neuroscientists can locate the regions of abnormal anatomical differences in the clinical population.

There are many techniques for obtaining the cortical thickness. The minimum Euclidean distance method (Fischl and Dale, 2000), Laplace equation method (Jones *et al.*, 2000), Bayesian construction (Miller *et al.*, 2000) and the automatic linkage method (MacDonald *et al.*, 2000; Kabani *et al.*, 2000) are available.

7.2.1 *Cortical Thickness via Laplace Equation*

The popular method of Jones *et al.* (2000) computes thickness directly from the volumetric data by assuming the gray matter to be inside of two conducting boundaries. The distribution of fictional charges within the two boundaries sets up a scalar potential field Ψ, which satisfies the Poisson equation

$$\Delta \Psi = \frac{\partial^2 \Psi}{\partial x^2} + \frac{\partial^2 \Psi}{\partial y^2} + \frac{\partial^2 \Psi}{\partial z^2} = \frac{\rho}{\epsilon_0},$$

where ρ is the total charge within the boundaries. If we set up the two boundaries at different potential, say at Ψ_0 and Ψ_1, without any enclosing charge, we have the Laplace equation

$$\Delta \Psi = 0.$$

By solving the Laplace equation with the two boundary condition, we obtain the potential field Ψ. Then the electric field perpendicular to the isopotential surfaces is given by $-\nabla \Psi$. The Laplace equation is mainly solved using the finite difference scheme. The electric field lines radiate from one conducting surface to the other without crossing each other. By tracing the electric field line, we computes cortical thickness. The underlying framework is identical to the Laplace equation based surface flattening given in Section 7.1.

Without using the finite difference scheme, we can use an analytic approach for solving the Laplace equation in an arbitrary manifold $\mathcal{M}$, where the manifolds can be a 2D patch of cortical surfaces or 3D gray matter regions. The proposed method is essentially Galerkin's method (Kirby, 2000). Galerkin's method usually discretize partial differential equations and integral equations as a collection of linear equations involving basis functions. The linear equations are then usually solved in the least squares fashion. The iterative residual fitting (IRF) algorithm (Chung *et al.*, 2007) can be considered as a special case of Glerkin's method.

We will use the eigenfunctions ψ_j of the Laplace-Beltrami operator defined in $\mathcal{M}$ as a basis: We need to solve the eigenfunction equation

$$\Delta \psi_j = \lambda_j \psi_j, \tag{7.4}$$

to obtain the basis. For 3D image, assuming image dimension to be $L1 \times L2 \times L3$, with the indexing for eigenfunctions $l = (l_1, l_2, l_3)$, the eigenfunctions are

$$\psi_l(p) = \left(\frac{\sqrt{2}}{L_1} \sin \frac{\pi l_1 p_1}{L_1} \right) \left(\frac{\sqrt{2}}{L_2} \sin \frac{\pi l_2 p_2}{L_2} \right) \left(\frac{\sqrt{2}}{L_3} \sin \frac{\pi l_3 p_2}{L_3} \right)$$

and the eigenvalues are

$$\lambda_l = \left(\frac{l_1 \pi}{L_1} \right)^2 + \left(\frac{l_2 \pi}{L_2} \right)^2 + \left(\frac{l_3 \pi}{L_3} \right)^2.$$

The analytic solution of the Laplace equation is approximated as a finite expansion

$$f(p) = \sum_{j=0}^{k} c_j \psi_j(p).$$

Whenever we have a partial differential equation involving Laplacian, the use of the natural basis simplifies the discretization process substantially. Consider following boundary conditions

$$f(p) = 1,\ p \in \mathcal{M}_1,\ \text{and}\ f(p) = -1,\ p \in \mathcal{M}_{-1}, \tag{7.5}$$

where $\mathcal{M}_1$ and $\mathcal{M}_{-1}$ are subsets of $\mathcal{M}$. We may view $\mathcal{M}_1$ as the inner cortical surface and $\mathcal{M}_2$ as the outer cortical surface. The boundary conditions satisfy

$$1 = \sum_{j=0}^{k} c_j \psi_j(p_{2i}),\ p_{2i} \in \mathcal{M}_1 \tag{7.6}$$

and

$$-1 = \sum_{j=0}^{k} c_j \psi_j(p_{3i}),\ p_{3i} \in \mathcal{M}_{-1}. \tag{7.7}$$

In the interior regions $\mathcal{M} \backslash (\mathcal{M}_1 \cup \mathcal{M}_{-1})$, by taking the Laplacian on the both sides of (9.10), we have

$$0 = \sum_{j=0}^{k} c_j \lambda_j \psi_j(p_{1i}). \tag{7.8}$$

It is usually the case that the number of voxels or vertices in $\mathcal{M}_1$ and $\mathcal{M}_{-1}$ are substantially smaller than $\mathcal{M}$. So possibly we need to subsample the the interior region. We assume that there are a, b and c number of sampling voxels for equations (7.8), (7.6) and (7.7) respectively. We now combine linear equations (7.8), (7.6) and (7.7) together in a matrix form:

$$
\underbrace{\begin{pmatrix} 0 \\ \vdots \\ 0 \\ 1 \\ \vdots \\ 1 \\ -1 \\ \vdots \\ -1 \end{pmatrix}}_{\mathbf{y}} = \underbrace{\begin{pmatrix} \lambda_1\psi_1(p_{11}) & \cdots & \lambda_k\psi_k(p_{11}) \\ \vdots & \ddots & \vdots \\ \lambda_1\psi_1(p_{1a}) & \cdots & \lambda_k(p_{1a}) \\ \psi_1(p_{21}) & \cdots & \psi_k(p_{21}) \\ \vdots & \ddots & \vdots \\ \psi_1(p_{2b}) & \cdots & \psi_k(p_{2b}) \\ \psi_1(p_{31}) & \cdots & \psi_k(p_{31}) \\ \vdots & \ddots & \vdots \\ \psi_1(p_{3c}) & \cdots & \psi_k(p_{3c}) \end{pmatrix}}_{\mathbf{\Psi}} \underbrace{\begin{pmatrix} c_1 \\ c_2 \\ \vdots \\ c_{k-1} \\ c_k \end{pmatrix}}_{\mathbf{C}}. \tag{7.9}
$$

The above matrix equation can be solved by the least squares method:

$$\widehat{\mathbf{C}} = (\mathbf{\Psi'\Psi})^{-1}\mathbf{\Psi y}.$$

In order for the matrix $\mathbf{\Psi'\Psi}$ to have the inverse, the total number of sampling voxels $(a + b + c)$ should be larger than the total number of basis k, which is likely to be true for brain images so there is no need to use the pseudo-inverse here.

7.2.2 *Cortical Thickness vs. Gray Matter Density*

The cerebral cortex has a highly convoluted geometry and it is likely that the local difference in gray matter concentration can characterize a clinical population. Within the weighted Fourier representation framework that will be covered in the next chapter, gray matter density and cortical thickness can be compared. The main hypothesis of interest is if increased cortical thickness corresponds to increased gray matter locally.

Gray matter density is a 3D measure defined as the probability of a particular voxel belonging to gray matter. It has been used in various anatomical studies: normal development (Good *et al.*, 2001; Paus *et al.*, 1999), autism (Chung *et al.*, 2004), depression (Pizzagalli *et al.*, 2004), epilepsy (McMillan *et al.*, 2004) and Alzheimer's disease (Johnson *et al.*, 2004; Thompson *et al.*, 2003). There are many different techniques for obtaining the density depending on how it is defined. In VBM, it is modeled as a Gaussian mixture on tissue intensity values (Ashburner and Friston, 2000; Good *et al.*, 2001). In modulated-VBM (Good *et al.*, 2001), the density obtained from the standard VBM is rescaled by the Jacobian determinant of image registration to preserve the total amount of gray matter. This is related to the RAVENS (regional analysis of volumes examined in normalized space) approach (Davatzikos *et al.*, 2001).

Paus et al. modeled the density as a Bernoulli random variable taking value 1 inside the gray matter segmentation and 0 outside the segmented regions (Paus *et al.*, 1999). In a slightly different formulation, Thompson et al. computed the density as the fraction of gray matter within a ball of radius 15mm along a cortical surface (Thompson *et al.*, 2003). This approach is equivalent to convoluting the binary mask of the gray matter with a uniform probability distribution of radius 15mm and interpolating voxel values to the cortical surface mesh. This equivalence relation is the basis of how we project a 3D density map to a 2D cortical surface and compare them with cortical thickness.

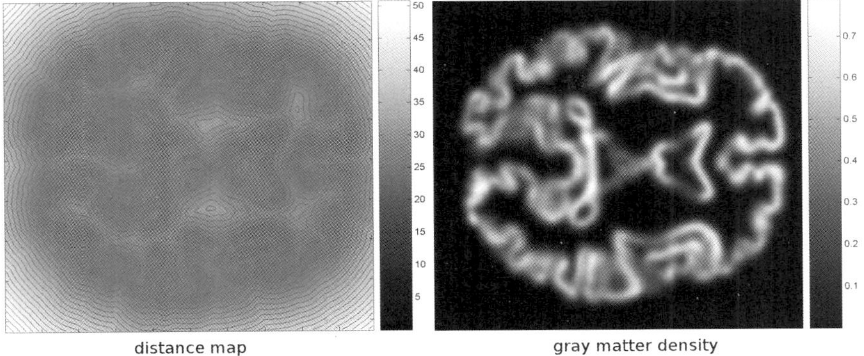

distance map   gray matter density

Fig. 7.5   Left: The average distance map of a cortical surface in mm scale. Gaussian kernel smoothing of the gray matter density map with 10mm FWHM.

7.2.3 *Distance Map*

We propose to construct the gray matter density using the 3D Euclidian distance map of the surfaces. For the outer surface $\mathcal{M}_o$, the distance map at each voxel x is defined as

$$\mathtt{dist}_o(x) = \min_{y \in \mathcal{M}_o} \|x - y\|,$$

where $\| \cdot \|$ is the Euclidian norm. The minimum is found using the nearest neighbor search algorithm on an optimized k-D tree (Friedman *et al.*, 1997). Similarly we denote the distance map for the inner surface $\mathcal{M}_i$ as $\mathtt{dist}_i(x)$. Then the average distance map is defined as

$$\mathtt{dist}(x) = \frac{\mathtt{dist}_o(x) + \mathtt{dist}_i(x)}{2}.$$

The average distance map for a subject is shown in Figure 7.5. The minimum of the average distance is always obtained in the middle of the outer and inner surfaces, where the probability of a voxel belong to the gray matter class should be the highest. Then we define the gray matter density as

$$\mathtt{density}(x) = \exp\left[-\frac{\mathtt{dist}^2(x)}{2\rho^2} \right], \tag{7.10}$$

where parameter ρ^2 controls the spread of density ($\rho^2 = 3$ in our study). The gray matter density is always between 0 and 1 and it obtains its maximum in the interior of the gray matter region, where the average distance map obtains the minimum. The density map is further convoluted with the

3D Gaussian kernel K with 10mm FWHM to increase the smoothness and normality of data (Ashburner and Friston, 2000; Chung *et al.*, 2004) (Figure 7.5). Then the smoothed density map $K * \texttt{density}(x)$ is stochastically can be modeled as a Gaussian random field (Chung *et al.*, 2007).

The previously available approaches for computing the cortical thickness in discrete triangle meshes produce noisy thickness measures (Chung *et al.*, 2005a; Fischl and Dale, 2000; MacDonald *et al.*, 2000). So it is necessary to smooth the thickness measurements along the cortex using PDE based smoothing techniques (Andrade *et al.*, 2001; Cachia *et al.*, 2003a; Chung *et al.*, 2003c). The *weighted Fourier series* (WFS) representation, which will be covered in the next chapter, provides smooth functional representations of the outer and inner surfaces as the solution of heat diffusion. The WFS avoids this additional step of thickness smoothing done in most of thickness analysis literature (Chung *et al.*, 2005a, 2003c). Therefore, WFS can be used as a basis for comparing cortical thickness to gray matter density (Chung *et al.*, 2007).

Using the WFS-correspondence, we establish the homology between the outer and the inner surfaces in the least squares fashion (Chung *et al.*, 2007). The cortical thickness is then defined to be the Euclidean distance between the WFS-correspondence:

$$\texttt{thick}(p) = \left[\sum_{l=0}^{k} \sum_{m=-l}^{l} e^{-2l(l+1)\sigma} (g_{lm} - f_{lm})^2 \right]^{1/2},$$

where g_{lm}, f_{lm} are the spherical harmonic coefficients corresponding to the outer and inner cortical surfaces at degree l and order m. A similar approach has been proposed for measuring the closeness between two surfaces (Gerig *et al.*, 2001); however, this is the first study using harmonics in defining the cortical thickness. The cortical thickness obtained from the traditional approach introduces a lot of triangle mesh noise into its estimation while the WFS-correspondance approach does not. The spatial smoothness of the thickness is controlled by the bandwidth σ.

Most morphometric studies have never compared cortical thickness and gray matter density together so it is not clear if the two anatomical indices are positively correlated (Ashburner and Friston, 2000; Bookstein, 2001; Chung *et al.*, 2005a, 2003c; Fischl and Dale, 2000; Good *et al.*, 2001). Comparing density and thickness in Figure 7.7, no statistically significant regions overlap. Since both metrics have been assumed to be the indicators of the amount of gray matter, the result is paradoxical.

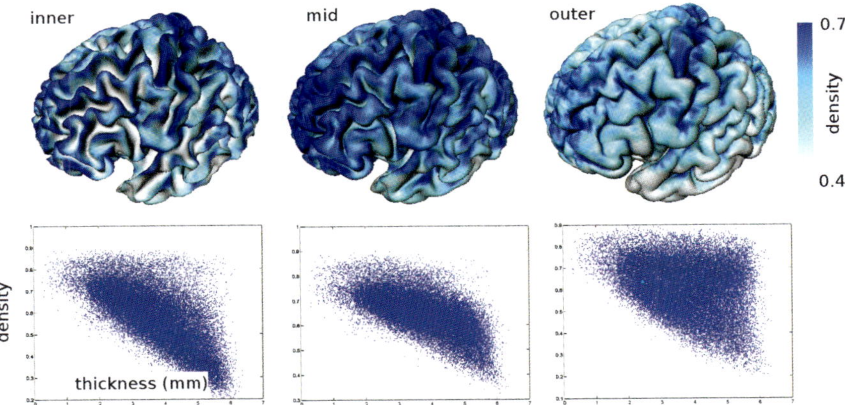

Fig. 7.6   Gray matter density projected onto inner, mid and outer surfaces for a single subject. On the inner surface, the deep sulcal regions show the low density while the gyral ridges show high density. On the outer surface, the pattern is opposite. The deep sulcal regions show high density while the gyral ridges show lower density. The middle surface shows high density. Bottom: Scatter plot of gray matter density over thickness. They show negative correlations.

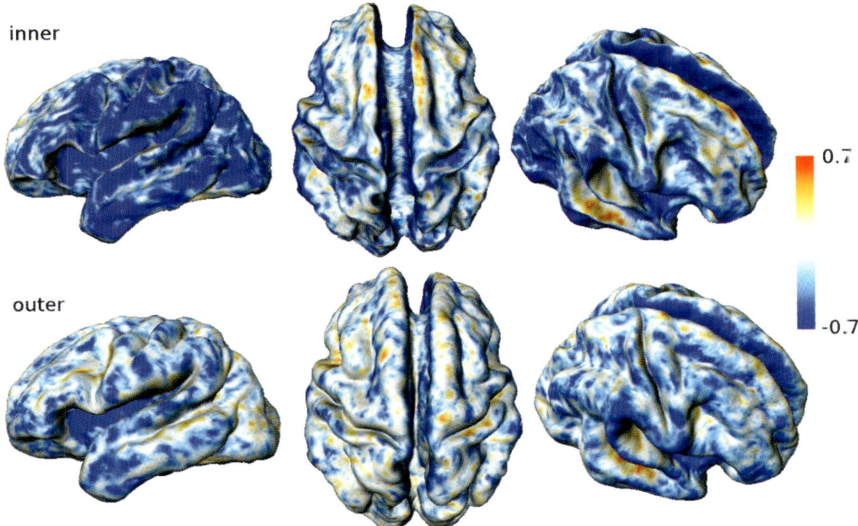

Fig. 7.7   Correlation of thickness and gray matter density for 24 subjects mapped on both the inner and the outer surfaces. Most of both inner and outer surfaces show negative correlation. Thicker cortical regions are less convoluted so the gray matter density tend do be lower.

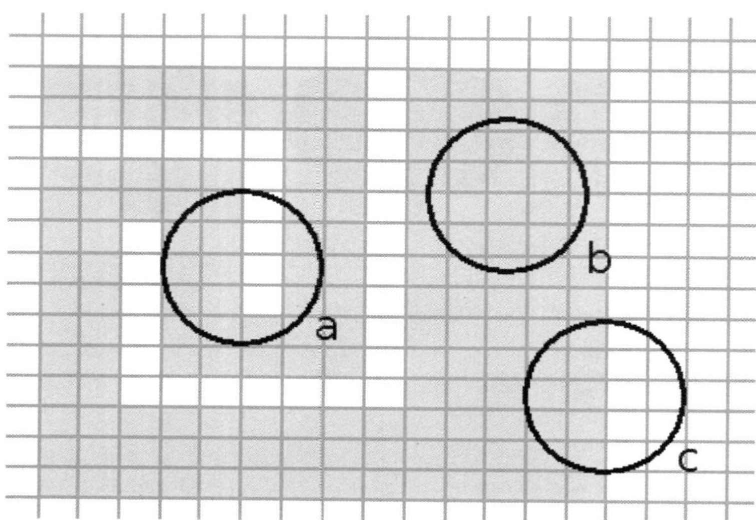

Fig. 7.8 Simple 2D schematic showing the negative correlation between thickness and gray matter density. Gray colored pixels are gray matter. The black circle is the contour of heat kernel. There are more gray matter pixels in region (a) than region (c) although the thickness in region (c) is thicker than that of region (a). The gray matter density in the middle of the gray matter (b) is 1 for almost all subject indicating very small between-subject and between-group variability. Because of the small between-group variability, VBM does not usually detect signal in the middle of the gray matter. Most of significant signal detected in VBM is near the tissue boundary where the between-group variability is high.

We have correlated these two metrics within a subject (Figure 7.6) and across subjects (Figure 7.7). Surprisingly the scatter plot in Figure 7.6 shows negative correlation. By assigning the density value of a voxel that contains a vertex of a cortical mesh to the vertex, we can project the gray matter density onto inner, middle and outer surfaces. The middle surface is obtained by averaging the inner and the outer surfaces in the WFS-correspondance. Figure 7.7 shows negatively correlated scatter plots. Figure 7.7 shows the complex pattern of nonuniformity of density. On the outer surface, deep sulci have higher density compared to gyri while on the inner surface, the pattern is opposite. The middle surface shows higher density compared to the outer and the inner surfaces as expected. These complex patterns of the nonuniformity of density is due to the folding pattern of the cortex. Since the sulci on the outer surface and the gyri on the inner surface are highly folded, these regions should have more gray matter within the sphere of fixed radius as illustrated in Figure 7.8. On the other hand, thin cortical regions will fold more than thick cortical regions. This inverse geometric relation is causing the negative correlation between density and thickness.

7.3 Partial Correlation Mapping

In this section, we present a partial correlation mapping technique for correlating behavioral measures to cortical thickness and detecting the regions of abnormal brain-behavior correlates. We correlate a facial emotion discrimination task score and its response time to cortical thickness measurements in a group of high functioning autistic subjects. Many previous correlation studies in brain imaging neglect to account for unwanted age effect and other variables and the subsequent statistical parametric maps may report spurious results. We demonstrate that the partial correlation mapping strategy presented here can remove the effect of age and global cortical area difference effectively while localizing the regions of high correlation difference. The advantage of the proposed correlation mapping strategy over the general linear model framework is that we can directly visualize more intuitive correlation measures across the cortex in each group.

Pearson's product-moment correlation (Fisher, 1915), in short simple correlation, has widely been used as a simple index for measuring dependency and the linear relationship between two variables. In human brain mapping research, it has been mainly used to map out functional or anatomical connectivity (Friston *et al.*, 1993b, 1996; Cao and Worsley, 1999a; Marrelec *et al.*, 2009; Worsley *et al.*, 2005b). In this framework, correlations between pairs of voxels are computed and thresholded via the random field theory to reveal the statistically significant regions of connectivity by testing the existence of correlation ρ on the template cortex $\partial \mathcal{M}$:

$$H_0 : \rho(p) = 0 \text{ for all } \text{ vs. } H_1 : \rho(p) \neq 0 \text{ for some .} \qquad (7.11)$$

In a different setting, Thompson *et al.* (2001) used the correlation between genetic factors and the amount of gray matter on the cortex via a linear model in mapping out the regions of genetic influence. Our use of correlation is somewhat similar to Thompson *et al.* (2001) in that we correlate anatomical index to non-anatomical index on the cortex. In this section, we map out the dependency of behavioral measures to an anatomical measure spatially over the cortex and localize the regions of abnormal correlation difference between groups. To remove unwanted covariates like age and total brain size difference, we use *partial correlation coefficient,* in short partial correlation. Chung *et al.* (2004) and Chung *et al.* (2005a) have already demonstrated the need for removing the effect of age and global brain size difference in morphometric analyses so it is crucial to use partial correlation rather than the usual simple correlation in our study. Although our correlation mapping strategy can be formulated in terms of a general linear model (GLM) as in the case of Thompson *et al.* (2001), our unified approach will provide a more intuitive alternative that is visually comprehensive.

As an application, we applied our method in characterizing abnormal brain-behavior correlation in autism. We correlated two behavioral measures with the anatomical measure, *cortical thickness*. The cortical thickness measures the thickness of the gray matter shell bounded by the both outer and inner cortical surfaces (MacDonald *et al.*, 2000; Chung *et al.*, 2003c, 2005a). The first behavioral measure is the emotional face recognition task score. The task score counts the number of correct responses when judging whether a subject is viewing an emotional (happy, fear and anger) or neutral face (Dalton *et al.*, 2005). The second behavioral measure is the time required to produce a response. The response time is measured in ms. Each behavioral measure was correlated with the cortical thickness measure at each point on the cortex for the both autistic and control groups, and a statistical test was performed to determine the regions of differing correlation pattern between groups.

7.3.1   *Partial Correlations*

Let $Y = (Y_1, Y_2)$ be two variables of interests and $X = (X_1, \cdots, X_p)$ be a row vector of variables that should be removed in a data analysis. For instance, we may let Y_1 be the cortical thickness, Y_2 be the response time, and X_1 and X_2 be the age and total surface area respectively. The covariance matrix of $(Y, X)'$ is denoted by

$$\mathbb{V}(Y, X)' = \begin{pmatrix} \Sigma_{YY} & \Sigma_{YX} \\ \Sigma_{XY} & \Sigma_{XX} \end{pmatrix} \tag{7.12}$$

Note Σ_{XY} is the cross-covariance matrix of X and Y. Σ_{YX} and Σ_{XX} are defined similarly. Then the partial covariance of Y given X is

$$\Sigma_{YY} - \Sigma_{YX}\Sigma_{XX}^{-1}\Sigma_{XY} = (\sigma_{ij}).$$

The *partial correlation* $\rho_{Y_i,Y_j|X}$ is the correlation between variables Y_i and Y_j while removing the effect of variables X and it is defined as

$$\rho_{Y_i,Y_j|X} = \frac{\sigma_{ij}}{\sqrt{\sigma_{ii}\sigma_{jj}}}.$$

The *conditional* notation $|$ is used in defining the partial correlation since the partial correlation is equivalent to *conditional correlation* if

$$\mathbb{E}(Y|X) = a + BX$$

for some vector a and matrix B, which is true under the normality of data. This is the formulation we used to compute the partial correlation. If vector X consists of a single measurement, i.e. $X = X_1$, the partial correlation can be computed from the simple correlation via

$$\rho_{Y_1,Y_2|X} = \frac{\rho_{Y_1,Y_2} - \rho_{Y_1,X}\rho_{Y_2,X}}{\sqrt{(1 - \rho_{Y_1,X}^2)(1 - \rho_{Y_2,X}^2)}}.$$

The *sample partial correlation* $r_{Y_1,Y_2|x}$ is defined similarly by replacing the covariance with the sample covariance in (7.12).

7.3.2 *Statistical Inference on Correlations*

Let ρ_k be the partial correlation for group k (autism $= 1$, control $= 2$ for instance).

One Sample Case. For each fixed $p \in \partial\mathcal{M}$, one may test the significance of correlation in a group:

$$H_0^A : \rho_k(p) = 0 \text{ vs. } H_1^A : \rho_k(p) \neq 0. \tag{7.13}$$

Inference type (7.13) is useful if only one sample is available or determining high correlation regions within a group. Assuming the normality of measurements X and Y, the partial correlation $r = r_{Y_i,Y_j|X}$ can be transformed to be distributed as:

$$T = \frac{r\sqrt{n - 2}}{\sqrt{1 - r^2}} \sim t_{n-2},$$

the t distribution with $n - 2$ degrees of freedom. This test statistic can be used for testing a one-sample inference type (7.13).

Two Sample Case. Suppose we are interested in testing the equality of correlations between the groups. So at each fixed point $p \in \partial \mathcal{M}$, we are interested in testing

$$H_0^B : \rho_1(p) = \rho_2(p) \text{ vs. } H_1^B : \rho_1(p) \neq \rho_2(p). \tag{7.14}$$

For two sample inference type (7.14), one approach is based on the *Fisher transform* (Fisher, 1915), which shows the asymptotic normality:

$$r_k \to \operatorname{arctanh}(r_k) = \frac{1}{2} \ln\left(\frac{1+r_k}{1-r_k}\right) \sim N\left(\frac{1}{2}\ln\left(\frac{1+\rho_k}{1-\rho_k}\right), \frac{1}{n_k-3}\right).$$

The transform can be viewed as a variance stabilizing normalization process. Based on the Fisher transform, the test statistic under H_0^B is then given by:

$$W(p) = \frac{\ln\left(\frac{1+r_1}{1-r_1} \cdot \frac{1-r_2}{1+r_2}\right)}{2\sqrt{\frac{1}{n_1-3} + \frac{1}{n_2-3}}} \sim N(0, 1). \tag{7.15}$$

We further normalized the field $W(p)$ with mean $\mu(p) = \mathbb{E}W(p)$ and variance $S^2(p) = \mathbb{E}W^2(p) - \mu^2(p)$ by

$$Z(p) = \frac{W(p) - \mu(p)}{S(p)}.$$

μ and S^2 are estimated from random permutations. We can take the field Z to be Gaussian with zero mean and unit variance. To determine the null distribution of the test statistic, we permute two samples across the groups. For n_1 subjects for group 1 and n_2 subjects for group 2, we combine them together, do a random permutation, and partition the result into two groups with the same number of subjects. For this study, we generated 2000 random permutations out of $(n_1 + n_2)!$ possible permutations. Then for each permutation, we computed the statistic and based on the empirical distribution of the statistic, we estimated μ and S^2 (Figure 7.11).

Using Z as the test statistic, we tested:

$$H_0 : \rho_1(p) = \rho_2(p) \text{ for all } p \in \partial \mathcal{M}$$

$$\text{vs.}$$

$$H_1 : \rho_1(p) \neq \rho_2(p) \text{ for some } p \in \partial \mathcal{M}.$$

This is a usual multiple comparisons problem and Worsley's random field theory can be used. The resulting p-value maps are found in Figure 7.9 and 7.10.

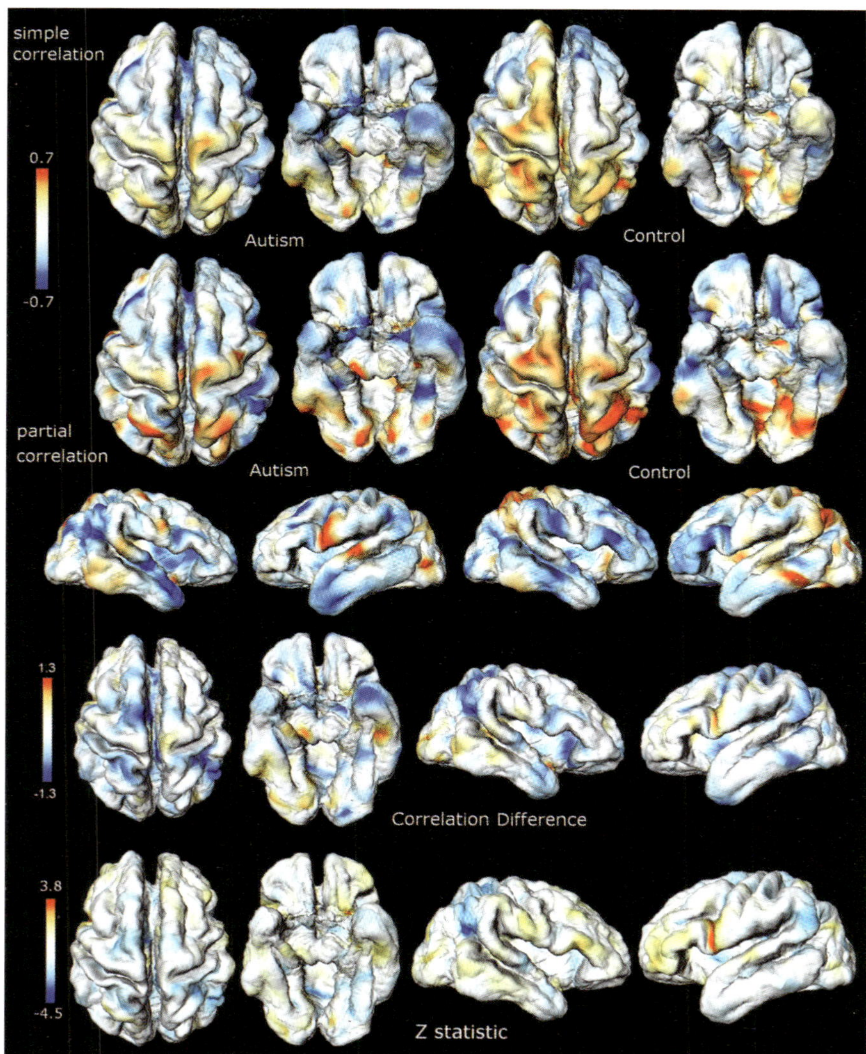

Fig. 7.9 Map of facial emotion discrimination task score correlated with thickness. The first raw is the simple correlation. The second and third rows are the partial correlation. The partial correlation tend to boost over all correlation values. The fourth row is the partial correlation difference between the two groups (autism − control). The last row shows the final Z-statistic map showing statistically significant correlation difference (P-value 0.03 for $z = 3.8$, and 0.002 for $z = -4.5$).

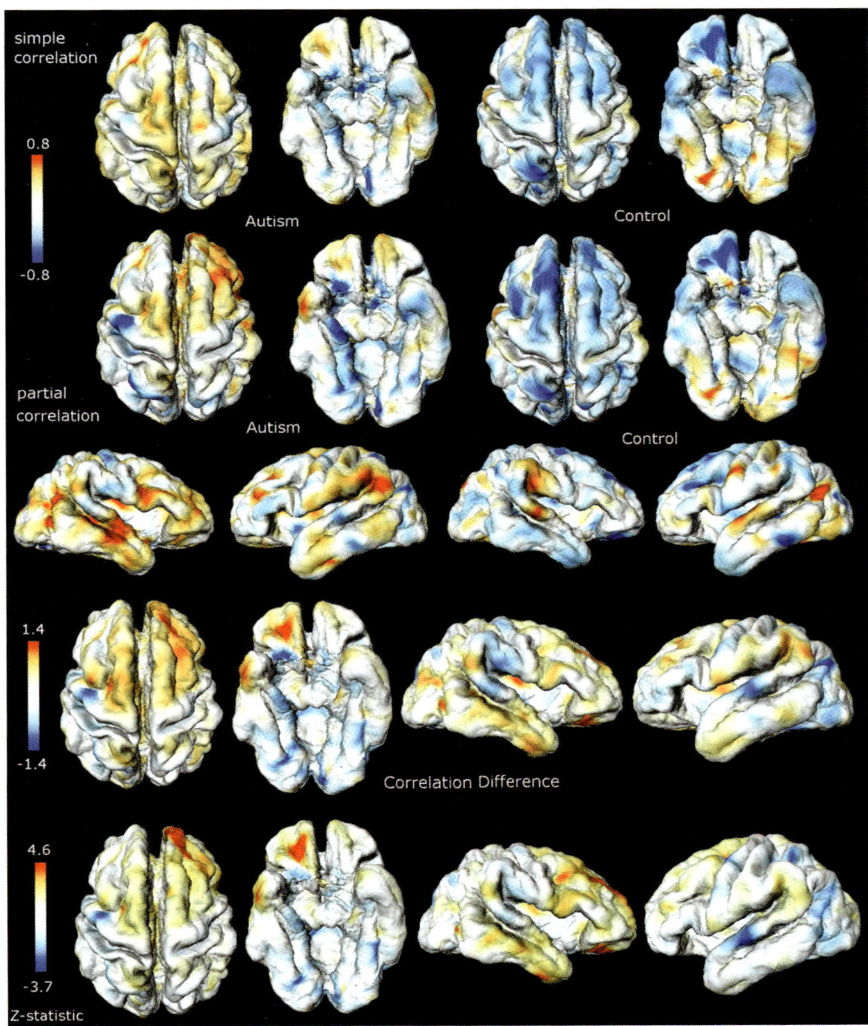

Fig. 7.10　Map of response time correlated with thickness. The first row shows the simple correlation. The second and third rows are the partial correlation removing the effect of age and cortical area differences. The fourth row shows the partial correlation difference. We are interested in testing the significance of this difference. The last row shows the final Z-statistic map showing statistically significant correlation difference (corrected P-value 0.04 for $z = -3.7$ and 0.001 for $z = 4.6$).

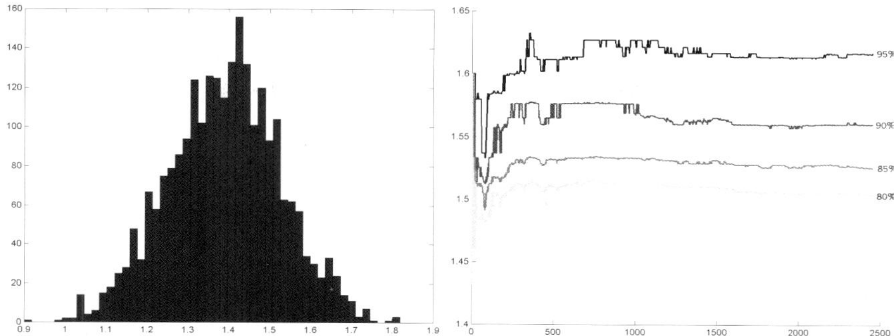

Fig. 7.11   Left: The empirical distribution of a test statistic under the null hypothesis based on 2400 permutations. Right: plots of 95%, 90%, 85% and 80% upper percentiles over the number of permutations showing the convergence after approximately 2000 permutations. Hence we used 2000 permutations for this study.

7.3.3   *Brain-Behavior Correlations*

We applied our methodology to detect the regions of abnormal brain-behavior correlates in autistic cortical regions. 14 high functioning autistic (HFA) and 12 normal control (NC) subjects used in this study were screened to be right-handed males. Age distributions for HFA and NC are 15.93 ± 4.71 and 17.08 ± 2.78 respectively. This is the same data set used in previous studies Chung *et al.* (2004, 2005a); Dalton *et al.* (2005).

High resolution anatomical magnetic resonance images (MRI) were obtained using a 3-Tesla GE SIGNA (General Electric Medical Systems, Waukesha, WI) scanner with a quadrature head RF coil. A three-dimensional, spoiled gradient-echo (SPGR) pulse sequence was used to generate T_1-weighted images. The imaging parameters were TR/TE = 21/8 ms, flip angle = $30°$, 240 mm field of view, 256x192 in-plane acquisition matrix (interpolated on the scanner to 256x256), and 128 axial slices (1.2 mm thick) covering the whole brain.

Following image processing steps described in Chung *et al.* (2005a), both the outer and inner cortical surfaces were extracted for each subject via deformable surface algorithm (MacDonald *et al.*, 2000). Surface normalization is performed by minimizing an objective function that measures the global fit of two surfaces while maximizing the smoothness of the deformation in such a way that the pattern of gyral ridges are matched smoothly (Robbins, 2003; Chung *et al.*, 2005a). To increase the signal-to-noise ratio, we applied a surface based smoothing method called heat kernel smoothing was applied for each subject (Chung *et al.*, 2003c, 2005a) with a relatively large 30mm FWHM. This is an improved formulation over the previously developed *diffusion smoothing* (Andrade *et al.*, 2001; Chung *et al.*, 2003c; Cachia *et al.*, 2003a). In Andrade *et al.* (2001) and Cachia *et al.* (2003a), smoothing is done by solving an isotropic heat equation via the combination of the least squares estimation of the Laplace-Beltrami operator and the finite difference method (FDM). In Chung *et al.* (2003c), the heat equation is solved using the finite element method (FEM) and a similar FDM. The problem with these approaches to data smoothing is the complexity of setting up the FEM and making the FDM converge. Our heat kernel smoothing avoids all these problems.

7.3.4 *Facial Emotion Discrimination Tasks*

The subjects were asked to decide whether a picture of a human face was either emotional (happiness, fear or anger) or neutral (showing no obvious emotion) by pressing one of two buttons. The faces were black and white photographs taken from the Karolinska Directed Emotional Faces set (Dalton *et al.*, 2005). The task scores (maximum 40) for HFA and NC are 27.14 ± 15.34 and 39.42 ± 0.79 respectively, and the response time (ms) for HFA and NC are 1329.8 ± 206.7 and 1110.9 ± 182.3 and respectively. A more detailed description about the task can be found in (Dalton *et al.*, 2005).

The simple correlations between cortical thickness and both task score and response time were computed for each group and mapped onto the template cortex (Figure 7.9 and 7.10, first rows). The partial correlations were also computed while removing the effect of age and global area difference. (Figure 7.9 and 7.10, second and third rows). Comparing the partial correlation maps to the simple correlation maps, we see different patterns indicating that it is necessary to account for the age and the area terms for proper correlation analysis. The partial correlation difference maps (autism − control) show the regions of maximum correlation difference (Figure 7.9 and 7.10, fourth rows). To access the statistical significance of the correlation difference, the Fisher transformation and the normalization steps were used resulting in the Z-statistic maps (Figure 7.9 and 7.10, last rows).

Group difference between the autistic and control subjects were identified using brain-behavior correlations of task score and response time. Brain-behavior partial correlations of task score and cortical thickness identified group differences in mainly two cortical regions: right angular gyrus (area 39) and the left Broca's area (area 44). The area 39 shows the positive correlation for the control subjects while it shows the negative correlation for the autistic subjects (corrected P-value 0.002, z-value -4.5). The area 44 shows the negative correlation for the control subjects while it shows the positive correlation for the autistic subjects (corrected P-value of 0.03, z-value 3.8).

For time-thickness correlation, we found more statistically significant regions of difference that are consistent with previous studies. In general, the spatial patterns of behavioral response time and thickness correlation shows more negative correlation (blue) than positive correlation (red) in the control subjects and the pattern is opposite for the autistic subjects (Figure 7.10 second row). Faster response time in the control subject are related to a thicker right ventral and dorsal prefrontal cortex while they are related to thinning in the same area in the autistic subject (corrected P-value 0.001 z-value 4.6). We found correlation difference in the left superior temporal gyrus and superior temporal sulcus (corrected P-value 0.04, z-value -3.7) (Figure 7.10 last row). The autistic subjects show an aberrant spatial pattern of behavioral-thickness correlation in the right frontopolar region (BA10), which shows a direct correlation between response time duration and cortical thickness not seen in the control subjects. We also found that slower responses in controls are related to a thinner right inferior orbital frontal cortex but slower responses in the autistic subject are independent of right orbital prefrontal cortical thickness (corrected p-value 0.001, z-value 4.6).

7.4 Tensor-Based Surface Morphometry

So far cortical thickness is mainly used for the surface-based morphometry. In this section, tensor measures such as curvatures and area elements are used for quantifying cortical shape variations. This section summarizes the method first given in Chung *et al.* (2003b).

It is likely that different clinical population will show different differential geometric surface shape variations. By computing how surface metrics such as curvature and local surface area differ among different groups, brain shape differences can be quantified locally.

In modeling the surface deformation, that is required in comparing two different brain images, a proper mathematical framework might be found in both differential geometry and fluid dynamics. The concept of the evolution of phase-boundary in fluid dynamics (Drew, 1991; Gurtin and McFadden,

1991), which describes the geometric properties of the evolution of boundary layer between two different materials due to internal growth or external force, can be used to derive the mathematical formula for how the surface deform. It is natural to assume the cortical surfaces to be a smooth 2-dimensional Riemannian manifold parameterized by two parameters (Dale and Fischl, 1999; Davatzikos and Bryan, 1995). Surface parameterization of the cortical surface has been done previously by Joshi *et al.* (1995). From the surface parameterization, Gaussian and mean curvatures of the brain surface can be computed and used to characterize its shape (Griffin, 1994). In particular, Joshi *et al.* (1995) used the quadratic surface in estimating the Gaussian and mean curvature of the cortical surfaces. Surface parameterization enables us to compute surface metrics such as local area dilatation and curvature differences that characterize the surface shapes.

7.4.1 *Surface Deformation*

Let $u^i(x) = (u_1^i, u_2^i, u_3^i)'$ be the displacement vector required to deform the structure at $x = (x_1, x_2, x_3)$ in the gray matter of the template brain $\mathcal{M}_{atlas}$ to the homologous structure in subject brain $\mathcal{M}^i$. We assume that the whole gray matter volume in $\mathcal{M}_{atlas}$ will deform continuously and smoothly to $\mathcal{M}^i$ via the deformation $x \to x + u^i$ while the cortical boundary $\partial\mathcal{M}_{atlas}$ will deform to $\partial\mathcal{M}^i$. See Figure 7.12 for an illustration. The cortical surface $\partial\mathcal{M}^i$ may be considered as consisting of two parts: the outer cortical surface $\partial\mathcal{M}^i_{out}$ between the gray matter and CSF and the inner cortical surface

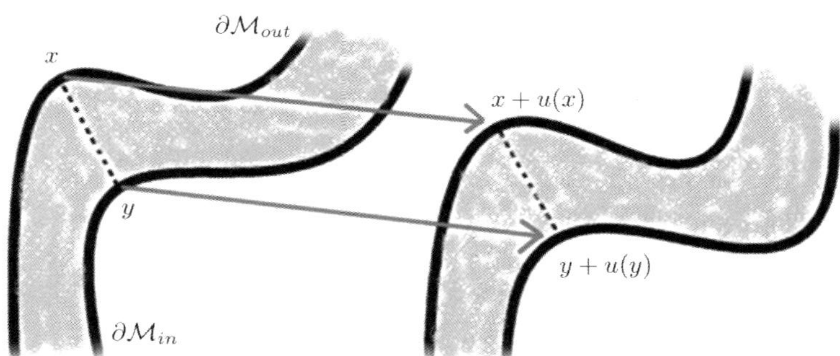

Fig. 7.12 Deformation of outer $\partial\mathcal{M}_{out}$ and inner $\partial\mathcal{M}_{out}$ cortical surfaces by the displacement u. The cortical thickness identified as $\|x - y\|$ will change to $\|x - y + u(x) - u(y)\|$. All other tensor measures will also change as a function of the displacement.

$\partial \mathcal{M}^i_{in}$ between the gray and white matter, i.e.

$$\partial \mathcal{M}^i = \partial \mathcal{M}^i_{out} \cup \partial \mathcal{M}^i_{in}.$$

Then we propose the following stochastic model on the displacement u^i:

$$u^i(x) = \mu(x) + \Sigma^{1/2}(x)\epsilon(x), \ x \in \mathcal{M}_{atlas}, \tag{7.16}$$

where μ is the mean displacement and $\Sigma^{1/2}$ is the covariance matrix, which allows for correlations between components of the displacement fields. The components of the error vector ϵ are are assumed to be independent and identically distributed as smooth stationary Gaussian random fields with zero mean and unit variance. This is the standard statistical model for displacement vector fields we have seen many occasions.

Estimating the surface displacement fields $u^{ij} : \partial \mathcal{M}^i \to \partial \mathcal{M}^j$ between two images i and j, and the surface extraction can be performed at the same time. This method works best in the case of matching two images of a single subject taken at different times. First, an ellipsoidal mesh placed outside the brain was shrunk down to the surface $\partial \mathcal{M}^i_{in}$. The vertices of the resulting inner mesh are indexed and the ASP algorithm will deform the inner mesh to fit the outer surface $\partial \mathcal{M}^i_{out}$ by minimizing a cost function that involves bending, stretch and other topological constrains (MacDonald *et al.*, 2000). The vertices indexed identically on both meshes will lie within a very close proximity and these define the automatic linkage in the ASP algorithm. To generate the outer surface $\partial \mathcal{M}^j_{out}$, we start with the inner surface $\partial \mathcal{M}^i_{in}$, and then deform it to match the outer surface $\partial \mathcal{M}^j_{out}$ by minimizing the same cost function. Starting with the same mesh in two outer surface extractions, each point on $\partial \mathcal{M}^i_{in}$ gets mapped to corresponding points on $\partial \mathcal{M}^i_{out}$ and $\partial \mathcal{M}^j_{out}$ giving us the outer surface deformation $u^{ij} : \partial \mathcal{M}^i_{out} \to \partial \mathcal{M}^j_{out}$. We do not use inner surface deformation in our study, estimating inner surface deformation can be done similarly. This method assumes that the shape of the cortical surface does not appreciably change between images i and j. This assumption is valid in the case of brain development for a short period of time, where it can be shown that the within-subject deformation field is substantially smaller than between-subject deformation.

Constructing surface template $\partial \mathcal{M}_{atlas}$, where statistical parametric maps (SPM) of surface metrics will be formed, is done by averaging the coordinates of corresponding vertices that have the same indices. This surface atlas construction method has been first introduced by MacDonald *et al.* (2000), where it is used to create the cortical thickness map for 150 normal subjects. The geometrical constraints such as stretch and bending terms in ASP algorithm enforces a relatively consistent correspondence on the cortical surface. The gyri of the subject matches the gyri of the atlas. Note the full anatomical details still presented in $\partial\mathcal{M}_{atlas}$ even after the vertex averaging. Major sulci such as the central sulcus and superior temporal sulcus are clearly identifiable. If there is no homology between corresponding vertices, one would only expect to see featureless dispersion of points.

Once we have extracted triangular surface meshes and established mapping from a vertex in $\partial\mathcal{M}^i$ to a corresponding vertex in $\partial\mathcal{M}^j$, the next step is modelling and computing the metric tensor differences between two surfaces. In order to compute metric tensors, *surface parameterization* is needed. We model the cortical surface as a smooth 2D Riemannian manifold parameterized by two parameters u^1 and u^2 such that any point $x \in \partial\mathcal{M}^i$ can be uniquely represented as $x = x(u)$ for some parameter space $\mathbf{u} = (u^1, u^2) \in D \subset \mathbb{R}^2$. A quadratic polynomial

$$z = \beta_1 u^1 + \beta_2 u^2 + \beta_3 (u^1)^2 + \beta_4 u^1 u^2 + \beta_5 (u^2)^2 \tag{7.17}$$

will be used as a local parameterization fitted via least-squares estimation on the tangent plane. Using the least-squares method, these coefficients β_i can be estimated. Slightly different quadratic surface parameterizations are used in estimating curvatures of a macaque monkey brain surface (Joshi *et al.*, 1997; Miller *et al.*, 1997). Once β_i are estimated,

$$x(u^1, u^2) = \left(u^1, u^2, z(u^1, u^2)\right)^t \tag{7.18}$$

becomes a local surface parameterizations of choice. Even thought metric tensors depend on the choice of parameterization, local surface area and curvature dilatation are independent of parameterization.

7.4.2 *Metric Tensor Computation on Surfaces*

We introduce the concepts of surface area and curvature dilatation before. These metrics can be used in quantifying surface shape differences. Suppose that $x = x(u)$ is the parameterization of surface $\partial\mathcal{M}$. Let

$$\mathbf{X}_i = \frac{\partial x}{\partial u^i}.$$

From (7.18), x_i are given in terms of coefficients β_i and the *Riemannian metric tensor* g_{ij} is given by the inner product between $\mathbf{X}_i$ and $\mathbf{X}_j$, i.e.

$$g_{ij} = \langle \mathbf{X}_i, \mathbf{X}_j \rangle.$$

The Riemannian metric tensor g_{ij} measures the amount of the deviation of the cortical surface from a flat Euclidean plane. The Riemannian metric tensor enables us to quantify lengths, angles and areas in the cortical surface. Let $g = (g_{ij})$ be a 2×2 metric tensor matrix. Then the total surface area of the cortex $\partial \mathcal{M}$ is given by

$$\|\partial \mathcal{M}\| = \int_D \sqrt{\det g}\; du,$$

where $D = X^{-1}(\partial \mathcal{M})$ is the parameter space (Kreyszig, 1959). The integrand $\sqrt{\det g}$ is called the *infinitesimal surface area element* and it measures the area of the unit square in the parameter space D, that has been transformed via $X : D \to \partial \mathcal{M}$. The infinitesimal surface area element is a generalization of Jacobian. The *local surface area dilatation* Λ_{area} from $\partial \mathcal{M}^i$ to $\partial \mathcal{M}^j$, whose metric tensor matrices are given by g_i and g_j, is then defined as

$$\Lambda_{area} = \frac{\sqrt{\det g_j} - \sqrt{\det g_i}}{\sqrt{\det g_i}}, \tag{7.19}$$

which measures percentage local area differences. The dilatation is invariant under parameterization, i.e. the area dilatation is the same no matter which parameterization is chosen.

Instead of using metric tensors g_{ij}, it is possible to formulate local surface area change in terms of the areas of the corresponding triangles. However, this formulation assign surface area change values to each face instead of each vertex and this causes problems in both surface-based smoothing and statistical analysis, where values are defined on vertices. Defining scalar values on vertices from face values can be done by the weighted average of face values, which should converge to (8.36). It is not hard to develop surface-based smoothing and statistical analysis on values defined on faces but traditionally surface metrics are computed on vertices. Our metric tensor approach will provides a basis of unifying surface metric computations, surface-based smoothing and statistical analysis together.

Curvatures of the surface can be also used to quantify the surface shape difference. The *principal curvatures* can characterize the shape and location of the sulci and gyri, which are the valleys and crests of the cortical surfaces (Joshi *et al.*, 1997; Miller *et al.*, 1997). By measuring the curvature changes, rapidly folding and cortical regions can be localized.

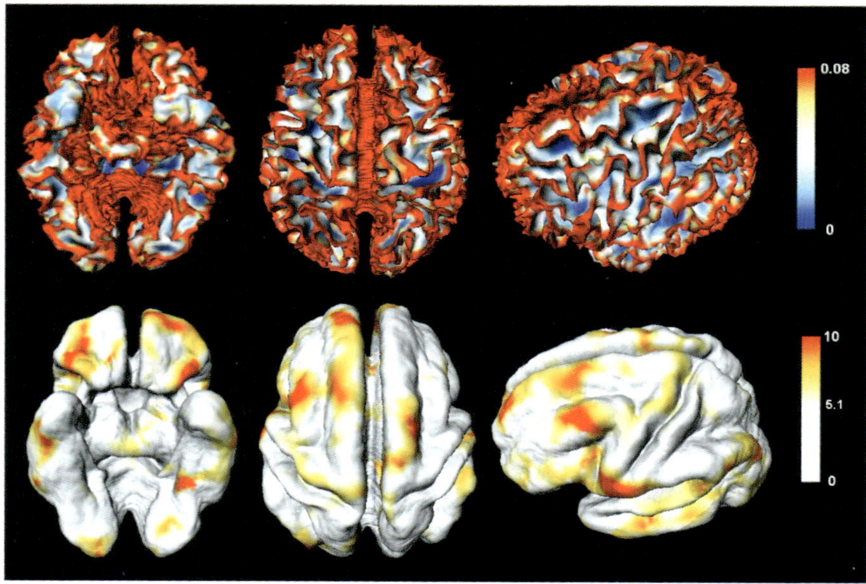

Fig. 7.13   Top: The thin-plate spline enery computed on the inner surface of a 14 year old subject. It measures the amount of folding in the cortical surface. Bottom: t statistical map showing statistically significant regions of curvature increase ($t > 5.1$) over time between ages 12 and 16. Most of curvature increase occurs on gyri while there is no significant change of curvature on most of sulci.

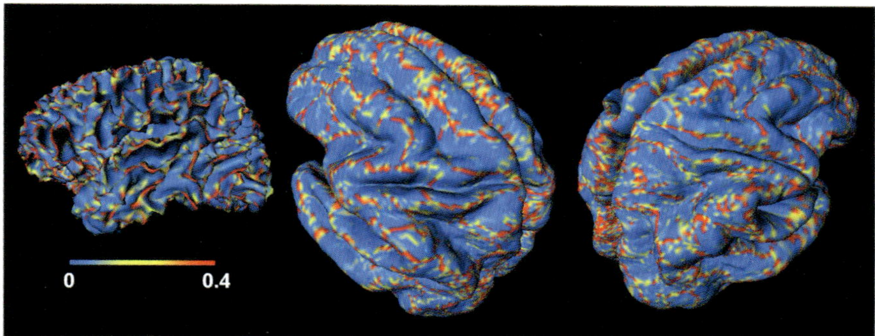

Fig. 7.14   Individual gyral patterns mapped onto the template surface The gyri of the subject match the gyri of the atlas illustrating a close homology between the surface of an individual subject and the template surface. The Gyri are extracted by thresholding the thin-plate spline energy on the inner surface. If there is no homology between the corresponding vertices, we would have complete misalignment.

Let κ_1 and κ_2 be the two principal curvatures as defined in Kreyszig (1959). The principal curvatures can be represented as functions of β_is in quadratic surface (7.17). To measure the amount of folding, we define curvature metric K as a function of the principal curvatures:

$$K = \frac{\kappa_1^2 + \kappa_2^2}{2} + \alpha.$$

We may arbitrarily set $\alpha = 0.001$. α is added to make sure that the curvature dilatation is well defined. The mean of the square of the principal curvatures is usually refereed as the thin-plate spline energy functional. If the cortical surface is flat, curvature metric K obtains the minimum 0.001. The larger the curvature metric, the more surface will be crested as shown in Figures 7.13 and 7.14. The *local curvature dilatation rate* $\Lambda_{curvature}$ is similarly defined as (8.36).

7.4.3 *Statistical Inference on Surfaces*

Under the assumption of stochastic model (7.16), it can be shown that the area dilatation is approximately distributed as Gaussian:

$$\Lambda(x) = \lambda(x) + \epsilon(x), \tag{7.20}$$

where

$$\lambda = \mathrm{tr}\left[g^{-1}(\nabla X)^t(\nabla \mu)\nabla X\right]$$

is the mean area dilatation and error ϵ is a mean zero Gaussian random field defined on the cortical surface. The curvature dilatation can be modeled similarly. These theoretical model assumptions have been verified using Lilliefors test at 0.05 level (Conover, 1980). From statistical model (7.20), we are interested in testing an hypothesis: $H_0 : \lambda(x) = 0$ for all $x \in \partial \mathcal{M}_{atlas}$., i.e. no structural difference between two groups. The maximum of T random field will be used as a test statistic (Worsley, 1994). The T random field on manifold $\partial \mathcal{M}_{atlas}$ is defined as

$$T(x) = \sqrt{n}\frac{M(x)}{S(x)}, \quad x \in \partial \mathcal{M}_{atlas}$$

where M and S are the sample mean and standard deviation of metric Λ. $T(\mathbf{x})$ is distributed as a student's t with $n - 1$ degrees of freedom at each voxel x. For simplicity, we are doing one sample or paired two-sample t test here but unpaired two-sample test is similar. The p-value of the test statistic can be approximated asymptotically. For high threshold y, it can be shown that

$$P\left(\max_{x\in\partial\mathcal{M}_{atlas}} T(x) \geq y\right) \approx \sum_{i=0}^{3} \phi_i(\partial\mathcal{M}_{atlas})\rho_i(y), \qquad (7.21)$$

where ρ_i is the i-dimensional EC-density and the Minkowski functional ϕ_i for $\partial\mathcal{M}_{atlas}$ are

$$\phi_0 = 2, \ \phi_1 = 0, \ \phi_2 = \|\partial\mathcal{M}_{atlas}\|, \ \phi_3 = 0$$

and $\|\partial\mathcal{M}_{atlas}\|$ is the total surface area of $\partial\mathcal{M}_{atlas}$. When diffusion smoothing with given FWHM is applied to metric Λ on surface $\partial\mathcal{M}_{atlas}$, the 0-dimensional and 2-dimensional EC-density becomes

$$\rho_0(y) = \int_y^\infty \frac{\Gamma(\frac{n}{2})}{((n-1)\pi)^{1/2}\Gamma(\frac{n-1}{2})}\left(1 + \frac{y^2}{n-1}\right)^{-n/2} dy,$$

$$\rho_2(y) = \frac{1}{\text{FWHM}^2}\frac{4\ln 2}{(2\pi)^{3/2}}\frac{\Gamma(\frac{n}{2})y\left(1 + \frac{y^2}{n-1}\right)^{-(n-2)/2}}{(\frac{n-1}{2})^{1/2}\Gamma(\frac{n-1}{2})}.$$

Therefore, the p-value can be approximated by

$$P\left(\max_{x\in\partial\mathcal{M}_{atlas}} T(x) \geq y\right) \approx 2\rho_0(y) + \|\partial\mathcal{M}_{atlas}\|\rho_2(y).$$

For one-sided α-level test, we numerically solve equation

$$2\rho_0(y) + \|\partial\mathcal{M}_{atlas}\|\rho_2(y) = \alpha$$

and reject H_0 if $T \geq y$ or $T \leq -y$.

7.4.4 *Quantifying Brain Growth*

As an illustration of the tensor-based surface morphometry, we will demonstrate how the surface-based statistical analysis can be applied in localizing the cortical regions of tissue growth and loss in brain images longitudinally collected in a group of children and adolescents.

Two T_1-weighted MR scans were acquired for 28 normal subject at different times on the GE Sigma 1.5-T superconducting magnet system. The first scan was obtained at the age $t_1 = 11.5 \pm 3.1$ years and the second scan was obtained at the age $t_2 = 16.1 \pm 3.2$ years. We are interested in detecting the regions of the cortical shape difference over time. We compute the total surface area $\|\partial\mathcal{M}_{atlas}\|$ by summing the area of each triangle in a triangulated surface. The total surface area of the average atlas brain is 275,800 mm^2, which is roughly the area of 53×53 cm^2 sheet. We also computed the local area and the curvature dilatations. Surface metrics are then filtered with 20mm FWHM diffusion smoothing. At 0.025 level, statistically significant regions of local area and curvature difference over time are detected. Figure 7.13 shows the superior frontal and middle frontal gyri curvature increase over time. We also detected local surface expansion in Broca's area in the left hemisphere and local surface shrinkage in the left superior frontal sulcus. Most of surface reduction are concentrated near the frontal region. It is interesting to note that between these two gyri we have detected local surface area decrease. It might be possible that local surface area shrinking in the superior frontal sulcus causes the bending in the neighboring middle and superior frontal gyri. While the gray matter is shrinking in both total surface area and volume, the cortex itself seems to get folded to give increasing curvature in brain development for children.

To verify that our modeling and analysis do not detect any false signal our methods have been checked on null data. The null data is created by reversing time for randomly chosen half of the subjects. In the null data, the mean time difference is $t_2 - t_1 = -0.24$ year so the statistical analysis presented here should not detect any morphological changes. In fact, we did not detect any statistically significant morphological changes.

7.4.5 *Tensor Computation via SPHARM*

Taking the weighted spherical harmonic representation (SPHARM) as a global parameterization for cortical surface $\mathcal{M}$, we can compute the Riemannian metric tensors that are needed in computing the local area element (Chung *et al.*, 2008a).

Spherical Parameterization. Let $\mathcal{M}$ and S^2 be a cortical surface and a unit sphere respectively. $\mathcal{M}$ and S^2 are realized as polygonal meshes with more than 80000 triangle elements. It is natural to assume the cortical surface to be a smooth 2-dimensional Riemannian manifold parameterized by two parameters (Davatzikos and Bryan, 1995). This parametrization is constructed in the following way. A point $u = (u_1, u_2, u_3) \in S^2$ is mapped to $p = (x, y, z) \in \mathcal{M}$ via the mapping U, which is obtained by a deformable surface algorithm that preserves anatomical homology and the topological connectivity of meshes. We will refer this mapping as the *spherical mapping*. Then we parameterize u by the spherical coordinates:

$$(u_1, u_2, u_3) = (\sin\theta\cos\varphi, \sin\theta\sin\varphi, \cos\theta)$$

with $(\theta, \varphi) \in \mathcal{N} = [0, \pi] \otimes [0, 2\pi)$. The polar angle θ is the angle from the north pole and the azimuthal angle φ is the angle along the horizontal cross section of a MRI.

The mapping from the parameter space $\mathcal{N}$ to the unit sphere S^2 will be denoted as X, i.e.

$$X : \mathcal{N} \to S^2.$$

Then we have a composite mapping Z from the parameter space to the cortical surface:

$$Z = U \circ X : \mathcal{N} \to \mathcal{M}.$$

Z is a 3D vector of surface coordinates and it will be stochastically modeled as

$$Z(\theta, \varphi) = \nu(\theta, \varphi) + \epsilon(\theta, \varphi), \tag{7.22}$$

where ν is a unknown true differentiable parametrization and ϵ is a random vector field on the unit sphere. The computation of the Riemannian metric tensors and the local area element require estimating differentiable function ν.

Metric Tensor Estimation.

The weighted-SPHARM estimation (Chung *et al.*, 2008a) $\widehat{\nu}$ of the unknown true parametrization μ is given by

$$\widehat{\nu}(\theta, \varphi) = \sum_{l=0}^{k} \sum_{m=-l}^{l} \lambda_{lm} Z_{lm} Y_{lm}$$

with $Z_{lm} = \langle Z, Y_{lm} \rangle$. The eigenvalues $\lambda_{lm} = e^{-l(l+1)\sigma}$ correspond to heat kernel. For detailed exposition of weighted-SPHARM, see the next chapter.

The Riemannian metric tensors g_{ij} will be computed by analytically differentiating the weighted-SPHARM. The estimation of the Riemannian metric tensors requires partial derivatives of $\widehat{\nu}$. Denoting the partial differential operators as $\partial_1 = \partial_\theta$ and $\partial_2 = \partial_\varphi$, we have

$$\partial_i \widehat{\nu} = \sum_{l=0}^{k} \sum_{m=-l}^{l} \lambda_{lm} Z_{lm} \partial_i Y_{lm}(\theta, \varphi).$$

The derivatives of spherical harmonics can be analytically computed. We start with the derivative for the associated Legendre polynomials.

$$\partial_\theta P_l^{|m|}(x) = l \cot \theta P_l^{|m|}(x) - (l + |m|) \sin^{-1} \theta P_{l-1}^{|m|}(x),$$

where $x = \cos\theta$. Note that $P_{l-1}^{|m|} = 0$ if $|m| \geq l$. The recursive formula introduces a numerical singularity at the north and south poles ($\theta = 0, \pi$) so we have chosen the poles to be the regions of non-interest that connect the left and the right hemispheres. Then the derivatives of spherical harmonics are expressed as the functions of spherical harmonics.

$$\partial_\theta Y_{lm} = l\cot\theta Y_{lm} - (l + |m|)\frac{c_{lm}}{c_{l-1,m}}\sin^{-1}\theta Y_{l-1,m}$$

with the convention $Y_{l-1,m} = 0$ if $|m| \geq l$. The constant in the second term can be further simplified as

$$(l + |m|)\frac{c_{lm}}{c_{l-1,m}} = \sqrt{\frac{2l+1}{2l-1}}(l^2 - m^2).$$

The derivative with respect to φ is simply given as

$$\partial_\varphi Y_{lm} = -mY_{l,-m}.$$

This recursive relation reduces the computational time by recycling the spherical harmonics used in estimating the SPHARM coefficients.

The 3×2 Jacobian matrix J of mapping from parameter space $\mathcal{N}$ to cortical surface $\mathcal{M}$ is given by

$$J = (\partial_\theta \hat{\nu}, \partial_\varphi \hat{\nu}).$$

The Riemannian metric tensors are

$$g = (g_{ij}) = J^t J.$$

The component is given by

$$g_{ij} = \partial_i \widehat{\nu} \cdot \partial_j \widehat{\nu}$$

with the vector inner product $\cdot$. The Riemannian metric tensors measure the amount of deviation of a cortical surface from a flat Euclidean plane. If the cortical surface is flat, we have $g_{ij} = \delta_{ij}$, the identity matrix.

Surface Area Element.

The Riemannian metric tensors enable us to compute the local *area element* $\sqrt{\det g}$. The area element measures the amount of the transformed area in $\mathcal{M}$ of the unit area in the parameterized space $\mathcal{N}$ via the mapping ν. Figure 7.15 shows the estimation of the metric tensors for a subject. Using the area element, the total surface area of $\mathcal{M}$ can be written as

$$\mu(\mathcal{M}) = \int_0^{2\pi} \int_0^{\pi} \sqrt{\det g}(\theta, \varphi)\, d\theta\, d\varphi.$$

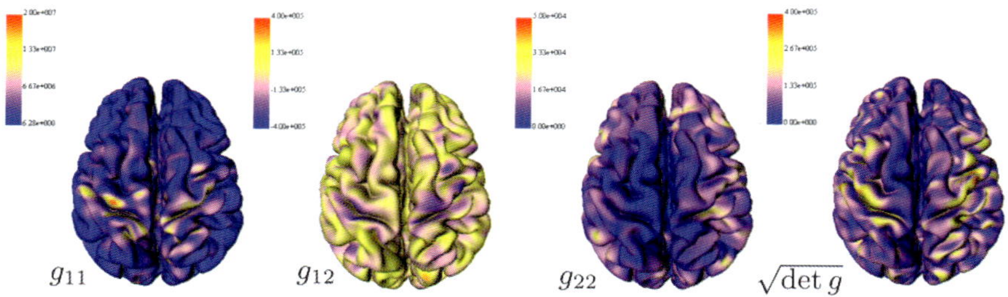

Fig. 7.15   Metric tensor estimation. The metric tensors g_{ij} are estimated by analytically differentiating the weighted-SPHARM representation. The local area element $\sqrt{\det g}$ measures the amount of area expansion and shrinking with respect to the parameter space $\mathcal{N}$.

Locally, surface deformation can be decomposed into the tangential and the normal components with respect to a surface normal vector (Chung *et al.*, 2003c). At each point p, we define *local gray matter volume* as

$$V(p) = \sqrt{\det g(p)} C(p),$$

where C is cortical thickness. Then the total gray matter volume is approximately given as $\int_{S^2} V(p) \, d\mu(p)$. The gray matter volume will change if either the area element increases (tangential expansion) or cortical thickness increases (normal expansion). Then the change in the gray matter volume is the sum of the change in local area and the change in cortical thickness (Chung *et al.*, 2003c):

$$\frac{dV}{V} = \frac{d\sqrt{\det g}}{\sqrt{\det g}} + \frac{dC}{C}.$$

The change in the local area element can be viewed as to contributing to the tangential component of the gray matter volume change.

The scale invariant area element is defined as $\sqrt{\det g}/\mu(\mathcal{M})$, where the total surface area $\mu(\mathcal{M})$ is estimated by summing the area of triangles in a mesh. Figure 7.16 shows the scale invariant area element for randomly selected 12 subjects. Although the scale invariant area element is invariant under affine scaling, it is not invariant under different parameterizations such as conformal mappings (Angenent *et al.*, 1999; Gu *et al.*, 2004; Hurdal and Stephenson, 2004), quasi-isometric mappings (Timsari and Leahy, 2000) and area preserving mappings (Brechbuhler *et al.*, 1995; Shen *et al.*, 2004; Styner *et al.*, 2006). Considering these parameterizations introduce area distortion, it is necessary to use a parameterization invariant metric for a stable statistical analysis. This can be obtained by directly

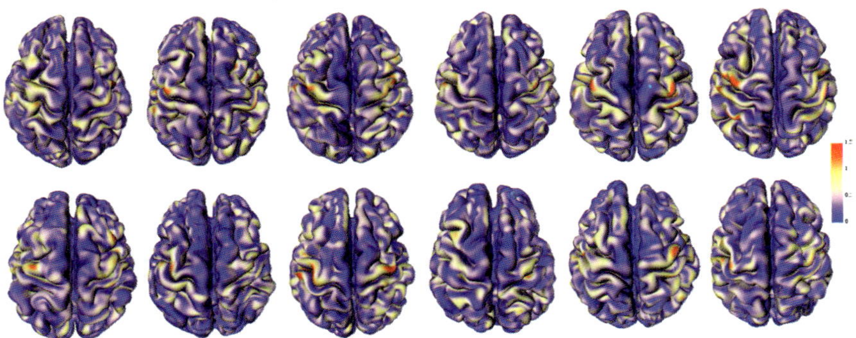

Fig. 7.16 Scale invariant area elements for randomly selected 6 control subjects (top) and 6 autistic subjects (bottom). The color scale is thresholded at 1.5 (150%) for better visualization. With respect to the parameter space $\mathcal{N}$, there is up to 300% area expansion.

measuring the area expansion rate with respect to a template surface $\mathcal{M}_0$ rather than the parameter space $\mathcal{N}$. Consider a mapping from the template $\mathcal{M}_0$ to the cortical surface $\mathcal{M}$. The Jocobian of this mapping will be noted as J_0. The Jacobian J_0 is expected to be invariant under different parameterizations and only depends on the registration between the two surfaces.

Let g_0 be the metric tensors of $\mathcal{M}_0$. The area element of $\mathcal{M}$ is

$$\sqrt{\det g} = \det J_0 \sqrt{\det g_0}.$$

Then the parameterization invariant measure is obtained by simply computing the percentage change of area expansion with respect to the template as

$$\frac{\sqrt{\det g} - \sqrt{\det g_0}}{\sqrt{\det g_0}} = \det J_0 - 1 \tag{7.23}$$

giving a local area related measure invariant under parameterization. This quantity is called the *surface area dilatation* and it is approximately the trace of the Jacobian determinant (Chung *et al.*, 2001a). Our methodology does not work for area-preserving mappings since the Jacobian determinant is 1. For this singular case, we can compute the Jacobian determinant directly from the surface registration result.

7.5 Multivariate General Linear Models

Multivariate general linear models (MGLM) generalize widely used univariate general linear models by incorporating vector valued response and explanatory variables (Anderson, 1984; Taylor and Worsley, 2008; Worsley *et al.*, 2004, 1996b). For instance, the hippocampus surface coordinates or displacement vector field can be taken as the response variable P (Figure 7.17 and 7.18). Consider the following MGLM at each fixed point along the template surface:

$$P_{n\times 3} = X_{n\times p}B_{p\times 3} + Z_{n\times r}G_{r\times 3} + U_{n\times 3}\Sigma_{3\times 3}, \tag{7.24}$$

where P is the matrix of coordinates, X is the matrix of contrasted explanatory variables, and B is the matrix of unknown coefficients. Nuisance covariates are in the matrix Z and the corresponding coefficients are in the matrix G. The subscripts denote the dimension of matrices. The components of Gaussian random matrix U are zero mean and unit variance. Σ accounts for the covariance structure of coordinates. Then we are interested in testing the null hypothesis

$$H_0 : B = 0.$$

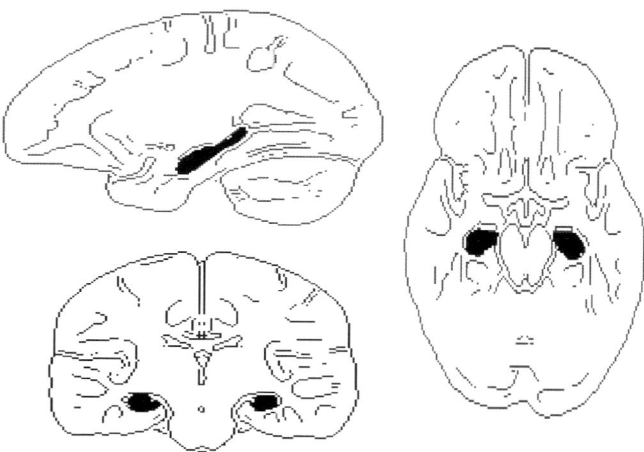

Fig. 7.17 Hippocampi binary segmentation in a template showing the relative location of the structures. A simple isosurfacing algorithm can be used to construct a triangular mesh out of the binary segmentation.The outline of the brain is obtained by detecting edges in the T1-weighted MRI using the Sobel method (Parker, 1996).

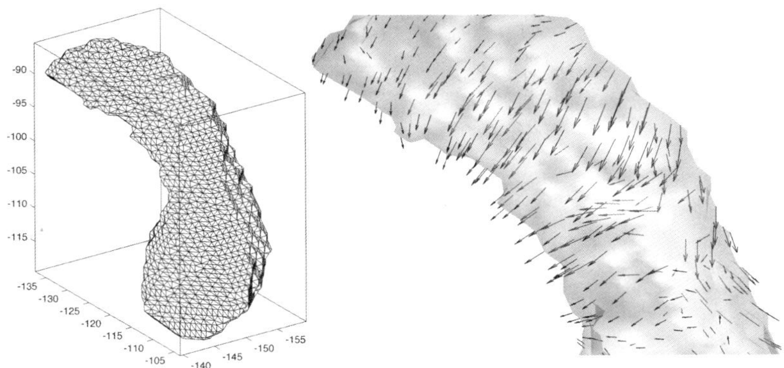

Fig. 7.18 The left hippocampus surface obtained from the binary segmentation showing approximate size of $30 \times 30 \times 15$ mm. The surface mesh consists of 2238 vertices and 4672 edges. The individual anatomical variability is encoded in the displacement vector fields on the template. The displacement vector field can be analyzed using the multivariate general linear models (Chung *et al.*, 2010d).

For the reduced model corresponding to $B = 0$, the least squares estimator of G is given by solving $P = ZG$. i.e.

$$\widehat{G}_0 = (Z'Z)^{-1}Z'P.$$

We will assume that there is more sample size n than the number of parameters r to be estimated. The residual sum of squares of the reduced model is

$$E_0 = (P - Z\widehat{G}_0)'(P - Z\widehat{G}_0).$$

For the full model, the parameters are estimated by solving

$$P_{n \times 3} = XB + ZG = [X, Z]_{n \times (p+r)} \begin{bmatrix} B \\ G \end{bmatrix}_{(p+r) \times 3}.$$

The least squares estimation is given by

$$\begin{bmatrix} \widehat{B} \\ \widehat{G} \end{bmatrix} = ([X, Z]'[X, Z])^{-1}[X, Z]'P.$$

The corresponding residual sum of squared error is

$$E = (P - X\widehat{B} - Z\widehat{G})'(P - X\widehat{B} - Z\widehat{G}).$$

By comparing how large the residual E is against the residual E_0, we can determine the significance of coefficients B. However, since E and E_0 are matrices, we take a function of eigenvalues of $E_0 E^{-1}$ as a statistic.

7.5.1 *Roy's Maximum Root*

Since we expect the sample size n to be larger than 3, there are three eigenvalues $\lambda_1, \lambda_2, \lambda_3$ satisfying

$$\det(E_0 - \lambda E) = 0.$$

This requires solving the generalized eigenvalue problem

$$E_0 v = \lambda E v$$

for eigenvectors v. The three eigenvectors give the orthogonal linear combinations of the responses that produces maximal univariate F statistics (Fox *et al.*, 2009). For instance, Lawley-Hotelling trace is given by the sum of eigenvalues $\lambda_1 + \lambda_2 + \lambda_3$, Wilks's Lambda is given by $(1+\lambda_1)^{-1}(1+\lambda_2)^{-1}(1+\lambda_3)^{-1}$ while *Roy's maximum root* R is the largest eigenvalue. The distributions of these multivariate test statistics are approximately F. In the case there is only one eigenvalue, all these multivariate test statistics simplify to *Hotelling's T-sqaure* statistic. The Hotelling's T-square statistic has been widely used in modeling 3D coordinates and deformations in brain imaging (Cao and Worsley, 1999b; Chung *et al.*, 2001a; Gaser *et al.*, 1999; Joshi, 1998; Thompson *et al.*, 1997). The random field theory for Hotelling's T-square statistic has been available for a while (Cao and Worsley, 1999b). However, the random field theory for the Roy's maximum root has not been developed until recently (Taylor and Worsley, 2008; Worsley *et al.*, 2004).

The inference for Roy's maximum root is based on the Roy's union-intersection principle (Roy, 1953; Worsley *et al.*, 2004), which simplifies the multivariate problem to a univariate linear model. Let us multiply an arbitrary constant vector $\nu_{3\times1}$ on both sides of (7.24):

$$P\nu = XB\nu + ZG\nu + U\Sigma\nu. \tag{7.25}$$

Obviously (7.25) is a usual univariate linear model with a Gaussian noise. For the univariate testing on $B\nu = 0$, the inference is based on the F statistic with p and $n - p - r$ degrees of freedom, denoted as F_ν. Then Roy's maximum root statistic can be defined as

$$R = \max_{\nu} F_\nu.$$

Now it is obvious that the usual random field theory can be applied in correcting for multiple comparisons. The only trick is to increase the search space, in which we take the supreme of the F random field, from the template surface to much higher dimension to account for maximizing over ν as well. Another way of defining Roy's maximum root is via maximal canonical correlations (Worsley *et al.*, 2004).

7.5.2 SurfStat

Keith Worsley's SurfStat package (http://www.math.mcgill.ca/keith/surfstat) has a built in MATLAB routines for determining the p-value for Roy's maximum root statistic so there is no need to worry about computational details for most users. SurfStat was developed to utilize a model formula and avoids the explicit use of design matrices and contrasts, which tend to be a hinderance to most end users not familiar with such concepts. SurtStat can import MNI (MacDonald *et al.*, 2000). FreeSurfer (surfer.nmr.mgh.harvard.edu) based cortical mesh formats as well as other volumetric image data. The model formula approach is implemented in many statistics packages such as Splus (www.insightful.com) R (www.r-project.org) and SAS (www.sas.com). These statistics packages accept a linear model like

$$P = Group + Age + Brain$$

as the direct input for linear modeling avoiding the need to explicitly state the design matrix. P is a $n \times 3$ matrix of coordinates, Age is the age of subjects, Brain is the total brain volume of subject and Group is the categorical group variable. This type of model formula has yet to be implemented in widely used SPM or AFNI packages.

Figure 7.19 shows an example of MGLM applied to brain and behavior association in autism (Chung *et al.*, 2010d). 10 control and 12 autistic subjects went through face emotion recognition task and a remote eye-tracking device was used to measure gaze fixation duration on eyes and faces during the task. It has been hypothesized that subjects with autism should exhibit diminished eye fixation duration relative to face fixation duration. We simply refer *gaze fixation* (Fixation) as the ratio of durations fixed on eyes over faces. Note that this is a unit less measure. The gaze fixation are 0.30 ± 0.17 (control) and 0.18 ± 0.16 (autism). Nacewicz *et al.* (2006) showed the gaze fixation duration correlate differently with amygdala volume between the two groups; however, it was not clear if the association difference is local or diffuse over all amygdala. The group variable Group is coded as a categorical dummy variable of either zero or one. The significance of the interaction between Group and Fixation can be determined using multivariate linear models. The reduced model is

$$P = Age + Brain + Group + Fixation$$

while the full model is

$$P = Age + Brain + Group + Fixation + Group * Fixation. \tag{7.26}$$

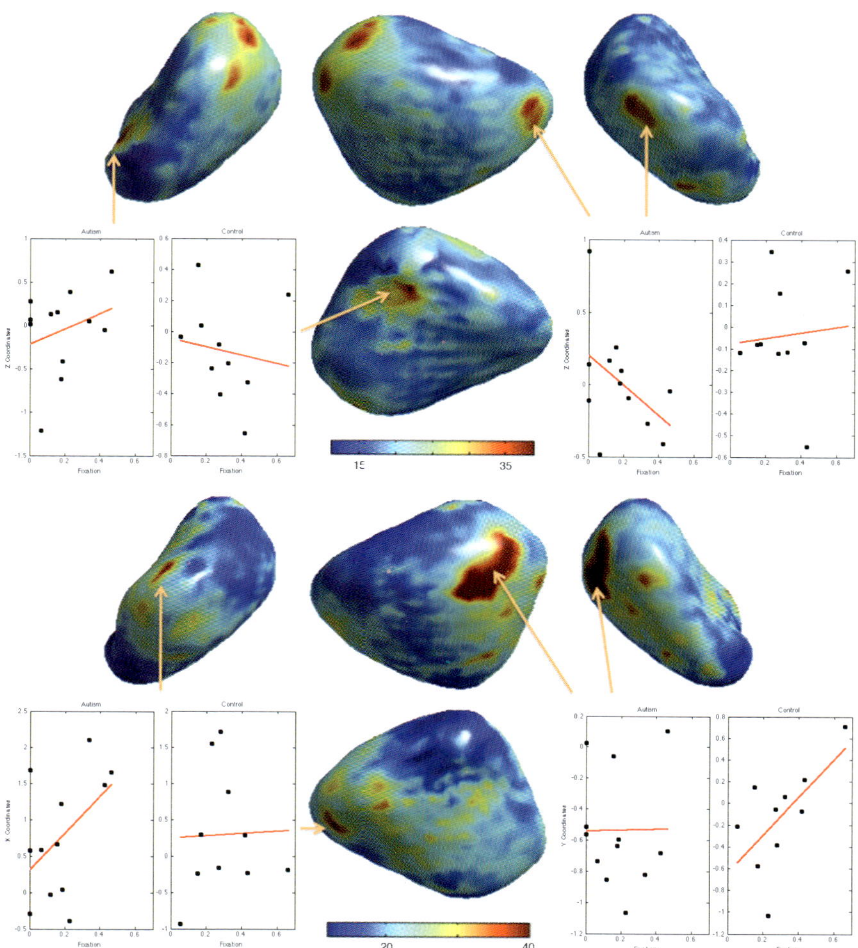

Fig. 7.19	F statistic map of significant interaction between group and gaze fixation duration on surface coordinate vector P (Chung *et al.*, 2010d). Red regions show significant interaction for left (top) and right (bottom) amygdale. The scatter plots show the particular coordinate over the gaze fixation duration. The red lines are linear regression lines.

We have obtained regions of significant interaction in the both left ($p <$ 0.05) and right ($p < 0.02$) lateral nuclei in amygdale. The largest cluster in the right amygdala shows highly significant interaction ($\max F = 65.68$, $p = 0.003$). The scatter plots of the z-coordinate of the displacement vector field vs. `Fixation` are shown at the two most significant clusters in each amygdala. The red lines are linear regression lines. The significance of interaction implies difference in regression slopes between groups in a multivariate fashion. Note that there are three different slopes corresponding to x, y and z coordinates but we only showed one coordinate at a time.

The total number of unknown parameters in our most complicated model (7.26) is $6 \times 3 = 18$ including the constant terms. This is a large number of parameters to estimate if (7.26) was a univariate linear model. However, in our multivariate setting, it is reasonable number of parameters since we are also tripling the number of measurements as well. Note that Roy's maximum root statistic is based on maximizing an F-statistic with 1 and $n - 1 - 5$ degrees of freedom. Since the number of subjects is $n = 22 + 24$, we have the sufficient degrees of freedom not to worry about the over-fitting problem. Unfortunately, practical power approximation for Roy's maximum root statistic does not exists although that of Lawley-Hotelling trace is available so the discussion of the parameter over-fitting is still an open statistical problem (Barton and Cramer, 1989; O'Brien and Muller, 1993).

7.6 Mixed Effect Models on Surface Shape Change

There are few studies that relate the longitudinal reduction in right hippocampus volume to stress and affective disorder. The severity of stress level in children negatively correlates with the change of right hippocampus volume in longitudinally collected images (Carrion *et al.*, 2007). Bipolar patients have significant smaller right hippocampus volume compared to normal control subjects (Swayze 2nd *et al.*, 1992). However, the limitation of these traditional volumetric studies is that even if we can determine the volume difference, there is no way of determining if the volume difference is diffuse over the whole hippocampus or localized within small regions of hippocampus. In this section, we introduce the mixed effect modeling framework that enables localized longitudinal hippocampus shape characterization and able to overcome the limitation of the traditional volumetric studies.

Extensive literature on mixed effect models are available (Fox, 2002; Milliken and Edland, 2000; Molenberghs and Verbeke, 2005; Pinehiro and Bates, 2002). There are three advantages of the mixed-effect model over the usual fixed-effect model. It explicitly models individual growth pattern. It accommodates an unequal number of follow-up image scans per subject and unequal intervals between scans.

7.6.1 *Longitudinal Imaging Data*

We applied the proposed method in determining the effect of family income on the growth of hippocampus in children. The data set is published in Chung *et al.* (2011b). T1-weighted MRIs were collected using a 3T GE SIGNA scanner on 124 children and adolescents from high- ($> 75000\$$; $n = 86$) and low-income ($< 35000\$$, $n = 38$) parents respectively. In addition to this cross-sectional data, longitudinal data was available for 82 of these subjects ($n = 66$, $> 75000\$$; $n = 16$, $< 35000\$$). This second MRI scan was acquired about 2 years later. The total number of MRI scans is 206.

Figure 7.21 scatter plots show the age distribution of the study. The first scans are taken at 11.6 ± 3.7 years while the second scans are taken at 14 ± 3.9 years. The symmetric diffeomorphic image normalization and template construction was performed on MRI (Avants *et al.*, 2008). The left and right hippocampi were manually segmented in the template using the protocol outlined in Rusch *et al.* (2001). The marching cubes algorithm was then used to obtain the surface mesh model. On the template surface, we have displacement vector field of mapping from the template to individual subject (Figure 7.18). The length of the displacement vector measures the amount of growth from the template. Since the length measurement is noisy, surface-based smoothing is necessary. We have used heat kernel smoothing (Figure 7.20). Other than deformation fields, we have the following variables available in the data set:

(1) `subject`: an identification number keeping tract of which scans belong to which subject.
(2) `age`: the subject's age in months.
(3) `income`: a factor indicating whether the subject is from high- or low-income families.

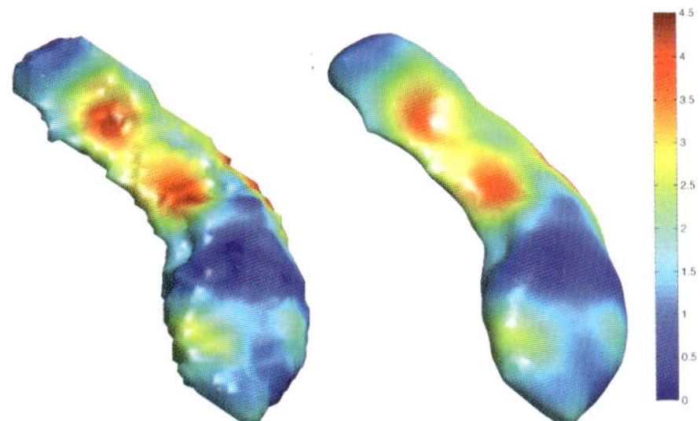

Fig. 7.20   Left: the length of displacement vector field on a template. Right: heat kernel smoothing with bandwidth $\sigma = 0.5$ and degree $k = 500$.

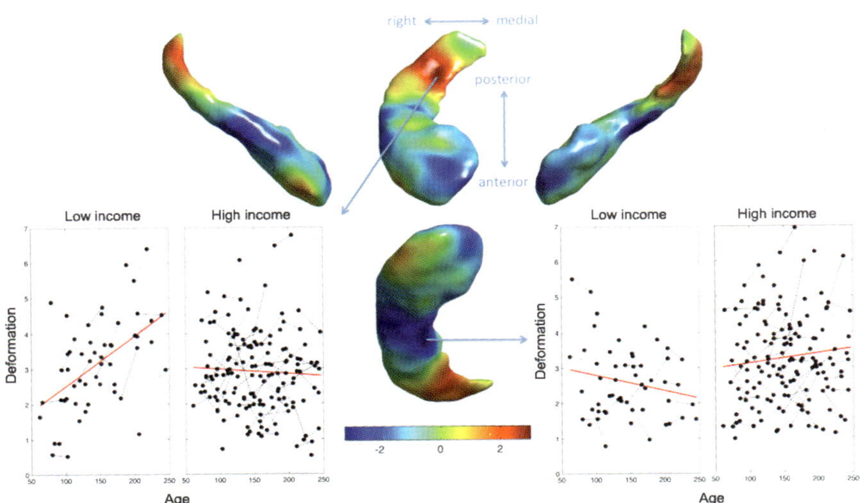

Fig. 7.21   *T*-statistic map showing significant growth rate difference between children from low-income and high-income families. The significance of the growth rate difference is determined by the interaction term in a linear model. Highly focalized regions of group difference were detected in the right hippocampus (corrected p-value $=0.03$). The posterior region is enlarging while the midbody and the anterior parts are shrinking in children from low-income families. On the other hand the pattern is opposite for children from high-income families.

7.6.2 *Mixed Effect Models*

Let us follow notations given in Milliken and Edland (2000). Longitudinal data on the i-th subject will be modeled as

$$Y_i = X_i\beta + Z_i\gamma_i + e_i, \tag{7.27}$$

where Y_i is the longitudinal outcome from an image, β are fixed effects shared by all subjects, γ_i are subject specific random effects and $e_i \sim N(0, \sigma^2)$ are independent and identically distributed noise. X_i and Z_i are design matrix corresponding to the fixed and random effects. For our application, we have $Z_i = (1, age)$ and $\gamma_i = (\gamma_{i1}, \gamma_{i2})'$. The linear mixed effect model assumes the individual growth trend with an individualized linear model

$$Z_i\gamma_i = \gamma_{i1} + \mathsf{age} \cdot \gamma_{i2}.$$

Since 82 subjects have the second scans after about 2 years later, it is necessary to explicitly model the within-subject variability. We assume the i-th subject have repeated scans $y_{i1}, \cdots, y_{in_i}$ at a given fixed mesh vertex. Since each subject has only one or two scans, n_i is either 1 or 2. If the data is balanced (identical number of scans per subject), the mixed effect model is straightforward but the complication arises when the data is not balanced.

Fixed Effect Model. In the fixed effect model, we simply treat the within-subject repeated scans as statistically independent. So we have a linear model containing fixed effect term age_{ij}:

$$y_{ij} = \beta_0 + \beta_1\mathsf{age}_{ij} + \epsilon_{ij}, \tag{7.28}$$

where ϵ_{ij} is assumed to follow Gaussian. The population average is modeled modeled linearly linearly with intercept β_0 and slope β_1.

Random Effect Model. In the model (7.28), every subjects have identical growth trajectory $\beta_0 + \beta_1\mathsf{age}$, which is unrealistic. Biologically every subjects are expected to have its own unique growth trajectory. So we assume each subject to have its own intercept $\beta_0 + \gamma_{i0}$ and slope $\beta_1 + \gamma_{i1}$:

$$y_{ij} = \beta_0 + \gamma_{i0} + (\beta_1 + \gamma_{i1})\mathsf{age}_{ij} + \epsilon_{ij}. \tag{7.29}$$

It is reasonable to assume $\gamma = (\gamma_{i0}, \gamma_{i1})'$ to be multivariate normal. The model (7.29) can be decomposed into fixed and random effect terms:

$$y_{ij} = (\beta_0 + \beta_1\mathsf{age}_{ij}) + (\gamma_{i0} + \gamma_{i1}\mathsf{age}_{ij}) + \epsilon_{ij}. \tag{7.30}$$

Matrix Form. The mixed effect model can be written in a more compact matrix form. Consider the general model (7.27), where $Y_i = (y_{i1}, \cdots, y_{in_i})'$, $\beta = (\beta_0, \beta_1)'$ and $\gamma_i = (\gamma_{i0}, \gamma_{i1})'$. X_i and Z_i are $n_i \times 2$ design matrices corresponding to the fixed and the random effect respectively for the i-th subject. (7.27) can be also written in a single matrix form:

$$Y = X\beta + Z\gamma + \epsilon,$$

We assume $\gamma_i \sim N(0, \Gamma)$ and $\epsilon_i \sim N(0, \Sigma_i)$. Hierarchically we can also model (7.27) as

$$Y_i | \gamma_i \sim N(X_i\beta + Z_i\gamma_i, \Sigma_i), \ \gamma_i \sim N(0, \Gamma).$$

The size of the covariance matrix is $n_i \times n_i$. The within-subject variability is expected to be smaller than between-subject variability and explicitly modeled by Σ_i. The covariance of γ_i and ϵ are expected to have block diagonal structure such that there is no correlation among the scans of different subjects while there is high correlation between the scans of the same subject:

$$\mathbb{V}\begin{pmatrix} \gamma_i \\ \epsilon_i \end{pmatrix} = \begin{pmatrix} \Gamma & 0 \\ 0 & \Sigma_i \end{pmatrix}.$$

The covariance of Y_i is given by

$$\mathbb{V}Y_i = Z_i \Gamma Z_i' + \Sigma_i.$$

The random-effect contribution is $Z_i \Gamma Z_i'$ while the within-subject contribution is Σ_i.

7.6.3 *Restricted Maximum Likelihood Estimation*

The parameters and the covariance matrices are estimated by maximizing the likelihood function. Let $f(y_i|\gamma_i)$ and $f(\gamma_i)$ are density functions for $Y_i|\gamma_i$ and γ_i. The marginal density of Y_i is then given by

$$f(y_i) = \int f(y_i|\gamma_i) f(\gamma_i) \, d\gamma_i.$$

It can be shown that Y_i is again a multivariate normal

$$Y_i \sim N(X_i\beta, V_i),$$

where $V_i(\alpha) = Z_i \Gamma Z_i' + \Sigma_i$. The covariance V_i is given by some parameters α. The likelihood function is given by

$$L(\alpha, \beta) \propto \prod_{i=1}^{n} |V_i|^{-1/2} exp\left[-\frac{1}{2}(y_i - X_i\beta)'V_i^{-1}(y_i - X_i\beta) \right]. \quad (7.31)$$

For any parameters α, the estimate

$$\widehat{\beta}(\alpha) = \left(\sum_{i=1}^{n} X_i V_i^{-1} X_i' \right)^{-1} \sum_{i=1}^{n} X_i V_i^{-1} Y_i,$$

maximizes the likelihood (7.31). It can be shown that

$$\mathbb{E}\,\widehat{\beta}(\alpha) = \beta$$

and

$$\mathbb{V}\,\widehat{\beta}(\alpha) = \left(\sum_{i=1}^{n} X_i V_i^{-1} X_i' \right)^{-1}.$$

Maximizing the restricted likelihood without β produces the *restricted maximum likelihood* (REML) estimates for covariance parameters α (Fox, 2002; Pinehiro and Bates, 2002).

The REML estimate of α is as follows. Consider any full rank matrix K satisfying $KX = 0$. Then the marginal distribution of $Z = KY$ does not depend on β:

$$Z = K\epsilon \sim N(0, KVK).$$

Once V is estimated by REML, β is estimated by plugging $\widehat{V}$.

The most widely used tools for fitting mixed effect model is the `nlme` library in R statistical package, which has been extensively covered in (Pinehiro and Bates, 2002). However, tere is no need to use R to fit the mixed effect model. Keith Worsley has implemented REML procedure in `SurfStat` package that runs on top of `MATLAB` (Worsley *et al.*, 2009; Chung *et al.*, 2010d).

7.6.4   *Longitudinal Hippocampus Shape Model*

We will take the length of the surface displacement with respect to the template as the response variable (Figure 7.20). If we have age information in a cross-sectional data, we can still set up a linear model involving the age term `age` like

$$\texttt{deformation} = \beta_0 + \beta_1\texttt{age} + \beta_2\texttt{group} + \epsilon.$$

However, this is not truly a longitudinal model but a cross-sectional model. Having the age term in the model does not make the model longitudinal. The main difference between the longitudinal and cross-sectional models is whether if we can explicitly able to incorporate the dependence of repeated measurements (multiple scans of the same subject). This can be done by introducing a random effect term the above fixed effect model.

Since 82 subjects have the second scans after about 2 years later, it is necessary to explicitly model the within-subject variability that is expected to be smaller than between-subject variability. For each scan at a given mesh vertex p, we have the following mixed effect model containing fixed effect terms (`age`, `group`) and a random effect term (`subject`):

$$\texttt{deformation} = \beta_0 + \beta_1 \texttt{age} + \beta_2 \texttt{group} + \beta_3 \texttt{age} \cdot \texttt{group} + \gamma \texttt{subject} + \epsilon,$$

where ϵ and γ are Gaussian noise. The covariance of γ and ϵ are expected to have block structures such that there is no correlation among the scans of different subjects while there is high correlation between the scans of the same subject. The parameters are estimated using the restricted maximum likelihood (REML) method (Pinehiro and Bates, 2002; Fox, 2002). The REML method is implemented in `SurfStat` package (Chung *et al.*, 2010d).

We did not detect any statistically significant group difference (β_2) at 0.01 level (corrected) in the both left and right hippocampi. However, we obtained highly focalized regions of group difference in the growth rate (interaction term β_3) in the right hippocampus (corrected pvalue =0.03). The posterior region is enlarging while the midbody and the anterior parts are shrinking in children from low-income families (Figure 7.21). On the other hand the pattern is opposite for children from high-income families.

This is the first study localizing the regions of hippocampus growth difference in children from high- and low- income families. Note that the right hippocampus is involved in the active maintenance of associations with spatial information (Piekema *et al.*, 2006). Future studies investigating the relation between family socioeconomic status and spatial information processing measures are warranted.

7.6.5 *Functional Mixed Effect Models*

It is possible to extend a linear mixed effect model to incorporate more complex nonlinear growth pattern by taking functional covariates into the model. Goldsmith *et al.* (2011) modeled the clinical outcome Y_i of the i-th subject as

$$Y_i = X\beta + \int_0^1 W_i(p)f(p)\, dp + \epsilon_i, \tag{7.32}$$

where $W_i(p)$ is the functional observation at position p and f is the smooth functional parameter that has to be estimated. β is the fixed effect shared by all subjects. (7.32) is related to the standard impulse-response model, which has been often used in modeling fMRI responses. In the standard impulse-response model, the impulse function W_i is usually discrete and the response Y_i is continuous. The fixed-effect model (7.32) is further generalized by incorporating the subject specific random effect terms in Goldsmith *et al.* (2012).

Let the j-th measurement of the i-th subject be Y_{ij}. We also have the corresponding functional observations $W_{ij}(p)$. Then Y_{ij} is modeled as

$$Y_{ij} = X_{ij}\beta + Z_{ij}\gamma_i + \int_0^1 W_{ij}(p)f(p)\, dp + \epsilon_i, \tag{7.33}$$

where X_i is the fixed effects and Z_i is the subject specific random effects. $f(p)$ is the vector of functional effect that has to be estimated. The functional effect $f(p)$ are population level parameters and do not vary across different subjects.

Using the Karhunen-Loeve (KL) expansion, $W_{ij}(p)$ is decomposed as

$$W_{ij}(p) = \sum_k c_{ijk}\psi_k(p), \tag{7.34}$$

where c_{ijk} are uncorrelated random variables and ψ_k are KL-basis. The main limitation of this model is that the model is based on a single scalar outcome per subject. So this is not a true functional mixed-effect model.

On the other hand, Zipunnikov *et al.* (2011a) and Zipunnikov *et al.* (2011b) are proposing a more general functional mixed effect model:

$$Y_{ij}(p) = \mu(p) + W_{ij}(p), \tag{7.35}$$

where $\mu(p)$ is the population level fixed functional effect and $W_i(p)$ is the subject specific random functional effect. W_{ij} is then decomposed using the similar KL-decomposition (7.34).

7.7 Sparse Surface Shape Recovery

So far we explained how to construct the Laplace-Beltrami (LB) eigenfunctions on cortical manifolds. Traditionally, the LB-eigenfunctions are used as a basis for intrinsically representing surface shapes by forming a Fourier series expansion. To reduce high frequency noise, only the first few terms are used in the expansion and higher frequency terms are simply thrown away. However, some lower frequency terms may not necessarily contribute significantly in reconstructing the surfaces. Motivated by this idea, we propose to filter out only the significant eigenfunctions by incorporating L_1 norm penalty term in the least squares estimation. The method is used in investigating the influence of age and gender on amygdala and hippocampus shapes in an elderly normal population. The sparse surface shape modeling framework was first introduced in (Kim *et al.*, 2012a).

The atrophy of brain tissues associated with the increase of age is extensively examined in many *in-vivo* magnetic resonance imaging (MRI) studies (Chung *et al.*, 2001a; Good *et al.*, 2001; Thompson *et al.*, 2000). However, the age effect on subcortical structures has been somewhat controversial (Sullivan *et al.*, 2005; Walhovd *et al.*, 2009). In the previous volumetric studies, the total volume of subcortical structures such as amygdala and hippocampus was typically estimated by tracing the region of interest (ROI) and counting the number of voxels within the ROI. The limitation of the ROI-based volumetry is that it cannot determine if the volume difference is diffuse over the whole ROI or localized within specific regions of the ROI (Chung *et al.*, 2010d).

The proposed sparse shape representation can localize the volume difference up to the mesh resolution at each surface mesh vertex. The sparse shape modeling flow is as follows:

(1) Starting with the 3D deformation field derived from the spatial normalization, obtain a mean volume of a subcortical structure by averaging the spatially normalized binary masks.

(2) Extract a template surface from the averaged binary volume.

(3) Interpolate the 3D displacement vector field onto the vertices of the surface meshes.

(4) Estimate a sparse representation of Fourier coefficients with L_1-norm penalty for the displacement length along the template surface to reduce noise.

(5) Apply a general linear model (GLM) testing the effect of age and gender on the displacement.

The proposed framework can be subsequently used in examining the effect of age and gender on amygdala and hippocampus shapes in the normal aging population, contrasting the traditional volumetric analysis (Kim *et al.*, 2012a).

7.7.1 *Sparse Regression on Surface Data*

Consider a real-valued functional measurement Y on a manifold $\mathcal{M} \subset \mathbb{R}^3$. We assume the following additive model:

$$Y(p) = \theta(p) + \epsilon(p),$$

where θ is the unknown mean signal to be estimated and ϵ is a zero-mean Gaussian random field. The Laplace-Beltrami (LB) eigenfunctions can be used in parametrically representing the surface data Y and this is taken as the estimate for the unknown signal θ.

In previous LB-eigenfunction and spherical harmonic (SPHARM) expansion approaches only the first few terms are used in the expansion and higher frequency terms are simply thrown away to reduce the high frequency noise (Chung *et al.*, 2007; Qiu *et al.*, 2006; Seo *et al.*, 2010; Styner *et al.*, 2006). However, some lower frequency terms may not necessarily contribute significantly in reconstructing the surfaces. So it is necessary to sparsely filter out insignificant eigenfunctions by imposing the L_1-norm penalty (Kim *et al.*, 2008; Tibshirani, 1996). For this motivation in mind, we present a new framework that sparsely filter out signal using the LB-eigenfunction expansion using the L_1-norm penalty, which is often used in compressed sensing and sparse regression.

Solving

$$\Delta \psi_j = \lambda_j \psi_j,$$

on $\mathcal{M}$, we find the eigenvalues λ_j and eigenfunctions ψ_j. The eigenfunctions ψ_j form an orthonormal basis in $L^2(\mathcal{M})$, the space of square integrable functions on $\mathcal{M}$ (Chung *et al.*, 2007; Lévy and Inria-Alice, 2006). We may order eigenvalues as

$$0 = \lambda_0 < \lambda_1 \leq \lambda_2 \cdots$$

and corresponding eigenfunctions as $\psi_0, \psi_1, \psi_2, \cdots$.

Since the closed form expression for the eigenfunctions of the LB-operator on an arbitrary curved surface is unknown, the eigenfunctions are numerically estimated by discretizing the LB-operator. Using the Cotan discretization (Chung and Taylor, 2004; Qiu *et al.*, 2006; Seo *et al.*, 2010), we obtained the eigenfunctions ψ_j. Then we can parametrically estimate the unknown mean signal θ as

$$\theta(p) = \sum_{i=0}^{k} \beta_j \psi_j,$$

where β_j is the Fourier coefficients to be estimated. Traditionally, the truncation degree k is usually low. For example, in Styner *et al.* (2006), up to degree 15 SPHARM expansions were used for hippocampus and caudate respectively The Fourier coefficients can be obtained by the usual least squares estimation (LSE) by solving

$$\mathbf{Y} = \boldsymbol{\psi}\boldsymbol{\beta}. \tag{7.36}$$

$\mathbf{Y} = (Y(p_1), \cdots, Y(p_n))'$ is the measurement at mesh vertex p_i. $\boldsymbol{\beta} = (\beta_1, \cdots, \beta_k)'$ is the Fourier coefficients. $\boldsymbol{\psi} = (\psi_i(p_j))$ is an $n \times k$ matrix of eigenfunctions evaluated at all mesh vertices. Here, the notation follows Chung *et al.* (2007). The LSE is given by

$$\widehat{\boldsymbol{\beta}} = (\boldsymbol{\psi}'\boldsymbol{\psi})^{-1}\boldsymbol{\psi}'\mathbf{Y}. \tag{7.37}$$

assuming $k \ll n$.

However, the estimation may include low degree coefficients that do not contribute significantly. Therefore, instead of using LSE, we introduce the additional L_1-norm penalty to sparsely filter out insignificant low degree coefficients by minimizing

$$||\mathbf{Y} - \boldsymbol{\psi}\beta||_2^2 + \lambda||\beta||_1, \tag{7.38}$$

where the parameter $\lambda > 0$ controls the amount of sparsity (Kim *et al.*, 2012a; Seo *et al.*, 2011a).

We have used $\lambda = 1$ for this study. This results in 73 non-zero coefficients out of 1310 in average for amygdale (5.6%), and 133 non-zero coefficients out of 2499 in average for hippocampi (5.3%). Figure 7.22 shows the comparison between LSE and the sparse estimation. The sparse method shrinks the estimated coefficients toward zero.

Basically, the sparse regression approach penalizes insignificant low degree LB-coefficients while the LSE does not. Then only about 5-6% non-zero coefficients were used to reconstruct the surface. As a result, the sparse regression smooth out the resulting statistical map whereas LSE does not. Therefore, LSE probably needs an additional pre-smoothing step to guarantee the smoothness for the random field theory.

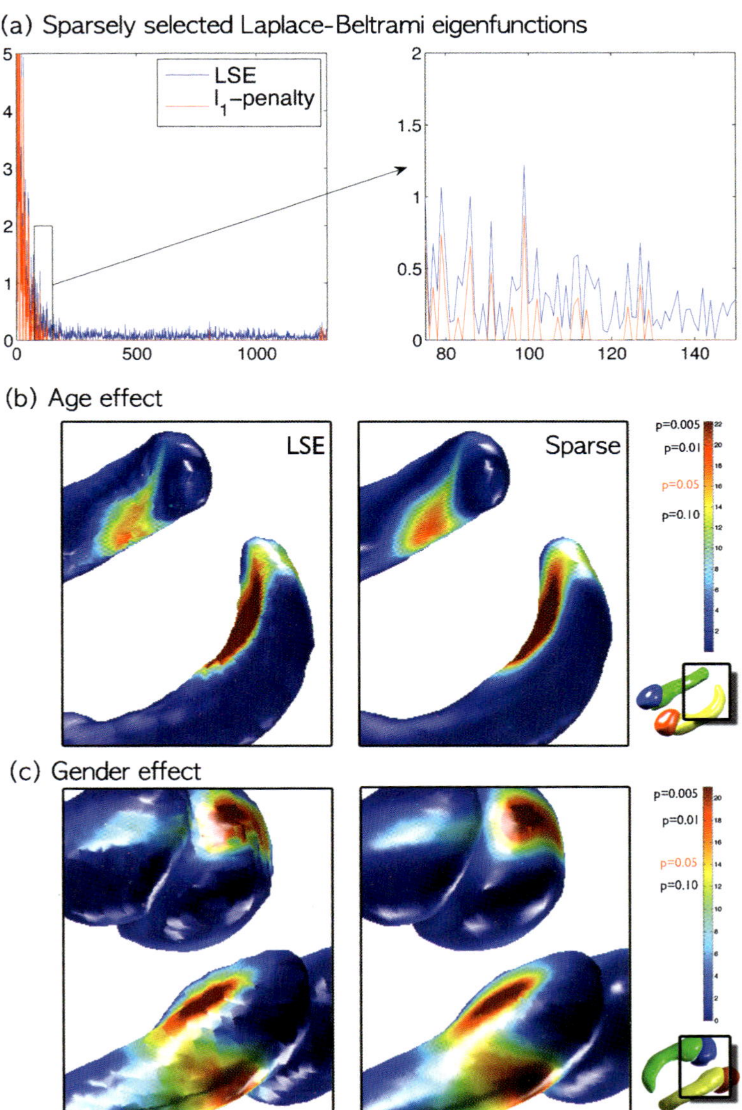

Fig. 7.22　(a) Sparsely selected Laplace-Beltrami eigenfunctions. Absolute values of the corresponding coefficients are shown. Age (b) and gender (c) effects are shown. The details of the study can be found in Kim *et al.* (2012a). The figure was generated by Seung-Goo Kim of Seoul National University.

7.7.2 *Effect of Aging on Hippocampus Shape*

The sparse shape modeling framework can be used in determining the effects of age and gender on the shape of amygdala and hippocampus. Here, we demonstrate that the proposed L_1-penalty approach can detect the localized anatomical difference within the subcortical structures while the traditional method cannot.

Image Processing. We have high-resolution T1-weighted inverse recovery fast gradient echo MRI, collected in 124 contiguous 1.2-mm axial slices (TE=1.8 ms; TR=8.9 ms; flip angle = 10°; FOV = 240 mm; 256 × 256 data acquisition matrix) of 52 middle-age and elderly adults ranging between 37 to 74 years (mean age = 55.52 ± 10.40 years). There are 16 men and 36 women in the study. Trained raters manually segmented the amygdala and hippocampus structures from T1-weighted images. Brain tissues in the MRI scans were automatically segmented using Brain Extraction Tool (BET) (Smith, 2002). Then we performed a nonlinear image registration using the diffeomorphic shape and intensity averaging technique with the cross-correlation as the similarity metric using Advanced Normalization Tools (ANTS) (Avants *et al.*, 2008). Using the deformation field obtained from warping the individual image to the template, we aligned the amygdala and hippocampus binary masks to the template space. The normalized masks were then averaged to produce the subcortical structure template. The isosurfaces of the subcortical structure template were extracted using the marching cube algorithm (Lorensen and Cline, 1987).

Surface Displacement. The displacement vector field is defined on each voxel, while the vertices of mesh are located within a voxel. So we linearly interpolated the vector field on mesh vertices from the voxels. The length of the displacement vector at each vertex is computed and used as a feature to measure the local shape variation with respect to the template space. Since the lengths of displacement defined on mesh vertices are expected to be noisy due to errors associated with image acquisition and preprocessing, it is necessary to smooth out the noise and increase the signal-to-noise ratio (SNR) (Chung *et al.*, 2003c, 2010d). Further, smoothing is desirable in satisfying the assumptions of the random field theory, which is used in correcting for multiple comparisons (Adler, 2000; Worsley *et al.*, 1996b). Gaussianness and sufficient smoothness of random fields are needed. Therefore, it is crucial so smooth the displacement along the subcotical surfaces.

Many previous surface data smoothing approaches have used heat diffusion type of smoothing to reduce surface noise (Andrade *et al.*, 2001; Chung *et al.*, 2003b; Malladi and Ravve, 2002; Perona and Malik, 1990; Sochen *et al.*, 1998; Tang *et al.*, 1999; Taubin, 2000). However, such approaches tend to have numerical instability that has been amply discussed in previous chapters.

Volume Difference. In the traditional approach, the volume of a structure is simply computed by counting the number of voxels within the binary mask. In order to account for the effect of inter-subject variability in brain size, the brain volume excluding cerebellum was estimated and covariated in a general linear models (GLM). The brain volume is significantly correlated with the amygdala (p-value < 0.0001) and the hippocampus volumes (p-value < 0.00001). Since amygdala and hippocampus volumes are related to the brain volume, it is crucial to factor out the brain volume in GLM. So we model $\mathtt{Volume}$ of amygdala and hippocampus as

$$\mathtt{Volume} = \beta_1 + \beta_2 \cdot \mathtt{Brain} + \beta_3 \cdot \mathtt{Age} + \beta_4 \cdot \mathtt{Gender} + \epsilon,$$

where $\mathtt{Brain}$ is the total brain volume, $\mathtt{Age}$ and $\mathtt{Gender}$ are age and gender of subjects. We did not find a significant age effect on the amygdala and hippocampus at $\alpha = 0.05$. However, we found a significant gender effect on the left hippocampus (p-value $= 0.04$), Since the results are based on the whole volume of the amygdala and hippocampus, it is still unclear if the there are any localized shape differences within the parts of the subcortical structures. Therefore, we performed a localized deformation-based morphometry (DBM) on the surfaces of the substructures.

Deformation-Based Surface Morphometry. The length of displacement vector field on the template surface was estimated using the sparse framework. $\mathtt{Length}$ is regressed over the total brain volume and other variables:

$$\mathtt{Length} = \beta_1 + \beta_2 \cdot \mathtt{Brain} + \beta_3 \cdot \mathtt{Age} + \beta_4 \cdot \mathtt{Gender} + \epsilon.$$

The age and gender effects were determined by testing the significance of the estimated parameters β_3 and β_4 at $\alpha = 0.05$. The results are displayed in Figure 7.22.

We found the region of significant effect of age on the posterior part of hippocampi (left: max $F = 33.5, p < 0.0002$; right: max $F = 18.5, p = 0.016$). Particularly, on the caudal regions of the left and right hippocampi, we found highly localized effect. It is consistent with other shape modeling studies on hippocampus (Qiu and Miller, 2008; Xu *et al.*, 2008). We did not find any age effects on the amygdala surface at $\alpha = 0.05$. We also found the localize regions of gender effect on the amygdalae (left max $F = 16.90, p = 0.02$; right max $F = 26.41, p < 0.001$) and the left hippocampus (max $F = 25.35, p < 0.002$).

Chapter 8

Weighted Fourier Representation

There are extensive literature on local cortical shape modeling and analysis (Chung *et al.*, 2005a; Fischl and Dale, 2000; Joshi *et al.*, 1997; Taylor and Worsley, 2008; Thompson and Toga, 1996; Lerch and Evans, 2005; Luders *et al.*, 2006b; Miller *et al.*, 2000)). The medial representation (Pizer *et al.*, 1999) has been also successfully used in modeling various subcortical structures including the cross sectional images of the corpus callosum (Joshi *et al.*, 2002), hippocampus and amygdala complex (Styner *et al.*, 2003), ventricle and brain stem (Pizer *et al.*, 1999). In the medial representation, the binary object is represented using the finite number of atoms and links that connect the atoms together to form a skeletal representation of the object. The medial representation is mainly used with the principal component analysis type of approach for shape classification and group comparison.

Unlike the medial representation, which is in a discrete representation, there is a continuous parametric approach called the spherical harmonic representation (Gerig *et al.*, 2001; Gu *et al.*, 2004; Kelemen *et al.*, 1999; Shen *et al.*, 2004). The spherical harmonic representation has been mainly used as a data reduction technique for compressing global shape features into small number of coefficients. The main global geometric features are encoded in low degree coefficients while the noise will be in high degree spherical harmonics (Gu *et al.*, 2004). The method has been used to model various subcortical structures such as ventricles (Gerig *et al.*, 2001), hippocampi (Shen *et al.*, 2004) and cortical surfaces (Chung *et al.*, 2007). The spherical harmonics have global support. So the spherical harmonic coefficients contain only the global shape features and it is not possible to directly obtain local shape information from the coefficients only. However, it is still possible to obtain local shape information by evaluating the representation at each fixed point, which gives the smoothed version of the coordinates of surfaces. In this fashion, the spherical harmonic representation can be viewed as mesh smoothing (Chung *et al.*, 2007). Instead of using the global basis of spherical harmonics, there have been attempts of using the local wavelet basis for parameterizing cortical surfaces (Nain *et al.*, 2007; Yu *et al.*, 2007).

Other shape modeling approaches include distance transforms (Leventon *et al.*, 2000), deformation fields (Miller *et al.*, 1997) obtained by warping individual substructures to a template, and the particle-based method (Cates *et al.*, 2008). A distance transform is a function that for each point in the image is equal to the distance from that point to the boundary of the object (Golland *et al.*, 2001). The distance map approach has been applied in classifying a collection of hippocampus (Golland *et al.*, 2001). The deformation fields based approach has been somewhat popular and has been applied to modeling whole 3D brain volume (Ashburner *et al.*, 1998; Chung *et al.*, 2001a; Gaser *et al.*, 1999), cortical surfaces (Chung *et al.*, 2003c; Thompson *et al.*, 2000), hippocampus (Joshi *et al.*, 1997) and cingulate gyrus (Csernansky *et al.*, 2004). The particle-based method uses a nonparametric, dynamic particle system to simultaneously sample object surfaces and optimize correspondence point positions (Cates *et al.*, 2008).

In this chapter, we presented the unified mathematical theory of the Fourier representation which encompasses the spherical harmonic representation as a special case in $\mathbb{R}^3$. The representation can be used for cortical surface parameterization, smoothing and registration in a unified Hilbert space framework. The weighted version of the Fourier representation is also developed to address many shortcomings of the traditional spherical harmonic representation (Chung *et al.*, 2007). The weighted version differs from the traditional spherical harmonic representation in many ways. Although the truncation of the series expansion in the spherical harmonic representation can be viewed as a form of smoothing, there is no direct equivalence to the full width at half maximum (FWHM) usually associated with kernel smoothing. So it is difficult to relate the unit of FWHM widely used in brain imaging to the degree of spherical harmonic representation. On the other hand, the weighted representation can easily relate to FWHM of smoothing kernel so we have a clear sense of how much smoothing we are performing beforehand. The traditional representation suffers from the Gibbs phenomenon (ringing artifacts) (Gelb, 1997) that usually happens in representing rapidly changing or discontinuous data with smooth periodic basis. The weighted representation can substantially reduce the amount of

Gibbs phenomenon by weighting the coefficients of the spherical harmonic expansion.

8.1 Fourier Series in Hilbert Space

Consider a compact differentiable manifold $\mathcal{M} \in \mathbb{R}^d$ that will be our anatomical object of interest. Let $L^2(\mathcal{M})$ be the space of square integrable functions in $\mathcal{M}$ with inner product

$$\langle g_1, g_2 \rangle = \int_{\mathcal{M}} g_1(p)g_2(p)\, d\mu(p), \tag{8.1}$$

where μ is the Lebegue measure such that $\mu(\mathcal{M})$ is the total volume of $\mathcal{M}$. The norm $\| \cdot \|$ is defined as

$$\|g\| = \langle g, g \rangle^{1/2}.$$

The partial differential operator $\mathcal{L}$ is *self-adjoint* if

$$\langle g_1, \mathcal{L}g_2 \rangle = \langle \mathcal{L}g_1, g_2 \rangle$$

for all $g_1, g_2 \in L^2(\mathcal{M})$. The eigenvalues λ_j and eigenfunctions ψ_j of the operator $\mathcal{L}$ are obtained by solving

$$\mathcal{L}\psi_j = \lambda_j \psi_j. \tag{8.2}$$

Without the loss of generality, we can order eigenvalues

$$0 = \lambda_0 < \lambda_1 \leq \lambda_2 \leq \cdots$$

and make the eigenfunctions to be orthonormal with respect to the inner product (8.1).

Let $\mathcal{H}_k$ be the subspace

$$\mathcal{H}_k = \Big\{ \sum_{j=0}^{k} \beta_j \psi_j(p) : \beta_j \in \mathbb{R} \Big\} \subset L^2(\mathcal{M}),$$

which is spanned by the finite number of basis up to degree k. We are interested in finding a function $h \in \mathcal{H}_k$ that is the closest to f in L_2-norm. Obviously, from the property of Hilbert space $L^2(\mathcal{M})$, we have

$$\sum_{j=0}^{k} f_j \psi(p) = \arg \min_{h \in \mathcal{H}} \|f - h\|^2,$$

where $f_j = \langle f, \psi_j \rangle$ are Fourier coefficients. Figure 8.1 shows an example of representing amygdala surface coordinates using the Fourier series expansion with the spherical harmonic basis.

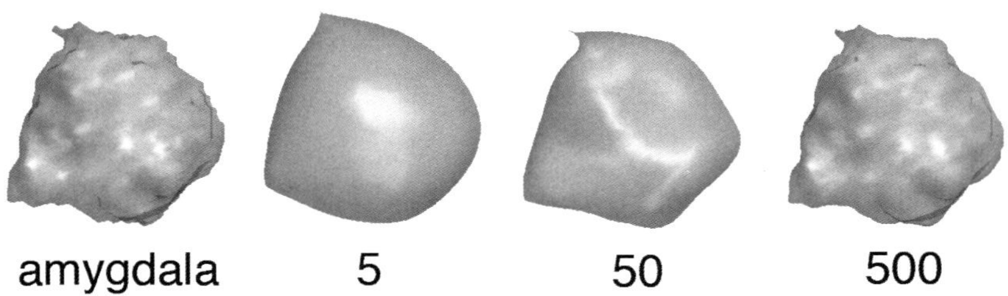

Fig. 8.1   Fourier representation of left amygdala using the Laplace-Beltrami eigenfunctions. The geometric feature of sharp corner at the top is preserved in the representations. This is possibly caused by segmentation and need to be reduced by mesh smoothing.

There are three main methods for computing Fourier coefficients.

(1) The first method numerically integrates the Fourier coefficients over a high resolution triangle mesh (Chung, 2006). Although this approach is the simplest to implement numerically and possibly the most accurate, the computation is extremely slow, due to the brute force nature of the technique. This is not a recommended approach.

(2) The second method is based on the fast Fourier transform (FFT) (Bulow, 2004; Gu *et al.*, 2004). The drawback of FFT is the need for a predefined regular grid system so if the mesh topology is different for different surfaces, a time consuming interpolation is needed. Cortical meshes obtained from FreeSurfer (Fischl and Dale, 2000) produces topologically different meshes for different subjects so FFT is also not recommended.

(3) The third method is based on solving a system of linear equations (Gerig *et al.*, 2001; Shen *et al.*, 2004; Shen and Chung, 2006) in a least squares fashion. This is the most widely used numerical technique in the spherical harmonic representation literature. However, the direct application of the least squares estimation is not desirable when the size of the linear equation is extremely large.

For extremely large least squares problems, new iterative strategies such as the *iterative residual fitting* (IRF) is required (Chung *et al.*, 2007). Suppose f is observed at the finite number of points $p_1, \cdots, p_n \in \mathcal{M}$. Then we wish to find $h \in \mathcal{H}_k$ that minimizes the sum of the squared distance

$$\|f - h\|^2 \approx \sum_{i=1}^{n} \left[f(p_i) - \sum_{j=0}^{k} \beta_j \psi_j(p_i) \right]^2. \tag{8.3}$$

The minimum of (8.3) is obtained when

$$f(p_i) = \sum_{j=0}^{k} \beta_j \psi_j(p_i), i = 1, \cdots, n \tag{8.4}$$

The equation (8.4) is referred as the *normal equation* and is usually solved by matrix inversion as follows. Let $f = (f(p_1), \cdots, f(p_n))'$ and $\beta = (\beta_0, \cdots, \beta_k)'$. Also let

$$\Psi = \begin{bmatrix} \psi_0(p_1) & \cdots & \psi_k(p_1) \\ \vdots & \ddots & \vdots \\ \psi_0(p_n) & \cdots & \psi_k(p_n) \end{bmatrix}$$

be a $n \times (k+1)$ matrix consisting of basis functions evaluated at mesh vertices. Then (8.4) can be rewritten in the following matrix form:

$$f = \Psi\beta. \tag{8.5}$$

The solution of the matrix equation is

$$\beta = (\Psi'\Psi)^{-}\Psi'f, \tag{8.6}$$

where $(\Psi'\Psi)^{-}$ is the generalized inverse. The problem with this widely used formulation is that the size of the matrix Ψ can be fairly large and for very large n and k. So it may become impractical to perform matrix operation (8.6) directly. This is mainly true for FreeSurfer (Fischl and Dale, 2000) which produces more than $200,000$ nodes for each cortical hemisphere. This computational bottleneck can be overcome by breaking the least squares problem in the subspace $\mathcal{H}_k$ into smaller subspaces using the IRF-algorithm (Shen and Chung, 2006; Chung *et al.*, 2007).

8.2　Weighted Fourier Representation

The *weighed Fourier representation* generalizes the usual Fourier representation with additional exponential weights. This new representation is both a global hierarchical parameterization and an explicit data smoothing technique formulated as a solution to a self-adjoint partial differential equation (PDE). The exponentially decaying weights make the representation converges faster and reduce the Gibbs phenomenon (ringing artifacts) significantly (Gelb, 1997). When the self-adjoint operator $\mathcal{L}$ is the Laplace-Beltrami operator, the representation becomes heat kernel smoothing (Chung *et al.*, 2007).

8.2.1 *Cauchy Problem*

Consider a Cauchy problem

$$\frac{\partial g}{\partial \sigma} + \mathcal{L}g = 0, \, g(p, \sigma = 0) = f(p). \tag{8.7}$$

The initial functional data $f(p)$ can be further stochastically modeled as

$$f(p) = \eta(p) + \epsilon(p), \tag{8.8}$$

where ϵ is a mean zero Gaussian random field and η is the unknown signal to be estimated. The partial differential equation (8.7) diffuses initial data f over time and the solution is given as the estimate for η. The time σ controls the amount of smoothing and will be termed as the *bandwidth*. Using the eigenfunctions (9.10), the unique solution to equation (8.7) is given by

$$g(p, \sigma) = \sum_{j=0}^{\infty} e^{-\lambda_j \sigma} f_j \psi_j(p) \tag{8.9}$$

with Fourier coefficients $f_j = \langle f, \psi_j \rangle$. For each fixed σ, g has expansion

$$g(p, \sigma) = \sum_{j=0}^{\infty} c_j(\sigma) \psi_j(p). \tag{8.10}$$

Substitute equation (8.10) into (8.7). Then we obtain

$$\frac{\partial c_j(\sigma)}{\partial \sigma} + \lambda_j c_j(\sigma) = 0. \tag{8.11}$$

The solution of equation (8.11) is given by $c_j(\sigma) = b_j e^{-\lambda_j \sigma}$. So we have solution

$$g(p, \sigma) = \sum_{j=0}^{\infty} b_j e^{-\lambda_j \sigma} \psi_j(p).$$

At $\sigma = 0$, we have

$$g(p, 0) = \sum_{j=0}^{\infty} b_j \psi_j(p) = f(p).$$

The coefficients b_j must be the Fourier coefficients $\langle f, \psi_j \rangle$ and this proves our claim. The solution (8.9) decreases exponentially as time σ increases and smoothes out high spatial frequency noise much faster than low frequency noise. This is the basis of many of PDE-based image smoothing methods. Partial differential equations involving self-adjoint linear partial differential operators such as the Laplace-Beltrami operator or iterated

Laplacian have been widely used in medical image analysis as a way to smooth either scalar or vector data along anatomical boundaries (Andrade *et al.*, 2001; Bulow, 2004; Cachia *et al.*, 2003a; Chung *et al.*, 2001b). These methods directly solve the PDE using standard numerical techniques such as the finite difference method or the finite element method. However, the main problem with directly solving PDE is the numerical instability and the complexity of setting up the numerical scheme.

8.2.2 *Heat Kernel Smoothing*

In Section 6.3, we have introduced heat kernel smoothing which has been numerically implemented as a sequence of iterated kernel convolutions. Heat kernel K_σ is approximated linearly using Gaussian kernel in the tangent space. This process bounds to compound the linearization error. The linearization problem can be avoided if we can determine heat kernel precisely. Motivated by the solution (8.9), we define the *weighted Fourier representation* of f as

$$\sum_{j=0}^{\infty} e^{-\lambda_j \sigma} f_j \psi_j(p). \tag{8.12}$$

By rearranging the inner product in (8.12), we have

$$\sum_{j=0}^{\infty} e^{-\lambda_j \sigma} f_j \psi_j(p) = \sum_{j=0}^{\infty} e^{-\lambda_j \sigma} \psi_j(p) \int_{\mathcal{M}} f(q) \psi_j(q) \, d\mu(q)$$

$$= \int_{\mathcal{M}} K_\sigma(p, q) f(q) \, d\mu(q)$$

with the positive definite symmetric kernel K_σ given by

$$K_\sigma(p, q) = \sum_{j=0}^{\infty} e^{-\lambda_j \sigma} \psi_j(p) \psi_j(q).$$

This shows that the solution of the Cauchy problem (8.7) can be interpreted as kernel smoothing

$$K_\sigma * f = \sum_{j=0}^{\infty} e^{-\lambda_j \sigma} f_j \psi_j(p).$$

When the differential operator $\mathcal{L} = \Delta$, the Laplace-Beltrami operator, the Cauchy problem (8.7) becomes an isotropic diffusion equation. For this particular case, K_σ is called the *heat kernel* with bandwidth σ (Chung *et al.*, 2005a; Chung, 2006). For an arbitrary cortical manifold, the basis functions ψ_j can be computed and the exact shape of heat kernel can be determined numerically. Although it can be done by setting up a huge finite element method (Qiu *et al.*, 2006), this is not a trivial numerical computation. A simpler approach is to use the first order approximation of the heat kernel for small bandwidth and iteratively apply it up to the desired bandwidth (Chung *et al.*, 2005a).

8.2.3 *Kernel Regression*

The weighted Fourier representation can be reformulated as a kernel regression problem (Fan and Gijbels, 1996). We restrict the function space $L^2(\mathcal{M})$ to a finite subspace that is more useful in numerical implementation. Let

$$\mathcal{H}_k = \left\{ \sum_{j=0}^{k} \beta_j \psi_j(p) : \beta_j \in \mathbb{R} \right\}$$

be the subspace spanned by basis $\psi_0, \cdots, \psi_l$. We claim that the k-th degree expansion of (8.12) satisfies

$$\sum_{j=0}^{k} e^{-\lambda_j \sigma} f_j \psi_j = \arg \min_{h \in \mathcal{H}_k} \int_{\mathcal{M}} \int_{\mathcal{M}} K_\sigma(p,q) \big| f(q) - h(p) \big|^2 \, d\mu(p) \, d\mu(q).$$

This can be seen by letting $h = \sum_{j=0}^{k} \beta_j \psi_j(p)$. Let the inner integral be

$$I = \int_{\mathcal{M}} K_\sigma(p,q) \Big| f(q) - \sum_{j=0}^{k} \beta_j \psi(p) \Big|^2 \, d\mu(q).$$

Simplifying the expression, we obtain

$$I = \sum_{j=0}^{k} \sum_{j'=0}^{k} \psi_j(p) \psi_{j'}(p) \beta_j \beta_{j'} - 2 K_\sigma * f(p) \sum_{j=0}^{k} \psi_j(p) \beta_j + K_\sigma * f^2.$$

Since I is an unconstrained positive semidefinite qudratic program (QP) in β_j, there is no unique global minimizer of I without additional linear constraints. Integrating I further with respect to $\mu(p)$, we collapses the QP to a positive definite QP, which yields a unique global minimizer as

$$\int_{\mathcal{M}} I \, d\mu(p) = \sum_{j=0}^{k} \beta_j^2 - 2 \sum_{j=0}^{k} e^{-\lambda_j \sigma} f_j \beta_j + \text{ const.}$$

The minimum of the above integral is obtained when all the partial derivatives with respect to β_j vanish, i.e.

$$\int_{\mathcal{M}} \frac{\partial I}{\partial \beta_j} \, d\mu(p) = 2\beta_j - 2 e^{-\lambda_j \sigma} f_j = 0$$

for all j. Hence $\sum_{j=0}^{k} e^{-\lambda_j \sigma} f_j \psi_j$ is the unique minimizer in $\mathcal{H}_k$.

We can also show that the weighted spherical harmonic representation is related to previously available surface-based isotropic diffusion smoothing (Andrade *et al.*, 2001; Cachia *et al.*, 2003a; Chung *et al.*, 2003c, 2005a). When $\mathcal{L} = \Delta$, the weighted Fourier representation (8.9) is the solution of the isotropic heat diffusion. Then from the property of the generalized Fourier series, the finite expansion is the closest to the infinite series in $\mathcal{H}_k$ in the least squares fashion (Rudin, 1991). This can be formally stated as

$$\sum_{j=0}^{k} e^{-\lambda_j \sigma} f_j \psi_j = \arg\min_{h \in \mathcal{H}_k} \|h - h_0\|,$$

where h_0 is the solution to the isotropic heat diffusion

$$\frac{\partial h_0}{\partial \sigma} = \Delta h_0, \tag{8.13}$$

with the initial value condition $h_0(p, \sigma = 0) = f(p)$ in the manifold $\mathcal{M}$.

8.2.4 *Iterative Residual Fitting Algorithm*

We present an iterative technique for solving (8.5) for extremely large number of basis k. Decompose the subspace $\mathcal{H}_k$ into smaller subspaces as the direct sum:

$$\mathcal{H}_k = \mathcal{I}_0 \oplus \mathcal{I}_1 \cdots \oplus \mathcal{I}_k,$$

where subspace $\mathcal{I}_l$ is the the projection of $\mathcal{H}_k$ along the k-th basis. Other way of decomposing $\mathcal{H}_k$ is to use more than one basis for $\mathcal{I}_l$. For instance, for the collection of spherical harmonics Y_{lm}, at each degree l, there are $2l + 1$ basis $Y_{l,-l}, \cdots, Y_{l,l}$. So we define $\mathcal{I}_l$ as the $2l + 1$ dimensional subspace generated by all l-th degree spherical harmonics. Then the algorithm estimates the Fourier coefficients β_j in each subspace $\mathcal{I}_l$ iteratively from increasing the degree from 0 to k. Suppose we estimated the coefficients up to degree $l - 1$ somehow. The estimated coefficients are denoted as $\widehat{\beta}_0, \cdots, \widehat{\beta}_{l-1}$. Then the residual r_{l-1} of the fit is given by

$$r_{l-1} = f - \sum_{j=0}^{l-1} \widehat{\beta}_j \psi_j. \tag{8.14}$$

At the next degree l, we estimate the coefficients β_l by minimizing the difference between the residual r_{l-1} and $\beta_l \psi_l$, i.e.

$$\widehat{\beta}_l = \arg\min_{\beta_l} \|r_{l-1} - \beta_l \psi_l\|^2.$$

The minimization is achieved in the least squares fashion with a smaller normal equation. Let $\Psi_l = (\psi_l(p_1), \cdots, \psi_l(p_n))'$. Then

$$\widehat{\beta}_l = (\Psi_l'\Psi_l)^{-1}\Psi_l' r_{l-1}.$$

The model for given functional data f is then $\sum_{j=0}^{l} \widehat{\beta}_j \psi_j$. In this fashion, the algorithm hierarchically builds the Fourier expansion from lower to higher degree. To speed up the computation, we can decompose $\mathcal{H}_k$ such that each subspace $\mathcal{I}_k$ is spanned by more than one basis if necessary. The iterative procedure presented here is refereed to as the *iterative residual fitting (IRF)* algorithm since we are iteratively fitting a linear equation to the residuals obtained from the previous iteration (Chung *et al.*, 2007). However, one limitation with IRF is that it was known that the stepwise regression always underestimate the Fourier coefficients in absolute value.

8.2.5 *Best Model Selection*

In many spherical harmonic representation literature (Bulow, 2004; Gerig *et al.*, 2001; Gu *et al.*, 2004; Shen and Chung, 2006; Shen *et al.*, 2004), the optimal degree is simply selected based on a pre-specified error bound that depends on the size of anatomical structure. Although increasing the degree of the representation increases the goodness-of-fit, it also increases the number of coefficients to be estimated quadratically. So it is necessary to find the optimal degree where the goodness-of-fit and the number of parameters balance out. The stepwise model selection framework offers a way to automatically determine the optimal degree (Chung *et al.*, 2007).

From (8.8), we can have

$$f(p_i) = \sum_{j=0}^{k-1} e^{-\lambda_j \sigma} \beta_j \psi_j(p_i) + \epsilon(p_i), \tag{8.15}$$

where $\epsilon(p_i)$ is a zero mean Gaussian random variable. Then we determine if adding the k-th degree terms in the $(k-1)$-th degree model (8.15) is statistically significant by testing the null hypothesis

$$H_0 : \mu_k = 0.$$

Let the k-th degree *sum of squared errors* (SSE) be

$$\mathrm{SSE}_k = \sum_{i=1}^{n} r_k^2(p_i).$$

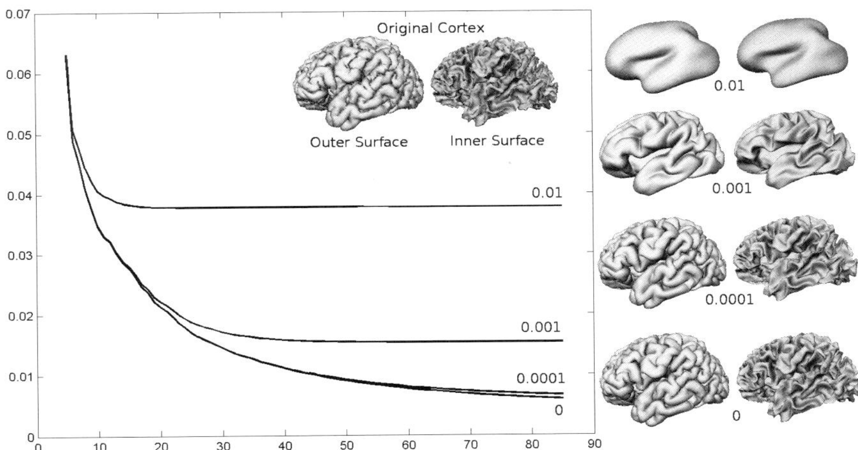

Fig. 8.2 Plots of the RMSE for the weighted spherical harmonic representation with varying σ $(0.01, 0.001, 0.0001, 0)$. When $\sigma = 0$, we have the traditional spherical harmonic representation. The cortical surfaces correspond to the 85-th degree representation. As $\sigma \to 0$, the weighed representation converges to the traditional representation.

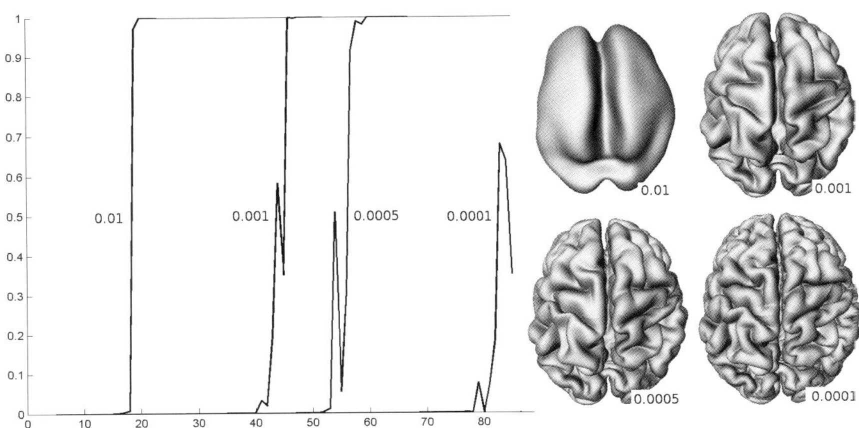

Fig. 8.3 Cortical thickness projected onto the average outer cortex for various t and corresponding optimal degree: $k = 18(t = 0.01), k = 42(t = 0.001), k = 52(t = 0.0005), k = 78(t = 0.0001)$. The average cortex is constructed by averaging the coefficients of the weighted-SPHARM. The highly noise first image shows thickness measurements obtained by computing the distance between two triangle meshes.

As the degree k increases, SSE keep decreasing until it flattens out. So it is reasonable to stop the iteration when the decrease in error is no longer significant. Figure 8.2 shows the plot of the *root mean squared errors* (RMSE), $\sqrt{\mathrm{SSE}_k/n}$. Under H_0, the test statistic is

$$F = \frac{\mathrm{SSE}_{k-1} - \mathrm{SSE}_k}{\mathrm{SSE}_{k-1}/(n-k-1)} \sim F_{1,n-k-1},$$

the F-distribution with 1 and $n-k-1$ degrees of freedom. We compute the F statistic at each degree and stop the IRF procedure if the corresponding P-value first becomes bigger than the pre-specified significance α which is usually set at 0.05 (Figures 8.2 and 8.3).

8.3 Weighted Spherical Harmonic Representation

8.3.1 *Spherical Harmonics*

The unit sphere S^2 can be parameterized by the polar angle θ and the azimuthal angel φ:

$$p = (\sin\theta\cos\varphi, \sin\theta\sin\varphi, \cos\theta) \qquad (8.16)$$

with $p = (\theta, \varphi) \in [0, \pi] \otimes [0, 2\pi)$. The spherical Laplacian Δ corresponding to the parametrization (8.16) is then given by

$$\Delta = \frac{1}{\sin\theta}\frac{\partial}{\partial\theta}\left(\sin\theta\frac{\partial}{\partial\theta}\right) + \frac{1}{\sin^2\theta}\frac{\partial^2}{\partial^2\varphi}.$$

There are $2l + 1$ eigenfunctions Y_{lm} $(-l \le m \le l)$, corresponding to the same eigenvalue $\lambda_l = l(l + 1)$ satisfying

$$\Delta Y_{lm} = \lambda_l Y_{lm}.$$

Y_{lm} is called the *spherical harmonic* of degree l and order m (Courant and Hilbert, 1953; Wahba, 1990). It is given explicitly as

$$Y_{lm} = \begin{cases} c_{lm} P_l^{|m|}(\cos\theta)\sin(|m|\varphi), & -l \le m \le -1, \\ \frac{c_{lm}}{\sqrt{2}} P_l^0(\cos\theta), & m = 0, \\ c_{lm} P_l^{|m|}(\cos\theta)\cos(|m|\varphi), & 1 \le m \le l, \end{cases}$$

where $c_{lm} = \sqrt{\frac{2l+1}{2\pi}\frac{(l-|m|)!}{(l+|m|)!}}$ and P_l^m is the associated Legendre polynomials of order m. The spherical harmonics are shown in Figure 8.4. Unlike many previous imaging literatures on spherical harmonics that used the complex-valued spherical harmonics (Bulow, 2004; Gerig *et al.*, 2001; Gu *et al.*, 2004;

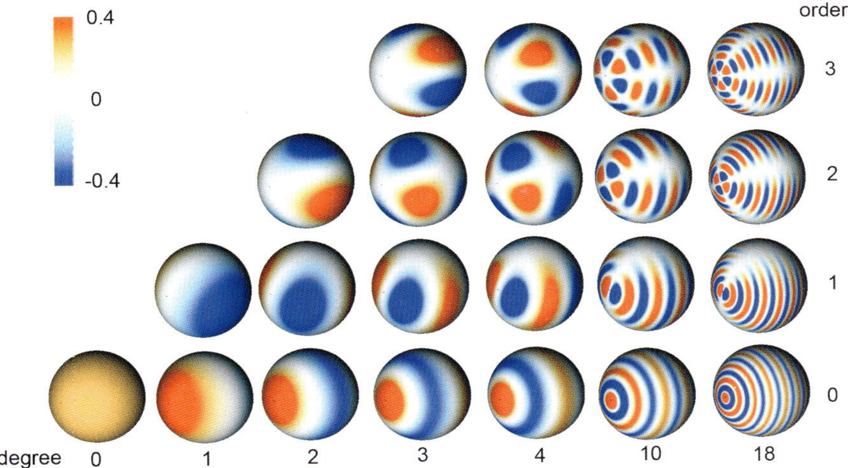

Fig. 8.4 Spherical harmonics for various degree and order. Only nonnegative orders are shown. For the l-th degree, there are $2l + 1$ different orders. Using the spherical harmonic basis, the spherical harmonic representation construct a function as a Fourier expansion.

Shen *et al.*, 2004), only real-valued spherical harmonics are used throughout the book for convenience in setting up a real-valued stochastic model.

For $f, h \in L^2(S^2)$, we define the inner product as

$$\langle f, h \rangle = \int_{\varphi=0}^{2\pi} \int_{\theta=0}^{\pi} f(p)h(p) \, d\mu(p),$$

where Lebesgue measure $d\mu(p) = \sin\theta d\theta d\varphi$. Then with respect to the inner product, the spherical harmonics satisfies the orthonormal condition

$$\int_{S^2} Y_{ij}(p)Y_{lm}(p) \, d\mu(p) = \delta_{il}\delta_{jm},$$

where δ_{il} is the Kroneker's delta.

8.3.2 *Spherical Harmonic Representation*

The spherical harmonic (SPHARM) representation (Brechbuhler *et al.*, 1995) has been applied to subcortical structures such as the hippocampus and the amygdala (Gerig *et al.*, 2001; Gu *et al.*, 2004; Kelemen *et al.*, 1999; Shen *et al.*, 2004). In particular, Gerig *et al.* (2001) used the mean squared distance (MSD) of the SPHARM coefficients in quantifying ventricle surface shape in a twin study. Shen *et al.* (2004) used the principal component analysis technique on the SPHARM coefficients of schizophrenic hippocampal surfaces in reducing the data dimension. Recently it has begun to be applied to more complex cortical surfaces (Gu *et al.*, 2004; Shen and Chung, 2006). Gu *et al.* (2004) presented SPHARM as a surface compression technique, where the main geometric features are encoded in the low degree spherical harmonics, while the noises are in the high degree spherical harmonics. In the SPHARM representation, all measurements are assigned equal weights and the coefficients of the series expansion is estimated in the least squares fashion. On the other hand, in the recently developed weighted version of SPHARM (Chung *et al.*, 2007), closer measurements are weighted more and the coefficients of the series expansion is estimated in the weighted least squares fashion. So weighted-SPHARM is more suitable than SPHARM when the realization of the cortical boundaries, as triangle meshes, are noisy and possibly discontinuous.

In SPHARM, spherical harmonics are used in constructing the Fourier series expansion of the mapping from cortical surfaces to a unit sphere. So SPHARM is more of an interpolation technique than a smoothing technique, and thus it will have the ringing artifacts (Gelb, 1997). On the other hand, the weighted version of SPHARM is a kernel smoothing technique given as a solution to a self-adjoint PDE (Chung *et al.*, 2007). The solution to the PDE is expanded in basis functions. In a similar spirit, Bulow (2004) used the spherical harmonics in isotropic heat diffusion via the Fourier transform on a unit sphere as a form of hierarchical surface representation. The weighted-SPHARM offers many advantages over the previous PDE-based smoothing techniques (Andrade *et al.*, 2001; Chung *et al.*, 2003c). The PDE-based smoothing methods tend to suffer numerical instability while the weighted-SPHARM has no such problem (Andrade *et al.*, 2001; Cachia *et al.*, 2003b,a; Chung *et al.*, 2003c). Since the traditional PDE-based smoothing gives an implicit numerical solution, setting up a statistical model is not straightforward. However, the weighted-SPHARM provides an explicit series expansion so it is easy to apply a wide variety of statistical modeling techniques such as the GLM (Friston., 2002), principal component analysis (PCA) (Shen *et al.*, 2004) and functional-PCA (Muller, 2005; Ramsay and Silverman, 1997). The SPHARM-based global parametrization is computationally expensive compared to the local quadratic polynomial fitting (Brechbuhler *et al.*, 1995; Chung *et al.*, 2003c; Dale and Fischl, 1999; Joshi *et al.*, 1995; Quicken *et al.*, 2000) while providing more accuracy and flexibility for hierarchical representation.

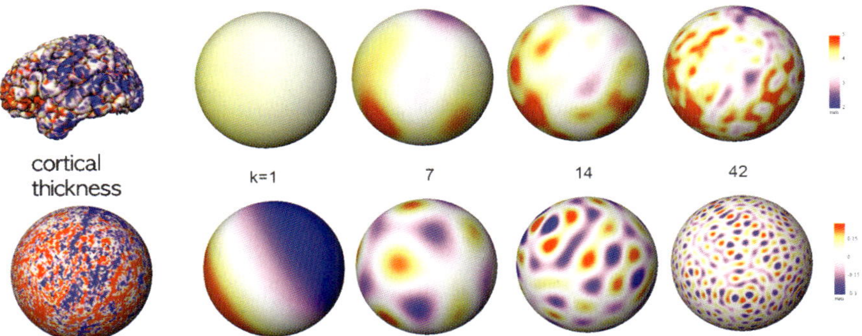

Fig. 8.5 Weighted spherical harmonic representation of cortical thickness. The second row sums all the k-th degree expansions $\sum_{m=-k}^{k} f_{km} Y_{km}$ while the first row sums up to k-th degree expansion from 0: $\sum_{l=0}^{k} e^{-l(l+1)\sigma} \sum_{m=-l}^{l} f_{lm} Y_{lm}$.

Let $\mathcal{M}$ be a cortical surface topologically equivalent to a sphere. The unit sphere S^2 is realized as a triangle mesh and deformed to match the surface in such a way that anatomical homology and the topological connectivity of meshes are preserved. The cortical surfaces can be assumed to be smooth 2-dimensional Riemannian manifolds parameterized by two parameters (Davatzikos and Bryan, 1995; Joshi *et al.*, 1995). Based on the deformable algorithm (MacDonald *et al.*, 2000) that establishes the homology between the S^2 mesh and the cortical surface, the Cartesian coordinates of the mapping are discretely parameterized by the spherical coordinates (8.16) as

$$v = (v_1(p), v_2(p), v_3(p)).$$

These discrete coordinate functions are further smoothed by the weighted-SPHARM:

$$v_i(p) = \sum_{l=0}^{k} \sum_{m=-l}^{l} e^{-l(l+1)\sigma} f_{lm}^i Y_{lm}(p). \tag{8.17}$$

In general, wiehgted-SPHARM representation can be applicable also to any scalar measurements along the cortex (Figure 8.5).

Since SPHARM is a special case when $\sigma = 0$, we will simply present a model for the weighted-SPHARM only. We model v_i stochastically as (6.3) by assuming f_{lm}^i to follow independent normal distribution $N(\mu_{lm}^i, \sigma_l^2)$ for coordinate i, degree l, and order m. This assumption is equivalent to modeling v_i as the sum of signal plus noise:

$$v_i(p) = \sum_{l=0}^{k} \sum_{m=-l}^{l} e^{-l(l+1)t} \mu_{lm}^i Y_{lm}(p) + \epsilon_i(p),$$

where ϵ_i is a zero mean Guassian random field with a certain isotropic covariance function. A similar stochastic modeling approach has been used in Miller *et al.* (1997), where the canonical expansion of a Gaussian random field is used to model the component of a deformation field.

The mean and the variance functions of the surface are then given by

$$\mathbb{E}v_i(p) = \sum_{l=0}^{k} \sum_{m=-l}^{l} e^{-l(l+1)\sigma} \mu_{lm}^i Y_{lm}(p), \tag{8.18}$$

$$\mathbb{V}v_i(p) = \sum_{l=0}^{k} \sum_{m=-l}^{l} e^{-2l(l+1)\sigma} \sigma_l^2 Y_{lm}^2(p)$$

The total variability of the surface is then measured by

$$\int_{S^2} \mathbb{V}v_i \, d\mu(p) = \sum_{l=0}^{k} \sum_{m=-l}^{l} e^{-2l(l+1)\sigma} \sigma_l^2$$

indicating the increase of smoothing bandwidth decreases the total variability. If

$$v_{ij}(\theta, \varphi) = \sum_{l=0}^{k} \sum_{m=-l}^{l} e^{-l(l+1)\sigma} f_{lm}^{ij} Y_{lm}(\theta, \varphi) \tag{8.19}$$

is the weighted-SPHARM for the j-th subject ($1 \leq j \leq s$), the unknown parameters μ_{lm}^i and σ_l^2 are estimated as the sample mean and the sample variance:

$$\widehat{\mu_{lm}^i} = \frac{1}{s} \sum_{j=1}^{n} f_{lm}^{ij}, \tag{8.20}$$

$$\widehat{\sigma_l^2} = \frac{1}{(2l+1)(s-1)} \sum_{m=-l}^{l} \sum_{j=1}^{s} (f_{lm}^{ij} - \mu_{lm}^i)^2.$$

8.3.3 *Iterative Residual Fitting on Spherical Harmonics*

For estimating the coefficients of the spherical harmonic expansion, we use the iterative residual fitting algorithm (IRF) that uses the special structure of the spherical harmonics.

For spherical harmonics, due to multiplicity, there are $2l + 1$ orthonormal basis corresponding to the l-th eigenvalue. So we can simultaneously estimate more than one coefficient at a time. The procedure is similar to estimating one coefficient at a time. Here we spell out the procedure for estimating the coefficients in the weighted Fourier representation. Suppose we have the normal equations

$$f(p_j) = \sum_{l=0}^{k} \sum_{m=-l}^{l} e^{-l(l+1)\sigma} f_{lm} Y_{lm}(p_j), \ j = 1, \cdots, n, \qquad (8.21)$$

where $f_{lm} = \langle f, Y_{lm} \rangle$. We rewrite (8.21) in the matrix form as

$$\mathbf{F} = \underbrace{\left[\mathbf{Y}_0, e^{-1(1+1)\sigma} \mathbf{Y}_1, \cdots, e^{-k(k+1)\sigma} \mathbf{Y}_k \right]}_{\mathbf{Y}} \beta, \qquad (8.22)$$

where the column vectors are

$$\mathbf{F} = \begin{pmatrix} f(p_1) \\ f(p_2) \\ \vdots \\ f(p_n) \end{pmatrix}, \beta = \begin{pmatrix} \beta_0 \\ \beta_1 \\ \vdots \\ \beta_k \end{pmatrix} \text{ and } \beta_l = \begin{pmatrix} f_{l,-l} \\ f_{l,-(l-1)} \\ \vdots \\ f_{l,l} \end{pmatrix}.$$

The length of the vector β is

$$1 + (2 \cdot 1 + 1) + \cdots + (2 \cdot k + 1) = (k+1)^2.$$

Each submatrix $\mathbf{Y}_l$ is given by

$$\mathbf{Y}_l = \begin{bmatrix} Y_{l,-l}(p_1), & \cdots & , Y_{l,l}(p_1) \\ \vdots & \ddots & \vdots \\ Y_{l,-l}(p_n), & \cdots & , Y_{l,l}(p_n) \end{bmatrix}.$$

We may tempted to directly estimate β in least squares fashion as

$$\widehat{\beta} = (\mathbf{Y}'\mathbf{Y})^{-1} \mathbf{Y}'\mathbf{F}.$$

However, since the size of matrix $\mathbf{Y}'\mathbf{Y}$ becomes $(k+1)^2 \times (k+1)^2$, for large degree k, it may be difficult to directly invert the matrix. Instead of directly solving the normal equations, we project the normal equations into a smaller subspace $\mathcal{I}_l$ and estimate $2l + 1$ coefficients in an iterative fashion.

At degree 0, we write

$$\mathbf{F} = \mathbf{Y}_0 \beta_0 + \mathbf{r}_0,$$

where $\mathbf{r}_0$ is the residual vector of estimating $\mathbf{F}$ in the subspace $\mathcal{I}_0$. Note that the residual vector $\mathbf{r}_0$ consists of residuals $r_0(p_1), \cdots, r(p_n)$. Then we estimate β_0 by minimizing the residual vector in least squares fashion:

$$\widehat{\beta}_0 = (\mathbf{Y}_0' \mathbf{Y}_0)^{-1} \mathbf{Y}_0' \mathbf{F} = \frac{\sum_{j=1}^n f(p_j) Y_{00}(p_j)}{\sum_{j=1}^n Y_{00}^2(p_j)}.$$

At degree l, we have

$$\mathbf{r}_{l-1} = e^{-l(l+1)\sigma} \mathbf{Y}_l \beta_l + \mathbf{r}_l, \tag{8.23}$$

where the residual vector $\mathbf{r}_{l-1}$ is obtained from the previous estimation as

$$\mathbf{r}_{l-1} = \mathbf{F} - \mathbf{Y}_0 \widehat{\beta}_0 \cdots - e^{-(l-1)l\sigma} \mathbf{Y}_{l-1} \widehat{\beta}_{l-1}.$$

The least squares minimization of $\mathbf{r}_l$ is then given by

$$\widehat{\beta}_l = e^{l(l+1)\sigma} (\mathbf{Y}_l' \mathbf{Y}_l)^{-1} \mathbf{Y}_l' \mathbf{r}_{l-1}.$$

The IRF-algorithm is similar to the *matching pursuit method* although they were developed independently (Mallat and Zhang, 1993). The IRF-algorithm was developed to avoid the computational burden of inverting a huge linear problem while the matching pursuit method was originally developed to compactly decompose a time frequency signal into a linear combination of pre-selected pool of basis functions called *dictionary*. In the usual least squares estimation with the design matrix Ψ of size $n \times k$ in (8.6), it is necessary to invert the $k \times k$ matrix $\Psi'\Psi$. Widely used matrix inversion algorithms such as Gauss-Jordan elimination, LU-decomposition and QR-decomposition, the running time is $\mathcal{O}(k^3) = \mathcal{O}(l^6)$, where

$$k = 1 + 3 + \cdots + 2l + 1$$

for using up to degree l (Stevens, 2003; Horn and Johnson, 1985). On the other hand, the IRF-algorithm, applied to spherical harmonics, requires to invert k number of submatrices of size $m \times m$ where $m = 1, 3, \cdots, 2l + 1$. The total running time is then

$$\mathcal{O}(1^3 + 3^3 + \cdots + (2l+1)^3) = \mathcal{O}(l^4),$$

which is a substantial reduction of running time.

In the IRF-algorithm, we minimize the residual component $\mathbf{r}_l$ in least squares fashion, i.e. minimizing the sum of squared residuals $\sum_{j=1}^n r_l^2(\Omega_j)$ over all mesh vertices. On the other hand, in the marching pursuit method, the norm $\|\mathbf{Y}_l \beta_l\|^2$ is maximized. Due to orthonormality, maximizing the norm is equivalent to minimizing the norm of the residual

$$\|\mathbf{r}_l\|^2 = \int_{\mathcal{M}} r_l^2(p) \, d\mu(p).$$

So there is a slight difference in how the residual is minimized. Although there is no limitation not to estimate multiple coefficients simultaneously in the matching pursuit method, Mallat and Zhang (1993) formulated it as the problem of estimating one coefficient at a time rather than multiple coefficients.

For the numerical implementation, the iterative residual fitting (IRF) algorithm can be used. The MATLAB codes are available at http://www.stat.wisc.edu/~mchung/softwares/weighted-SPHARM/weighted-SPHARM.html. For up to $k = 78$ degree, there are total $3(k+1)^2 = 18,723$ unknown Fourier coefficients corresponding to the three Cartesian coordinates of a cortical surface.

The IRF-algorithm result can be validated against the analytical solution of equation. For any arbitrary initial data of the form

$$f = \sum_{l=0}^{k} \sum_{m=-l}^{l} \alpha_{lm} e^{l(l+1)\sigma} Y_{lm}, \tag{8.24}$$

the weighted-SPHARM representation is given by

$$K_\sigma * f = \sum_{l=0}^{k} \sum_{m=-l}^{l} \alpha_{lm} Y_{lm}. \tag{8.25}$$

Comparing the analytical expression (8.25) to the numerical result obtained from the IRF-algorithm serves as the basis for validation. It is sufficient to use a single term in (8.24) for validation. For the initial data $f = e^{l(l+1)\sigma} Y_{lm}$, we have $K_\sigma * f = Y_{lm}$. Table 8.1 shows the comparison for various degrees and orders. The fourth column shows the mean absolute error between the theoretical value Y_{lm} and the numerical result obtained from the IRF-algorithm. The mean is taken over all mesh vertices. As expected, the mean absolute error decreases as the degree increases. For the 78th degree with $\sigma = 0.0001$, the error is smaller than 2 decimal places. We have also checked if $\langle Y_{lm}, Y_{lm} \rangle$ is close to 1 in the last column. The estimation is accurate up to 2 decimal places for all degrees. Table 8.1 shows that the IRF-algorithm provides sufficiently good numerical accuracy.

Table 8.1   The numerical accuracy of the weighted-SPHARM representation against the analytic solution f_{lm} for various bandwidth σ.

degree l	order m	bandwidth σ	mean absolute error	$\langle Y_{lm}, Y_{lm} \rangle$
18	17	0	0.0077	0.9979
18	17	0.0001	0.0078	0.9979
18	17	0.0005	0.0083	0.9981
18	17	0.01	0.0575	0.9995
42	41	0	0.0064	0.9977
42	41	0.001	0.0126	0.9992
52	51	0	0.0066	0.9972
52	51	0.0005	0.0101	0.9988
78	77	0	0.0060	0.9973
78	77	0.0001	0.0068	0.9984

8.4   Gibbs Phenomenon

The weakness of the traditional spherical harmonic representation is that it produces the Gibbs phenomenon (ringing artifacts) for discontinuous and rapidly changing continuous measurements (Gelb, 1997; Chung *et al.*, 2007). Gibbs phenomenon often arises in Fourier series expansion of discontinuous data. It is named after American physicist Josiah Willard Gibbs. In representing a piecewise continuously differentiable data using the Fourier series, the overshoot of the series happens at a jump discontinuity (Figure 8.6). The overshoot does not decease as the number of terms increases in the series expansion, and it converges to a finite limit called the Gibbs constant.

The Gibbs phenomenon was first observed by Henry Willbraham in 1848 but it did not attract any attention at that time (Wilbraham, 1848). Then a Nobel prize laureate Albert Michelson constructed an harmonic analyzer, one of the first mechanical analogue computers, that was used to plots Fourier series and observed the phenomenon. He thought the phenomenon was caused by mechanical error. Josiah W. Gibbs rediscovered the phenomenon in 1898 (Gibbs, 1898) and correctly explained the phenomenon as mathematical in 1899 (Gibbs, 1899). Later mathematician Maxime Bocher named it the Gibbs phenomenon and gave a precise mathematical analysis in 1906 (Bocher, 1906). The Gibbs phenomenon associated with spherical harmonics were first observed by Herman Weyl in 1968 (Gelb, 1997). The history and the overview of Gibbs phenomenon can be found in several literature (Foster and Richards, 1991; Jerri, 1998).

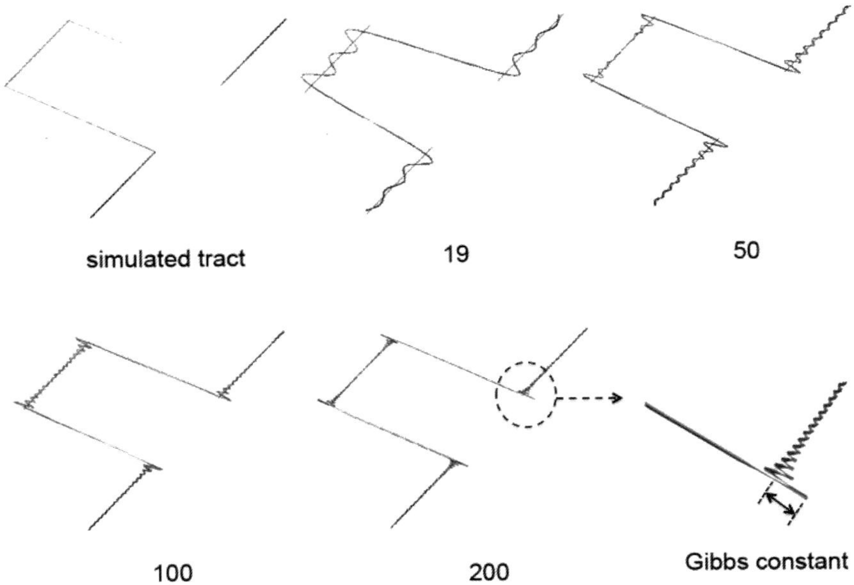

Fig. 8.6   Gibbs phenomenon on the cosine series representation of a simulated tract for degrees 19, 50, 100 and 200 (Chung *et al.*, 2010b). Increasing the number of basis does not reduce the overshoot at the corner. The maximum overshoot is proportional to Gibbs constant.

Consider the finite Fourier series expansion of 1D piecewise smooth function $f \geq 0$ with discontinuity at c given by

$$S_k(u) = \sum_{j=0}^{k} f_j \psi_j(u),$$

where $f_j = \langle f, \psi_j \rangle$. The basis is the usual sin and cosine functions. Let

$$d = \lim_{u \to c^+} f(u) - \lim_{u \to c^-} f(u) > 0$$

be the size of jump. Let $u_\circ$ be the first local maximum. Then the amount of overshoot associated with the k-th series expansion is given by

$$S_k(u_\circ) - \lim_{u \to c^+} f(u).$$

Then we can show that the limit of the overshoot is

$$\lim_{k \to \infty} S_k(u_\circ) - \lim_{u \to c^+} f(u) = \frac{d}{2}(g - 1),$$

where the Gibbs constant g is given by

$$g = \frac{2}{\pi} \int_0^\pi \frac{\sin x}{x}\, dx = 1.17897974\cdots.$$

Figure 8.6 shows the overshoot in the cosine series representation (Chung *et al.*, 2010b). In Figure 8.6, we have simulated 300 uniformly sampled control points along the parameterized curve $(x, y, z) = (t, 0, t)$ for $t \in [1, 100) \cup [200, 300)$ and $(x, y, z) = (t, 1, t)$ for $t \in [200, 300)$. The control points are fitted with the cosine representation with various degrees. As the degree increases to 200, the representation suffers from the severe ringing artifacts. The overshoot does not disappear even as the degree of expansion goes to infinity. Various neuroanatomical curvilinear structures are such as white matter fibers and corpus callosum boundaries are supposed to be smooth so we will not likely to encounter the severe Gibbs phenomenon.

8.4.1 *Reduction of Gibbs Phenomenon*

There are few available techniques for reducing Gibbs phenomenon (Brezinski, 2004; Gottlieb and Shu, 1997). Most techniques are variation on some sort of kernel methods. One of the standard method is to use the Fejer kernel which is defined as

$$K_n(u) = \frac{1}{n} \sum_{j=0}^{n-1} D_j(u),$$

where D_j is the Dirichlet kernel

$$D_j = \sum_{k=-j}^{j} e^{iku}.$$

Then it can be shown that

$$K_n(u) = \frac{1}{n}\left(\frac{\sin \frac{nu}{2}}{\sin \frac{u}{2}}\right)^2.$$

The kernel is symmetric and positive. Then we have

$$K_n * f \to f$$

for any $f \in L^2([-\pi, \pi])$ as $n \to \infty$. Since kernel is unimodal, it has the effect of smoothing the discontinuous signal f and in turn the convolution will not exhibit the ringing artifacts for sufficiently large n. Heat kernel smoothing and weighted Fourier representation behave similarly and can be used in reducing Gibbs phenomenon.

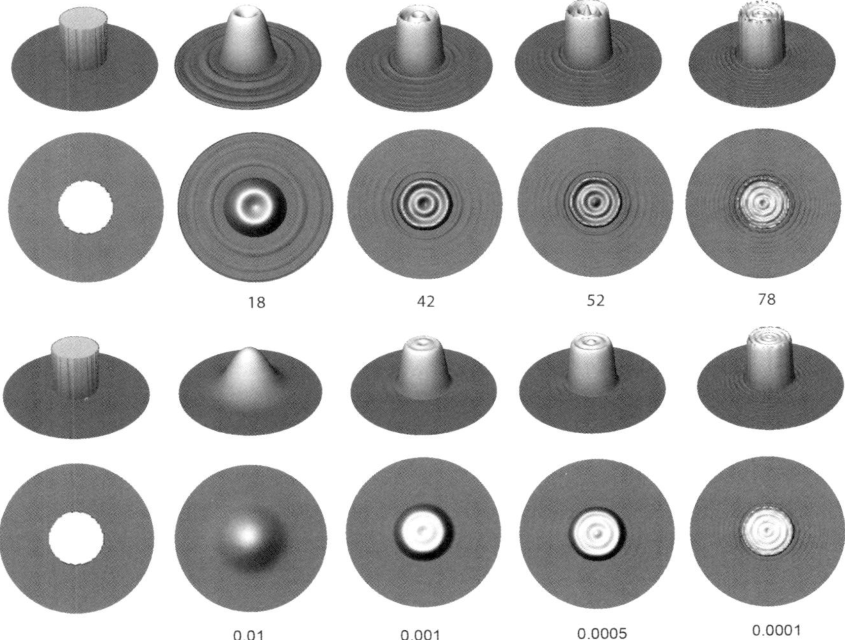

Fig. 8.7   Gibbs phenomenon on a hat shaped simulated surface. The SPHARM representation (top) of degrees 18, 42, 52 and 78 show severe ringing artifacts. One the other hand, the weighted-SPHARM representation (bottom) with bandwidths 0.01, 0.001, 0.0005, 0.0001 shows less ringing artifacts. The optimal degrees for the weighed representation is determined by the model selection procedure and found to be 18, 42, 52 and 78 respectively.

The Gibbs phenomenon will likely arise in modeling arbitrary anatomical objects with possible sharp corners. The Gibbs phenomenon can be effectively removed if the spherical harmonic representation converges faster as the degree goes to infinity. By weighting the spherical harmonic coefficients exponentially smaller, we can make the representation converges faster. This can be achieved by additionally weighting the spherical harmonic coefficients with the heat kernel. Figure 8.7 demonstrates the severe Gibbs phenomenon in the traditional spherical harmonic representation (top) on a hat shaped 2D surface. The hat shaped surface is simulated as $z = 1$ for $x^2 + y^2 < 1$ and $z = 0$ for $1 \leq x^2 + y^2 \leq 2$. On the other hand the weighted spherical harmonic representation (bottom) shows substantially reduced ringing artifacts. Due to very complex folding patterns,

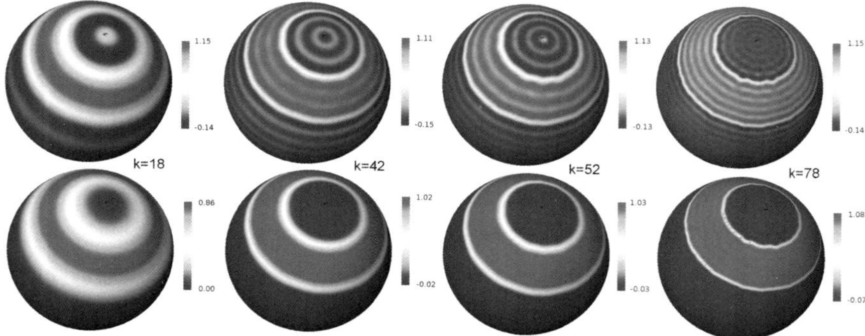

Fig. 8.8   Gibbs phenomenon in the SPHARM representation for degrees 18, 42, 52 and 78.   The traditional SPHARM (top) and the weighted representations (bottom) are performed on the discontinuous measurements on a unit sphere, which are defined as 1 in region $\frac{1}{8} < \theta < \frac{1}{4}$ and 0 in other regions. The SPHARM representation shows severe ringing artifacts while the weighted-SPHARM shows the negligible ringing effect.

sulcal regions of the brain exhibit more abrupt directional change than the simulated hat surface(upward of 180 degree compared to 90 degree in the hat surface) so there is a need for reducing the Gibbs phenomenon in the traditional spherical harmonic representation.

In Figure 8.8, a different example is given for Gibbs phenomenon. Discontinuous measurements are constructed as a step function of value 1 in the circular band $\frac{1}{8} < \theta < \frac{1}{4}$ and 0 outside of the band on a unit sphere. The SPAHRM representation of the step function resulted in significant ringing artifacts even for fairly high degrees up to $k = 78$. In comparison, the weighted-SPHARM representation does not exhibit any serious ringing artifacts. The superior performance of the weighted-SPHARM can be easily explained in terms of convergence. The weighted-SPHARM representation additionally weights Fourier coefficients with exponentially decaying weights, which contributes more rapid convergence even for discontinuous measurements. This robustness of weighted-SPHARM is also related to the fact that it is a PDE-based data smoothing technique while the traditional SPHARM is more of interpolation or reconstruction technique.

8.4.2   *The Overshoot of Gibbs Phenomenon*

The amount of the Gibbs phenomenon can be numerically quantified using the *overshoot* as the maximum of L_2 norm of the residual difference between

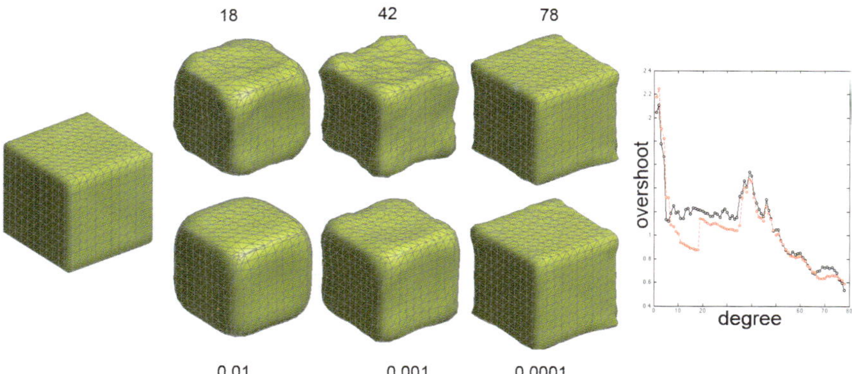

Fig. 8.9   The Gibbs phenomenon in the spherical harmonic representation (top) of a cube for degrees $k = 18, 42, 78$. The weighted spherical harmonic representation (bottom) at the same degrees but with bandwidth $\sigma = 0.01, 0.001, 0.0001$ respectively. The plots display the amount of overshoot for the traditional representation (black) vs. the weighted version (red). In almost all degrees, the traditional spherical harmonic representation shows more prominent Gibbs phenomenon compared to the weighted version.

the original and the reconstructed surface as

$$\sup_{(\theta,\varphi)\in S^2} \left\| p(\theta,\varphi) - \sum_{l=0}^{k} \sum_{m=-l}^{l} e^{-l(l+1)\sigma} f_{lm} Y_{lm}(\theta,\varphi) \right\|.$$

If surface coordinates are abruptly changing or their derivatives are discontinuous, the Gibbs phenomenon will severely distort the surface shape and the overshoot will never converge to zero. We have reconstructed a cube with various degree presentation and the bandwidth showing more ringing artifacts and overshoot in the traditional representation compared to the proposed weighted version (Figure 8.9). The exponentially decaying weights make the representation converge faster and reduce the Gibbs phenomenon significantly. The plots in Figure 8.9 display the amount of overshoot for the traditional representation (black) and the weighted version (red). The weighted spherical harmonic representation shows smaller overshoot compared to the traditional representation.

8.5   SPHARM Correspondance

Previously cortical surface normalization was performed by minimizing an objective function that measures the global fit of two surfaces while maximizing the smoothness of the deformation in such a way that the gyral patterns are matched smoothly (Chung *et al.*, 2005a; Robbins, 2003; Thompson and Toga, 1996). In the spherical harmonic representation, the surface normalization is straightforward and does not require any sort of optimization explicitly but at least requires some initial alignment. A crude alignment can be done by coinciding the first order ellipsoid meridian and equator in the SPHARM-correspondence approach (Gerig *et al.*, 2001; Styner *et al.*, 2006). For cortical meshes obtained using the anatomic segmentation using the proximities (ASP) algorithm (MacDonald *et al.*, 2000), such alignments are not needed. An approximate surface alignment is done during the cortical surface extraction process. The algorithm generates 40,962 vertices and 81,920 triangles with the identical mesh topology for all subjects. The vertices indexed identically on two cortical meshes will have a very close anatomic homology and this defines the surface alignment. This provides the same spherical parameterization at identically indexed vertices across different cortical surfaces.

Consider a surface $h = (h_1, h_2, h_3)$ obtained from the coordinates v_i measured at point p:

$$h_i(p) = \sum_{l=0}^{k} \sum_{m=-l}^{l} \langle v_i, Y_{lm} \rangle (p).$$

Consider another surface j_i obtained from coordinate functions w_i:

$$j_i(p) = \sum_{l=0}^{k} \sum_{m=-l}^{l} \langle w_i, Y_{lm} \rangle (p).$$

Suppose the surface h_i is deformed to $h_i + d_i$ under the influence of the displacement vector field d_i. We wish to find d_i that minimizes the discrepancy between $h_i + d_i$ and j_i in the finite subspace $\mathcal{H}_k$. This can be easily done by noting that

$$\sum_{l=0}^{k} \sum_{m=-l}^{l} (w_{lm}^i - v_{lm}^i) Y_{lm}(p) = \arg \min_{d_i \in \mathcal{H}_k} \left\| \widehat{h}_i + d_i - \widehat{j}_i \right\|. \qquad (8.26)$$

This implies that the optimal displacement in the least squares sense is obtained by simply taking the difference between two weighted spherical harmonic representation and matching coefficients of the same degree and order. Then a specific point $\widehat{h}_i(p_0)$ in one surface corresponds to $\widehat{j}_i(p_0)$ in the other surface. We refer to this point-to-point surface correspondence as the *spherical harmonic correspondence* (Chung *et al.*, 2007). The spherical harmonic correspondence shows that the optimal displacement in the least squares sense is obtained by simply taking the difference between two spherical harmonic representations. Unlike other surface registration methods used in warping surfaces between subjects (Chung *et al.*, 2005a; Robbins, 2003; Thompson and Toga, 1996), it is not necessary to consider an additional cost function that guarantees the smoothness of the displacement field since the displacement field $d = (d_1, d_2, d_3)$ is already a linear combination of smooth basis functions.

The previously available approaches for computing the cortical thickness in discrete triangle meshes produce noisy thickness measures (Chung *et al.*, 2005a; Fischl and Dale, 2000; MacDonald *et al.*, 2000). So it is necessary to smooth the thickness measurements along the cortex via surface-based smoothing techniques (Andrade *et al.*, 2001; Cachia *et al.*, 2003b,a; Chung *et al.*, 2003c). On the other hand, the weighted-SPHARM provides smooth functional representation of the outer and inner surfaces so that the distance measures between the surfaces should be already smooth.Hence, the weighted-SPHARM avoids the additional step of thickness smoothing done in most of thickness analysis literature (Chung *et al.*, 2005a, 2003c) while it is not necessary to perform data smoothing in the spherical harmonic formulation.

Cortical Thickness. The distance between the outer and inner cortical surfaces can be also determined using the spherical harmonic correspondence. Given the outer surface h_i and the inner surface j_i, the cortical thickness is defined to be the Euclidean distance between the two representations:

$$\texttt{thick}(p) = \sqrt{\sum_{i=1}^{3} \left[\sum_{l=0}^{k} \sum_{m=-l}^{l} \langle v_i - w_i, Y_{lm} \rangle \right]^2}.$$

A similar approach has been proposed for measuring the closeness between two surfaces (Gerig *et al.*, 2001). Figure 8.10 shows the comparison of cortical thickness computed from the traditional deformable surface algorithm (MacDonald *et al.*, 2000) and the spherical harmonic correspondence. The cortical thickness obtained from the traditional approach introduces a lot of triangle mesh noise into its estimation while the spherical harmonic correspondence approach does not. The spatial smoothness of the thickness is explicitly incorporated via the bandwidth σ.

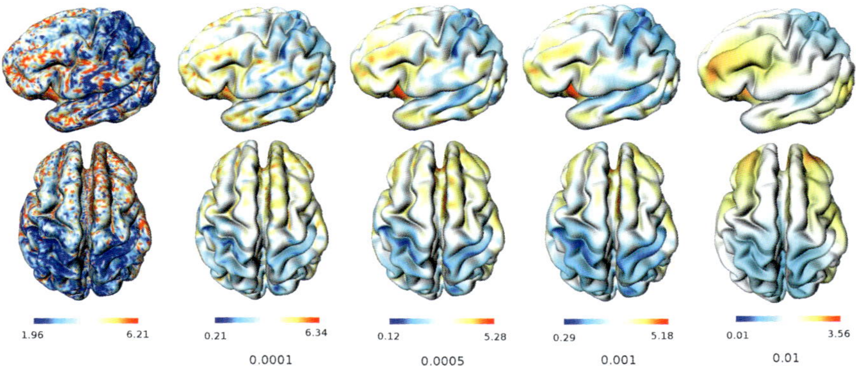

Fig. 8.10 Cortical thickness of a subject projected onto the surface template. The cortical thickness is computed from the spherical harmonic correspondence with heat kernel weights. As the bandwidth increases from $\sigma = 0.0001$ to 0.01, the amount of smoothing also increases. The first image shows the cortical thickness obtained from the traditional deformable surface algorithm (MacDonald *et al.*, 2000).

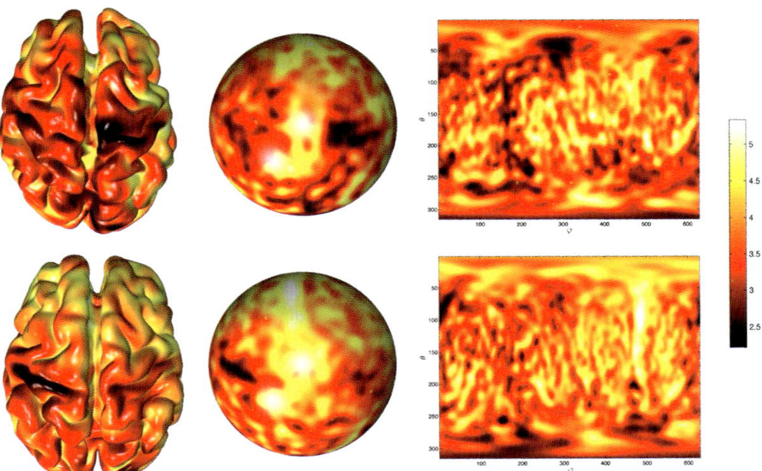

Fig. 8.11 Cortical thickness of two subjects. Cortical thickness has been smoothed using weighted-SPHARM with degree 42 and bandwidth $\sigma = 0.001$. The cortical surfaces are also smoothed using the same parameters. The cortical thickness maps can be easily projected onto a unit sphere and a rectangle using spherical harmonics.

8.6 Cortical Asymmetry

Previous neuroanatomical studies have shown left occipital and rigtht frontal lobe asymmetry, and left planum temporal asymmetry in normal controls (Barrick *et al.*, 2005; Kennedy *et al.*, 1999; Toga and Thompson, 2003). These studies mainly flip the whole brain 3D MRI to obtain the mirror reflected MRI with respect to the mid-saggital cross-section. Then the anatomical correspondence across the hemispheres is established and a subsequent statistical analysis is performed at each voxel in the 3D MRI. Although this approach is sufficient for the voxel-based morphometry (Ashburner and Friston, 2000), where we only need an approximate alignment of corresponding brain substructures, it may fail to properly align highly convoluted sulcal and gyral foldings of gray matter. In order to address this shortcoming inherent in 3D whole brain volume asymmetry analysis, we need a new 2D cortical surface based framework.

Asymmetry Index. As shown in the previous section, surface correspondence between two surfaces can be established using spherical harmonics. For asymmetry, we also need to establish hemispheric correspondence within a subject. However, it is not straightforward to establish a 2D surface-based hemispheric correspondence. Although there are many 3D volume-based brain hemisphere asymmetry analyses (Barrick *et al.*, 2005; Kennedy *et al.*, 1999), due to this simple reason, there is a lack of 2D surface-based asymmetry analyses. This will be the first unified mathematical framework on 2D cortical asymmetry. The inherent angular symmetry presented in the weighted spherical harmonic representation can be used to establish the inter-hemispheric correspondence. It turns out that the usual asymmetry index of (L-R)/(L+R) is expressed as the ratio between the sum of positive and negative order harmonics.

8.6.1 *Hemisphere Correspondence*

The spherical harmonic correspondence described in the previous section can be further used to establish the inter-hemispheric correspondence on cortical thickness. Suppose the weighted spherical harmonic representation of cortical thickness f is given by (Figure 8.11)

$$\widehat{g}(\theta, \varphi) = \sum_{l=0}^{k} \sum_{m=-l}^{l} e^{-l(l+1)\sigma} \langle f, Y_{lm} \rangle Y_{lm}(\theta, \varphi).$$

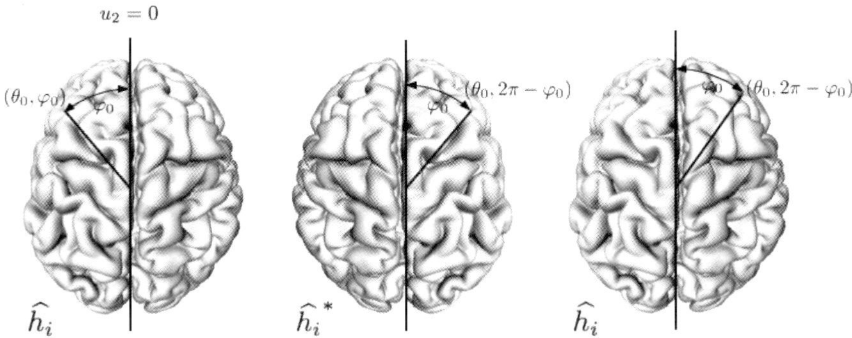

Fig. 8.12　The point $\widehat{h}_i(\theta_0, \varphi_0)$ (left) corresponds to $\widehat{h}_i^{\,*}(\theta, 2\pi - \varphi_0)$ (middle) after mirror reflection with respect to the midsaggital cross section $u_2 = 0$. From the spherical harmonic correspondence, $\widehat{h}_i^{\,*}(\theta, 2\pi - \varphi_0)$ corresponds to $\widehat{h}_i(\theta, 2\pi - \varphi_0)$ (right). This establishes the mapping from the left hemisphere to the right hemisphere in least squares fashion.

Let $\widehat{j}_i$ be the mirror reflection of $\widehat{h}_i$. The mirror reflection of $\widehat{h}_i$ with respect to the midsaggital cross section $u_2 = 0$ is simply given by

$$\widehat{j}_i(\theta, \varphi) = \widehat{h}_i^{\,*}(\theta, \varphi) = \widehat{h}_i(\theta, 2\pi - \varphi),$$

where $*$ denotes the mirror reflection operation. The specific point $\widehat{h}_i(\theta_0, \varphi_0)$ in the left hemisphere will be mirror reflected to $\widehat{j}_i(\theta_0, 2\pi - \varphi_0)$ in the right hemisphere. The spherical harmonic correspondence of $\widehat{j}_i(\theta_0, 2\pi - \varphi_0)$ is $\widehat{h}_i(\theta_0, 2\pi - \varphi_0)$. Hence, the point $\widehat{h}_i(\theta_0, \varphi_0)$ in the left hemisphere corresponds to the point $\widehat{h}_i(\theta_0, 2\pi - \varphi_0)$ in the right hemisphere. This establishes the inter-hemispheric anatomical correspondence. The schematic of obtaining this inter-hemispheric correspondence is given in Figure 8.12.

The inter-hemispheric correspondence is used to compare cortical thickness measurements f across the hemispheres. At a given position $\widehat{h}_i(\theta_0, \varphi_0)$, the corresponding cortical thickness is $\widehat{g}(\theta_0, \varphi_0)$, which should be compared with the thickness $\widehat{g}(\theta_0, 2\pi - \varphi_0)$ at position $\widehat{h}_i(\theta_0, 2\pi - \varphi_0)$:

$$\widehat{g}(\theta_0, 2\pi - \varphi_0) = \sum_{l=0}^{k} \sum_{m=-l}^{l} e^{-l(l+1)\sigma} \langle f, Y_{lm} \rangle Y_{lm}(\theta, 2\pi - \varphi). \qquad (8.27)$$

The equation (8.27) can be rewritten using the property of spherical harmonics:

$$Y_{lm}(\theta, 2\pi - \varphi) = \begin{cases} -Y_{lm}(\theta, \varphi), & -l \leq m \leq -1, \\ Y_{lm}(\theta, \varphi), & 0 \leq m \leq l, \end{cases}$$

$$\widehat{g}(\theta_0, 2\pi - \varphi_0) = \sum_{l=0}^{k} \sum_{m=-l}^{-1} e^{-l(l+1)\sigma} \langle f, Y_{lm} \rangle Y_{lm}(\theta_0, \varphi_0)$$

$$- \sum_{l=0}^{k} \sum_{m=0}^{l} e^{-l(l+1)\sigma} \langle f, Y_{lm} \rangle Y_{lm}(\theta_0, \varphi_0).$$

Symmetry Index. Comparing with the expansion for $\widehat{g}(\theta_0, \varphi_0)$, we see that the negative order terms are invariant while the positive order terms change sign. Hence we define the *symmetry index* as

$$S(\theta, \varphi) = \frac{1}{2} \left[\widehat{g}(\theta, \varphi) + \widehat{g}(\theta, 2\pi - \varphi) \right] = \sum_{l=0}^{k} \sum_{m=-l}^{-1} e^{-l(l+1)\sigma} \langle f, Y_{lm} \rangle Y_{lm}(\theta_0, \varphi_0),$$

and the *asymmetry index* as

$$A(\theta, \varphi) = \frac{1}{2} \left[\widehat{g}(\theta, \varphi) - \widehat{g}(\theta, 2\pi - \varphi) \right] = \sum_{l=0}^{k} \sum_{m=0}^{l} e^{-l(l+1)\sigma} \langle f, Y_{lm} \rangle Y_{lm}(\theta_0, \varphi_0).$$

Normalized Asymmetry Index. We normalize the asymmetry index by dividing it by the symmetry index as

$$N(\theta, \varphi) = \frac{\widehat{g}(\theta, \varphi) - \widehat{g}(\theta, 2\pi - \varphi)}{\widehat{g}(\theta, \varphi) + \widehat{g}(\theta, 2\pi - \varphi)}$$

$$= \frac{\sum_{l=1}^{k} \sum_{m=-l}^{-1} e^{-1(l+1)\sigma} \langle f, Y_{lm} \rangle Y_{lm}(\theta, \varphi)}{\sum_{l=0}^{k} \sum_{m=0}^{l} e^{-l(l+1)\sigma} \langle f, Y_{lm} \rangle Y_{lm}(\theta, \varphi)}.$$

We refer to this index as the *normalized asymmetry index* (Figure 8.13). The numerator is the sum of all negative orders while the denominator is the sum of all positive and the 0-th orders. Note that $N(\theta, 0) = N(\theta, \pi) = 0$. This index is intuitively interpreted as the normalized difference between cortical thickness in the left and the right hemispheres. Note that the larger the value of the index, the larger the amount of asymmetry. The index is invariant under the affine scaling of the human brain so it is not necessary to control for the global brain size difference in the later statistical analysis.

For each subject, its normalized asymmetry index $N(\theta, \varphi)$ is computed and modeled as a zero mean Gaussian random field. The null hypothesis is that $N(\theta, \varphi)$ is identical in the both groups for all (θ, φ), while the alternate hypothesis is that there is a specific point (θ_0, φ_0) at which the normalized asymmetry index is different. For the traditional group comparison between autistic and normal control subjects, the T statistic at each

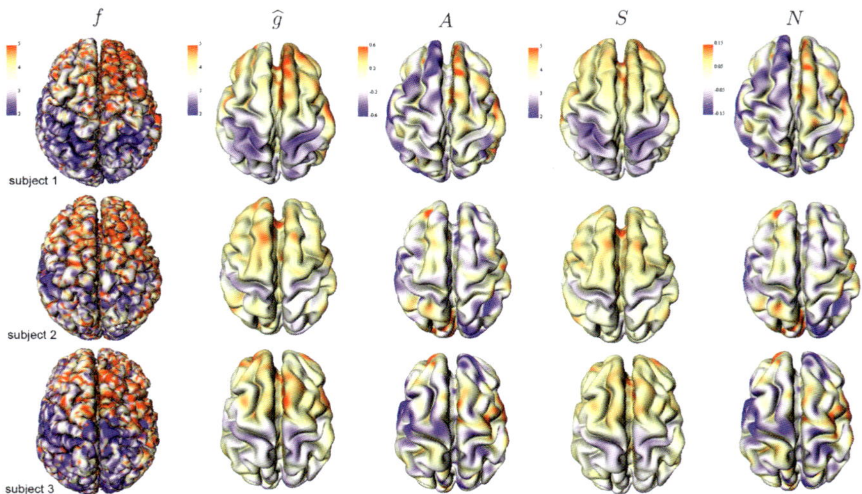

Fig. 8.13   Three representative subjects showing cortical thickness (f), the 42-th degree weighted-SPHARM representation ($\widehat{g}$), asymmetry index (A), symmetry index (S) and normalized asymmetry index (N). The cortical thickness is projected onto the original brain surface while all other measurements are projected onto the weighed-SPHARM.

point (θ, φ) would be constructed. Since T statistics at different points are correlated, it becomes a multiple comparison problem we covered in an earlier chapter (Benjamini and Hochberg, 1995; Benjamini and Yekutieli, 2001; Nichols and Hayasaka, 2003; Worsley *et al.*, 1996b). The corrected p-value accounting for spatially correlated test statistics is determined by computing the distribution of the supremum of T random field (Worsley *et al.*, 1996b), i.e.

$$P\left[\sup_{(\theta,\varphi)\in S^2} T(\theta, \varphi) > h \right]. \tag{8.28}$$

and the regions of abnormal asymmetry is localized.

8.6.2 *Abnormal Cortical Asymmetry in Autism*

Three Tesla T_1-weighted MR scans were acquired for 16 high functioning autistic and 12 control right handed males. The autistic subjects were diagnosed by a trained and certified psychologist at the Waisman center at the University of Wisconsin-Madison (Dalton *et al.*, 2005). The average ages were 17.1 ± 2.8 and 16.1 ± 4.5 for control and autistic groups respectively.

Intensity nonuniformity was corrected using a nonparametric nonuniform intensity normalization method (Sled *et al.*, 1988) and then the image was spatially normalized into the Montreal neurological institute stereotaxic space using a global affine transformation (Collins *et al.*, 1994). Afterward, an automatic tissue-segmentation algorithm based on a supervised artificial neural network classifier was used to segment gray and white matters (Kollakian, 1996).

Triangle meshes for outer cortical surfaces were obtained by a deformable surface algorithm (MacDonald *et al.*, 2000) and the mesh vertex coordinates were obtained. At each vertex, cortical thickness f was also measured. Once we obtained the outer cortical surfaces of all 28 subjects, the weighted spherical harmonic representations $\widehat{h}_i$ were constructed. We used bandwidth $\sigma = 0.001$ corresponding to $k = 42$ degrees. The normalized asymmetry index is used in localizing the regions of cortical asymmetry difference between the two groups. These normalized asymmetry index is projected on the average cortical surface (Figure 8.13). The average cortical surface is constructed by averaging the Fourier coefficients of all subjects within the same spherical harmonics basis following the spherical harmonic correspondence. The average surface serves as an anatomical landmark for displaying these indices as well as for projecting the final statistical analysis results in the next section.

For each subject, the normalized asymmetry index $N(\theta, \varphi)$ was computed and modeled as a Gaussian random field. The null hypothesis is that $N(\theta, \varphi)$ is identical in the both groups for all (θ, φ), while the alternate hypothesis is that there is a specific point (θ_0, φ_0) at which the normalized asymmetry index is different. The group difference on the normalized asymmetry index was tested using the T random field, denoted as $T(\theta, \varphi)$. Since we need to perform the test on every points on the cortical surface, it becomes a multiple comparison problem. We used the random field theory based t statistic thresholding to determine statistical significance (Worsley *et al.*, 1996b). The probability of obtaining false positives for the one-sided alternate hypothesis is given by

$$P\left[\sup_{(\theta,\varphi)\in S^2} T(\theta, \varphi) > h\right] \approx \sum_{d=0}^{2} R_d(S^2)\mu_d(h), \qquad (8.29)$$

where R_d is the d-dimensional Resel of S^2, and ρ_d is the d-dimensional Euler characteristic (EC) density of the T-field (Worsley *et al.*, 1996b), (Worsley *et al.*, 2004). The Resels are

$$R_0(S^2) = 2, R_1(S^2) = 0, R_2(S^2) = \frac{4\pi}{\text{FWHM}^2},$$

where FWHM is the full width at the half maximum of the smoothing kernel. Determining FWHM of heat kernel on a curved surface is not trivial and requires a numerical approach.

8.6.3   *FWHM of Heat Kernel*

For the random field-based inference on a sphere, it is necessary to estimate the full width at the half maximum (FWHM) of a heat kernel (Chung *et al.*, 2005a; Worsley *et al.*, 1996a). However, estimating the FWHM of the heat kernel is not trivial since there is no known close form expression for FWHM as a function of bandwidth σ on a curved surface. So it is necessary to estimate FWHM is numerically.

For $p, q, r \in S^2$, let us define the Cartesian inner product $\cdot$ as

$$p \cdot q = \cos(\theta),$$

where θ is an angle between p and q. The heat kernel (6.21) is symmetric along the geodesic circle. If $p \cdot q = p \cdot r$, we have

$$K_\sigma(p, q) = K_\sigma(p, r).$$

This property can be used to simplify the expansion (6.21) using the harmonic addition theorem (Groemer, 1996; Wahba, 1990), which states that

$$\sum_{m=-l}^{l} Y_{lm}(p) Y_{lm}(q) = \frac{2l+1}{4\pi} P_l^0(p \cdot q). \tag{8.30}$$

For any $p, q \in S^2$, the heat kernel can now be simplified as

$$K_\sigma(p, q) = \sum_{l=0}^{k} \frac{2l+1}{4\pi} e^{-l(l+1)\sigma} P_l^0(p \cdot q). \tag{8.31}$$

The expression (8.31) is used to plot the shape of the heat kernel by fixing p to be the north pole and by varying $\theta = \cos^{-1}(p \cdot q)$ (Figure 6.7). A similar result is also given in Bulow (2004).

The maximum of the heat kernel is obtained at $\theta = 0$. Then the FWHM is solved numerically for θ in the equation

$$\frac{1}{2} \sum_{l=0}^{k} \frac{2l+1}{4\pi} e^{-l(l+1)\sigma} = \sum_{l=0}^{k} \frac{2l+1}{4\pi} e^{-l(l+1)t} P_l^0(\cos\theta).$$

The FWHM is then 2θ. Figure 6.6 shows the nonlinear relationship between bandwidth σ and the corresponding FWHM. For instance, $\sigma = 0.0001$ corresponds to the FWHM of 0.0597mm.

In previous surface data smoothing techniques (Chung *et al.*, 2003c, 2005a), FWHM of between 20 to 30 mm was used for smoothing data directly along the brain surface. In our study, we used a substantially smaller FWHM since the analysis is performed on the unit sphere, which has smaller surface area. The compatible Resels of the unit sphere can be obtained by using the bandwidth of $\sigma = 0.001$, which corresponds to the FWHM of 0.0968 mm. Then, based on the formula (8.29), we computed the multiple-comparison corrected p-value and thresholded at $\alpha = 0.1$ (Figure 8.14). We found that the central sulci and the prefrontal cortex exhibits abnormal cortical asymmetry pattern in autistic subjects. The larger positive t-statistic value indicates thicker cortical thickness with respect to the corresponding thickness at the opposite hemisphere.

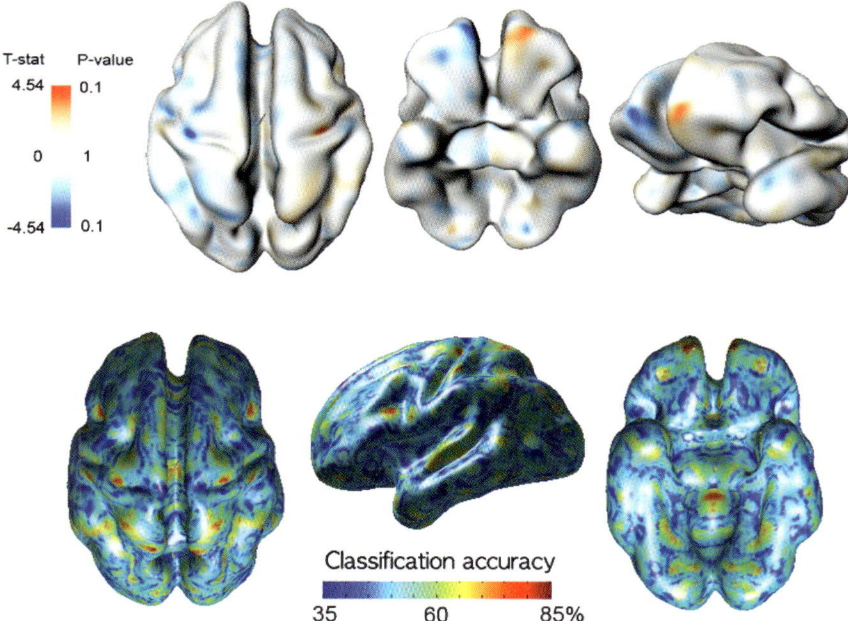

Fig. 8.14 Top: The statistically significant regions of cortical asymmetry thresholded at the corrected p-value of 0.1. The p-value has been corrected for multiple comparisons. Bottom: Classification accuracy in the logistic discriminant analysis on the normalized asymmetry index. The regions of significant regions closely match to the regions of high classification accuracy.

8.7 Logistic Discriminant Analysis on Cortical Surface

As another application of the spherical harmonic representation, we apply it to a discriminant analysis in localizing the regions of cortical asymmetry. Let us start with why the discriminant analysis is needed.

For multiple comparison corrections, it is necessary to compute the distribution of the supremum of a random field in (8.28). Unfortunately, computing the distribution of the supremum of the random field is not easy and requires satisfying many distributional assumptions that may not be true in the data. If we can come up with a different framework that does not use the traditional hypothesis testing paradigm, there is no need to compute the p-value. With this as a motivation, we can use a different approach called the *logistic discriminant analysis* that does not require computing the p-value and still be able to detect the regions of abnormal asymmetry pattern in a clinical population (Flury, 1997; Hastie *et al.*, 2003). Unlike previous discriminant techniques that tried to classify preselected feature vectors, our approach does not require any preselected feature vectors and performs the classification at each mesh vertex (Higdon *et al.*, 2004; Shen *et al.*, 2004; Thomaz *et al.*, 2006).

8.7.1 *Logistic Model*

Suppose we have p regressors $X_1, \cdots, X_p$. These can be both imaging and nonimaging biomarkers such as local area, cortical thickness, gender, age and behavioral measures at a voxel. Let $x_{i1}, \cdots, x_{ip}$ denote the measurements for the i-th subject. Let the response variable Y_i be the clinical state of the i-th subject modeled as a Bernoulli random variable with parameter π_i. $Y_i = 1$ if the i-th subject belongs to group 1 with probability π_i while $Y_i = 0$ if the subject belongs to group 2 with probability $1 - \pi_i$. π_i is the likelihood (probability) of a subject belong to the group 1, i.e. $\pi_i = P(Y_i = 1)$. For instance, Y_i can indicate the subject belongs to the elderly normal control or mild cognition impairment group respectively in an Alzheimer's disease study.

Consider a general linear model

$$Y_i = \mathbf{x}'_i \beta + \epsilon_i, \tag{8.32}$$

where

$$\mathbf{x}'_i = (1, x_{i1}, \cdots, x_{ip})$$
$$\beta' = (\beta_0, \cdots \beta_p).$$

We may assume $\mathbb{E}\epsilon_i = 0$ and $\mathbb{V}\epsilon_j = \sigma^2$. In this case, (8.32) is no longer appropriate since

$$\mathbb{E}Y_j = \pi_i = \mathbf{x}_i'\beta$$

but $\mathbf{x}_i'\beta$ may not be in the range $[0, 1]$. This inconsistency is caused by trying to match the continuous variables $x_{i1}, \cdots, x_{ip}$ to the categorical variable Y_i directly. To address this problem, we introduce the *logistic regression function g*:

$$\pi_i = g(\mathbf{x}_i) = \frac{\exp(\mathbf{x}_i'\beta_i)}{1 + \exp(\mathbf{x}_i'\beta_i)}.$$

Then using the *logit function*, we can write this as

$$\text{logit}(\pi_i) = \log \frac{\pi_i}{1 - \pi_i} = \mathbf{x}_i'\beta_i.$$

8.7.2 *Maximum Likelihood Estimation*

The unknown parameters β are estimated via the maximum likelihood estimation (MLE). The likelihood function is

$$L(\beta|y_1, \cdots, y_n) = \prod_{i=1}^{n} \pi_i^{y_i} (1 - \pi_i)^{1-y_i}$$

$$= \prod_{i=1}^{n} \left[\frac{\exp(\mathbf{x}_i'\beta_i)}{1 + \exp(\mathbf{x}_i'\beta_i)}\right]^{y_i} \prod_{i=1}^{n} \left[\frac{1}{1 + \exp(\mathbf{x}_i'\beta)}\right]^{1-y_i}.$$

The loglikelihood function is given by

$$\log L(\beta) = \text{const.} + \sum_{i=1}^{n} y_i \log \pi_i + (1 - y_i) \log(1 - \pi_i)$$

$$= \text{const.} + \sum_{i=1}^{n} y_i \mathbf{x}_i'\beta + \log(1 - \pi_i)$$

and its maximum is obtained when

$$\frac{\partial \log L(\beta)}{\partial \beta} = \sum_{i=1}^{n} \mathbf{x}_i(y_i - \pi_i) = 0.$$

In simplifying the expression, we used the following identities

$$\frac{\partial \pi_i}{\partial \beta_0} = \pi_i(1 - \pi_i)$$

and

$$\frac{\partial \pi_i}{\partial \beta_1} = x_i \pi_i(1 - \pi_i).$$

Since the logistic regression function π is in a complicated form, the maximum is obtained numerically. Define the *information matrix* to be

$$I(\beta) = -\frac{\partial^2 \log L(\beta)}{\partial \beta' \partial \beta} = \sum_{i=1}^{n} \pi_i(1 - \pi_i)\mathbf{x}_i\mathbf{x}_i'.$$

Then the Newton-Raphson algorithm is used to find the MLE in an iterative fashion. Starting with an arbitrary initial vector β^0, we estimate iteratively as

$$\beta^{j+1} = \beta^j + I(\beta^j)^{-1}\frac{\partial \log L(\beta)}{\partial \beta}(\beta^j).$$

Although we do not have the explicit formulas for the MLE, using the asymptotic normality of the MLE, the distributions of the estimators can be approximately determined. The distribution of MLE $\widehat{\beta}$ is approximately multivariate normal with means β with the covariance matrix $I(\widehat{\beta})^{-1}$.

Most statistical data analysis packages such as `R` and `MATLAB` has a built-in routine for estimating the parameters of the logistic regression.

8.7.3 *Best Model Selection*

Suppose we have the following logistic model

$$\mathrm{logit}(\pi_i) = \beta_0 + \beta_1 x_{i1} + \beta_2 x_{i2} + \cdots + \beta_p x_{ip}.$$

Among many possible logistic models over different p, we can determine the best model in the following fashion. Define the *deviance* D of a model as

$$D = -2\log L(\widehat{\pi}),$$

which is distributed asymptotically as χ^2_{n-p-1}. Let

$$\beta^{(1)} = (\beta_0, \cdots, \beta_q)'$$

and

$$\beta^{(2)} = (\beta_{q+1}, \cdots, \beta_p)'.$$

$\beta^{(1)}$ corresponds to the parameters of the *reduced model*. Then we are interested in testing $\beta^{(2)} = 0$. Let $\widehat{\pi}^{(p)}$ and $\widehat{\pi}^{(q)}$ be the estimated success probabilities for the full and reduced models. Let D_p and D_q be the associated deviances. Then the log-likelihood ratio statistic for testing $\beta^{(2)} = 0$ is

$$2(\log L(\widehat{\pi}^{(p)}) - \log L(\widehat{\pi}^{(q)})) = D_q - D_p \sim \chi^2_{p-q}.$$

Based on the χ^2-distribution, we can determine the best logistic model in a stepwise fashion.

8.7.4 Classification Accuracy

The discriminant analysis resulting from the estimated logistic model is called the *logistic discrimination*. We classify the i-th subject according to a *classification rule*. The simplest rule is to assign the i-th subject as group 1 if we have

$$P(Y_i = 1) > P(Y_i = 0).$$

This statement is equivalent to $\pi_i > 1/2$. Depending on the bias and the error of the estimation, the value $1/2$ can be adjusted. For the fitted logistic model, we classify the i-th subject as group 1 if $\mathbf{x}_i' \beta_i > 0$ and as 0 if $\mathbf{x}_i' \beta_i < 0$. The plane $\mathbf{x}_i' \beta = 0$ is the *classification boundary* that separates the two groups. The performance of classification technique is measured by the *error rate* γ, the overall probability of misclassification.

See Figure 8.15 for an example of classifying elderly controls (EC) from mild cognition impairment (MCI) subjects using the average cortical thickness and total cortical surface area.

Cross-Validation. The *cross-validation* is mainly used to estimate the error rate. This is done by randomly partitioning the data into the training and testing sets. In the *leave-one-out* scheme, the training set consists of $n - 1$ subjects while the testing set consists of one subject. Suppose the i-th subject is taken as the test set. Then using the training set, we determine the logistic model. Using the estimated model, we test if the i-th subject is correctly classified. It is classified correctly, we let the classification error $e_{-i} = 0$ and $e_{-i} = 1$ otherwise. The leave-one-out error rate is given by

$$\widehat{\gamma} = \frac{1}{n} \sum_{i=1}^{n} e_{-i}.$$

The *discriminant power* is then given as $1 - \widehat{\gamma}$. Figure 8.14 shows how to the localize the regions of abnormal asymmetry pattern in autistic subjects using the discriminant power.

p-value and Classification Accuracy. In order to show that the discriminant power can be used as an alternative to the usual *p*-value, the statistical significance of discriminant power is computed using Press's Q-statistic $n(2\widehat{\gamma} - 1)^2$, which is asymptotically distributed as χ_1^2 (Hair *et al.*, 1998). Larger discriminant power should correspond to smaller *p*-value.

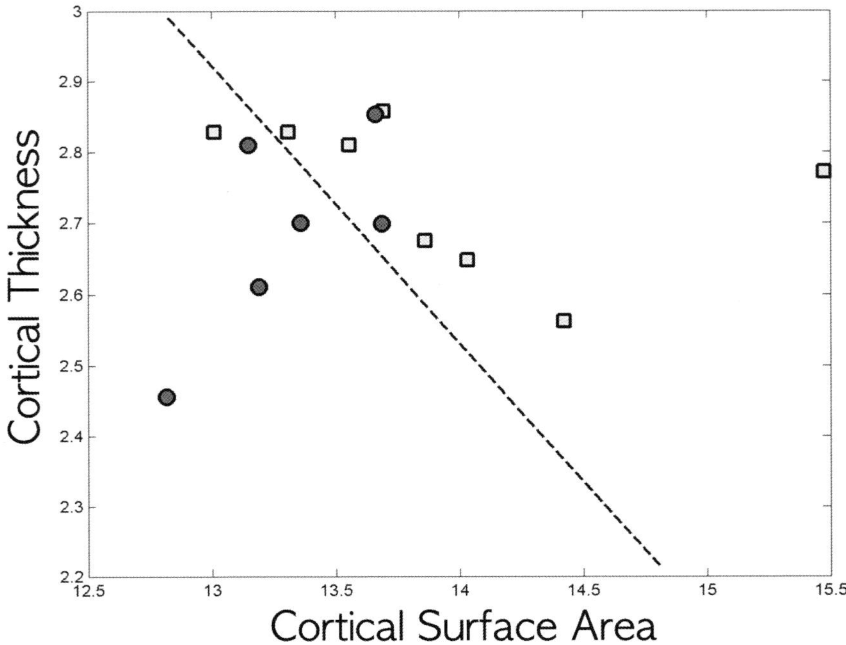

Fig. 8.15   Based on 8 elderly controls (EC) (square) and 6 mild cognition impairment (MCI) (circle) subjects, a logistic discrimination analysis was performed using the average cortical thickness and total outer cortical surface area. Using the cortical thickness alone results in 64.3% misclassification rate. On the other hand, using the both thickness and area results in significantly smaller misclassification rate of 28.6%. The rate is computed under the leave-one-out cross-validation scheme. This shows that the univariate analysis based on cortical thickness alone is not sufficient to discriminate between groups. On the other hand, analyzing data with cortical surface area reduces the error rate by 36%. Instead of performing many different univariate analyses, doing a single multivariate analysis can be a more effect way of discriminating the two groups. The dotted line in the figure is the classification boundary. The upper part is EC while the lower part is MCI. The analysis shows that EC has larger cortical surface area and cortical thickness consistent with previous literature on AD. The data is courtesy of Sterling C. Johnson of University of Wisconsin-Madison.

For instance, for $n = 28$ subjects, the discriminant power of 0.85 can correspond to the extremely small p-value of 0.0002. To account for multiple comparisons, this small p-value needed to be corrected by computing the probability of the supremum distribution of a test statistic similar to (8.28). However, this is not so trivial. On the other hand, the proposed discriminant power approach is much easier to compute numerically and interpret.

8.8 Tiling Surfaces with Orthonormal Basis

One main obstacle in building a sophisticated surface model along an arbitrary anatomical manifold is the lack of an easily available orthonormal basis. Although there are various numerical techniques available for constructing an orhonormal basis such as the Laplacian eigenfunction approach and the Gram-Smidth orthogonalization, they are computationally not so trivial and costly.

Gram-Smidth Orthogonalization. The well known Gram-Smidth orthogonalization procedure is inefficient for high resolution polygonal meshes (Gorski, 1994). In order to perform the Gram-Smidth orthogonalization as described in Gorski (1994), for a surface mesh with n vertices, we need to perform the Choleski decomposition as well as the inversion of matrix of size $n \times n$. For a cortical mesh generated with FreeSurfer (Fischl and Dale 2000), n can easily reach up to 400000.

Eigenfunctions of Laplace-Beltrami Operator. On the other hand, Qiu et al. Qiu *et al.* (2006) constructed an orthonormal basis as the eigenfunctions of the Laplace-Beltrami operator in a bounded regions of interest (ROI) on a cortical surface. The finite element method (FEM) is used to numerically construct the orthonormal basis by solving a system of large linear equations. The weakness of the FEM approach is the computational burden of inverting a matrix of size $n \times n$. One advantage of the eigenfunction approach is that since the eigenfunctions and eigenvalues are directly related to the Laplace-Beltrami operator, it is trivial and geometrically intuitive to construct the heat kernel analytically and perform a various heat kernel smoothing based modeling (Chung *et al.*, 2005a; Seo *et al.*, 2010).

Pullback Technique. In this section, we present a relatively simpler method that avoids the computational bottleneck by using a conceptually different machinery than available techniques. We assume an arbitrary manifold to be topologically equivalent to a sphere. Then we can establish a smooth mapping ζ from the manifold to the sphere using a surface flattening technique. On a unit sphere, a natural orthonormal basis is the spherical harmonics which can be easily computed. Using a smooth mapping ζ obtained we project the spherical harmonics to the anatomical surface. Obviously the projected spherical harmonics will no longer be orthonormal. However, if we correct the metric distortion introduced from the surface flattening using the Jacobian determinant, we can make the projected spherical harmonics orthonormal. This is the idea behind this simple method. The technique is very general enough that it can be applicable to other types of manifolds beyond anatomical surfaces.

8.8.1 *Orhonormal Basis on a Sphere*

It is assumed that the anatomical boundary $\mathcal{M}$ is a smooth 2-dimensional Riemannian manifold parameterized by two parameters. The one-to-one mapping ζ:

$$\zeta : \mathbf{p} = (p_1, p_2, p_3)' \in \mathcal{M} \to u = (u_1, u_2, u_3)' \in S^2,$$

can be obtained from various surface flattening techniques such as conformal mapping (Angenent *et al.*, 1999; Gu *et al.*, 2004; Hurdal and Stephenson, 2004), quasi-isometric mapping (Timsari and Leahy, 2000), area preserving mapping (Brechbuhler *et al.*, 1995; Shen *et al.*, 2004; Styner *et al.*, 2006) and the deformable surface algorithm (MacDonald *et al.*, 2000). Since the conformal mapping tend to introduce huge area distortion, most spherical harmonic literature tend to use area preserving mapping (Brechbuhler *et al.*, 1995; Shen *et al.*, 2004; Styner *et al.*, 2006).

Spherical Harmonics. Suppose a unit sphere S^2 is represented as a high resolution triangle mesh consisting of the vertex set $\mathcal{V}(S^2)$. Let us parameterize coordinates $u \in S^2$ with parameters θ, φ:

$$(u_1, u_2, u_3) = (\sin\theta\cos\varphi, \sin\theta\sin\varphi, \cos\theta),$$

where $(\theta, \varphi) \in \mathcal{N} = [0, \pi] \otimes [0, 2\pi)$. The polar angle θ is the angle from the north pole and φ is the azimuthal angle. The orthonormal basis on the unit sphere is given by the eigenfunctions of

$$\Delta f + \lambda f = 0,$$

where Δ is the spherical Laplacian. The eigenfunction Y_{lm} corresponding to the eigenvalue $l(l+1)$ is called the spherical harmonic of degree l and order m (Courant and Hilbert, 1953).

Continuous Inner Product. With respect to the inner product

$$\langle f, g \rangle_{S^2} = \int_{S^2} f(u)g(u)\, d\mu(u), \tag{8.33}$$

with measure $d\mu(u) = \sin\theta d\theta d\varphi$, Y_{lm} form the orthonormal basis in $L^2(S^2)$, the space of square integrable functions on S^2, i.e.

$$\langle Y_{lm}, Y_{l'm'}\rangle_{S^2} = \delta_{ll'}\delta_{mm'}. \tag{8.34}$$

The norm is defined as $\|f\| = \langle f, f\rangle^{1/2}$.

Discrete Inner Product. The inner product can be numerically computed as the Riemann sum over mesh vertices as

$$\langle Y_{lm}, Y_{l'm'}\rangle_{S^2} \approx \sum_{u_j \in \mathcal{V}(S^2)} Y_{lm}(u_j)Y_{l'm'}(u_j)D_{S^2}(u_j), \tag{8.35}$$

where $D_{S^2}(u_j)$ is the discrete approximation of $d\mu(u)$. Let $T_{u_j}^1, T_{u_j}^2, \cdots, T_{u_j}^{jm}$ be the area of triangles containing the vertex u_j. Then we estimate $D_{S^2}(u_j)$ as

$$D_{S^2}(u_j) = \frac{1}{3}\sum_{k=1}^{jm} T_{u_j}^k. \tag{8.36}$$

The summation is the total area of all triangles that contains vertex u_j. The discrete approximation (8.36) defines the area of triangles at a mesh vertex. The factor $1/3$ is chosen in such a way that

$$\sum_{u_j \in \mathcal{V}(S^2)} D_{S^2}(u_j) = 12.5514 = 4 \cdot 3.1378,$$

analogous to the relationship

$$\int_{S^2} d\mu(\mathbf{p}) = 4\pi.$$

The discrepancy between the integral and its discrete counter part is due to the mesh resolution and it should become smaller as the mesh resolution increases.

Based on the proposed discretization scheme, we have computed the inner product (8.35) for all degrees $0 \le l, l' \le 20$. Since for up to the k-th degree, there are total $(k+1)^2$ basis functions, we have total 441^2 possible inner product pairs, which is displayed as a matrix (Figure 8.16). For the diagonal terms, we obtained 0.9988 ± 0.0017 while for the off-diagonal terms, we have obtained 0.0000 ± 0.0005 indicating our basis and the discretization scheme is orthonormal with two decimal accuracy.

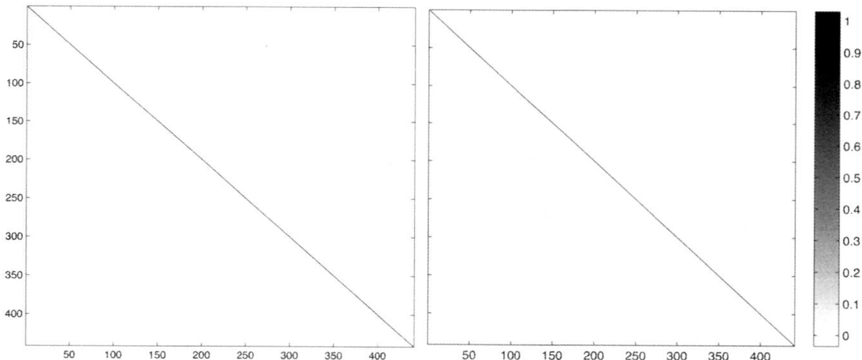

Fig. 8.16　Left: The inner products of eigenfunctions of the Laplace-Beltrami operator for every pairs. The pairs are rearranged from low to high degree. Right: The inner products of spherical harmonics computed using formula (8.33) for every pairs. The pairs are rearranged from low to high degree and order. There are total $(20 + 1)^2 = 441$ possible pairs for up to degree 20. Off-diagonal entries are not exactly zero but close to zero.

8.8.2　*Orthonormal Basis on Manifolds*

For $f, g \in L^2(\mathcal{M})$, the orthonormality is defined with respect to the inner product

$$\langle f, g \rangle_{\mathcal{M}} = \int_{\mathcal{M}} f(\mathbf{p}) g(\mathbf{p}) \, d\mu(\mathbf{p}).$$

Using the spherical harmonics in S^2, it is possible to construct an orthonormal basis in $\mathcal{M}$ numerically without the computational burden of solving the large matrix inversion associated with the eigenfunction method or the Gram-Smidth orthogonalization. Since the spherical harmonics are orthonormal in S^2 and, the manifolds S^2 and $\mathcal{M}$ can be deformed to each other by the mapping ζ, one would guess that the orthonormal basis in $\mathcal{M}$ can be obtained somehow using the spherical harmonics. Surprisingly this guess is not entirely wrong as we will show in this section.

For $f \in L^2(S^2)$, let us define the *pullback operation* $*$ as

$$\zeta^* f = f \circ \zeta.$$

While f is defined on S^2, the pullbacked function $\zeta^* f$ is defined on $\mathcal{M}$. The schematic of the pull back operation is given in Figure 8.17. Then even though we do not have orthonormality on the pullbacked spherical harmonics, i.e.,

$$\langle \zeta^* Y_{lm}, \zeta^* Y_{l'm'} \rangle_{\mathcal{M}} \neq \delta_{ll'} \delta_{mm'},$$

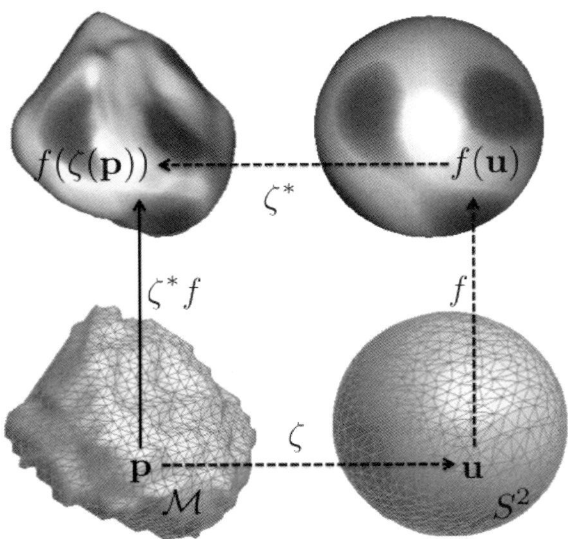

Fig. 8.17 A schematic showing how the pullback operation * is working. Point $\mathbf{p} \in \mathcal{M}$ is mapped to $u \in S^2$ via our new flattening technique. As an illustration $f = Y_{3,2} + 0.6Y_{2,1}$ is plotted on S^2. The function f is pulled back onto $\mathcal{M}$ by ζ.

we can make them orthonormal by using the Jacobian determinant of the mapping ζ somehow.

Consider the Jacobian J_ζ of the mapping $\zeta : \mathbf{p} \in \mathcal{M} \to u \in S^2$ defined as

$$J_\zeta = \frac{\partial u(\theta, \varphi)}{\partial \mathbf{p}(\theta, \varphi)}.$$

For functions $f, g \in L^2(S^2)$, we have the following change of variable relationship:

$$\int_{S^2} f \, d\mu(u) = \int_{\mathcal{M}} \zeta^* |\det J_\zeta| f \, d\mu(\mathbf{p}), \tag{8.37}$$

$$\langle f, g \rangle_{S^2} = \int_{\mathcal{M}} \zeta^* f(\mathbf{p}) \zeta^* g(\mathbf{p}) |\det J_\zeta| \, d\mu(\mathbf{p}). \tag{8.38}$$

Similarly we have the inverse relationship given as

$$\int_{\mathcal{M}} g \, d\mu(\mathbf{p}) = \int_{S^2} \zeta^{-1*} g |\det J_{\zeta^{-1}}| \, d\mu(u). \tag{8.39}$$

$$\langle \zeta^* f, \zeta^* g \rangle_{\mathcal{M}} = \int_{S^2} f(u) g(u) |\det J_{\zeta^{-1}}| \, d\mu(u). \tag{8.40}$$

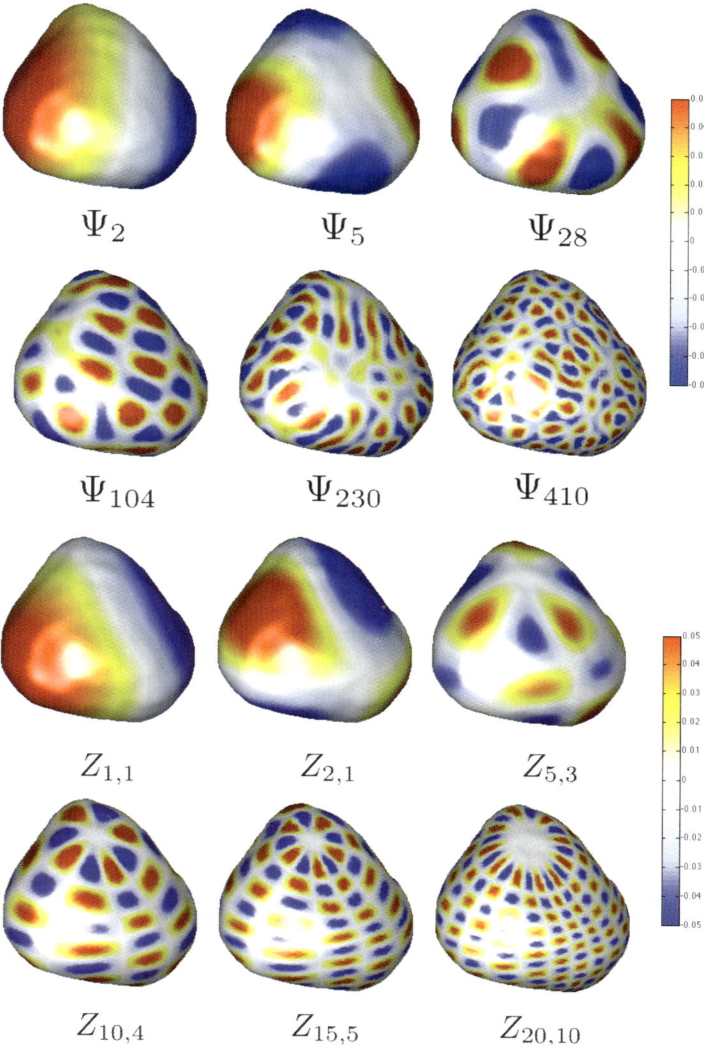

Fig. 8.18   Top: The eigenfunctions Ψ_j of the Laplace-Beltrami operator on the average amygdala surface. The eigenfunctions are provided by the courtesy of Anqi Qiu of National University of Singapore. Bottom: There can be infinitely many different orthonormal basis. A different orthonormal basis Z_{lm} is obtained by back projecting spherical harmonics onto the surface.

By letting $f = Y_{lm}$ and $g = Y_{l'm'}$ in (8.38), we obtain

$$\delta_{ll'}\delta_{mm'} = \int_{\mathcal{M}} \zeta^* Y_{lm}\zeta^* Y_{l'm'} |\det J_\zeta| \, d\mu(\mathbf{p}) \tag{8.41}$$

$$= \langle |\det J_\zeta|^{1/2}\zeta^* Y_{lm}, |\det J_\zeta|^{1/2}\zeta^* Y_{l'm'}\rangle_{\mathcal{M}}. \tag{8.42}$$

Equation (8.41) demonstrates that functions

$$Z_{lm} = |\det J_\zeta|^{1/2}\zeta^* Y_{lm} \tag{8.43}$$

are orthonormal in $\mathcal{M}$. We will refer l as degree and m as order of the basis function. Then using the Riesz-Fischer theorem (Kolmogorov and Fomin 1970), it is not hard to show that Z_{lm} form a complete basis in $L^2(\mathcal{M})$ (Figure 8.18).

In triangle meshes, the average area of adjacent triangles to a given vertex serves as the discrete estimation of the area element. The discrete estimation of the area elements would break down if the triangle mesh resolution is crude. However we are using using high resolution mesh with 2562 vertices for fairly small amygdala and a unit sphere.

8.8.3 *Numerical Implementation*

Although the expression (8.43) provides a nice analytical form for an orthonormal basis for an arbitrary manifold $\mathcal{M}$, it is not practical. If one want to use the basis (8.43), the Jacobian determinant needs to be numerically estimated somehow. We present a new discrete estimation technique for the surface Jacobian determinant that avoids estimating unstable spatial derivative estimation.

The Jacobian determinant J_ζ of the mapping ζ can be expressed in terms of the Riemannian metric tensors associated with the manifolds S^2 and $\mathcal{M}$. Consider determinants $\det g_{S^2}$ and $\det g_{\mathcal{M}}$ of the Riemannian metric tensors associated with the parameterizations $u(\theta, \varphi)$ and $\mathbf{p}(\theta, \varphi)$ respectively. Note that the integral of the area elements $\sqrt{\det g_{S^2}}$ and $\sqrt{\det g_{\mathcal{M}}}$ with respect to the parameter space $\mathcal{N}$ gives the total area of the manifolds, i.e.

$$\int_{\mathcal{N}} \sqrt{\det g_{S^2}} \, d\mu(\theta, \varphi) = 4\pi,$$

$$\int_{\mathcal{N}} \sqrt{\det g_{\mathcal{M}}} \, d\mu(\theta, \varphi) = \mu(\mathcal{M}).$$

Then we have the relationship

$$|\det J_{\zeta^{-1}}| = \frac{\sqrt{\det g_{\mathcal{M}}}}{\sqrt{\det g_{S^2}}},$$

$$|\det J_\zeta| = \frac{\sqrt{\det g_{S^2}}}{\sqrt{\det g_{\mathcal{M}}}}.$$

Note that the Jacobian determinant $\det J_\zeta$ measures the amount of contraction or expansion in the mapping ζ from $\mathcal{M}$ to S^2. So it is intuitive to have this quantity to be expressed as the ratio of the area elements. Consequently the discrete estimation of the Jacobian determinant at mesh vertex $u_j = \zeta(\mathbf{p}_j)$ is obtained as

$$|\det J_\zeta| \approx \frac{D_{S^2}(u_j)}{D_{\mathcal{M}}(\mathbf{p}_j)}.$$

Then our orthonormal basis is given by

$$Z_{lm}(\mathbf{p}_j) = \sqrt{\frac{D_{S^2}(\zeta(\mathbf{p}_j))}{D_{\mathcal{M}}(\mathbf{p}_j)}}\,\zeta^* Y_{lm}(\mathbf{p}_j). \tag{8.44}$$

The numerical accuracy can be determined by computing the inner product

$$\langle Z_{lm}, Z_{l'm'}\rangle_{\mathcal{M}} \approx \sum_{\mathbf{p}_j \in \mathcal{V}(\mathcal{M})} Z_{lm}(\mathbf{p}_j)Z_{lm}(\mathbf{p}_j)D_{\mathcal{M}}(\mathbf{p}_j).$$

$$= \sum_{\mathbf{p}_j \in \mathcal{V}(\mathcal{M})} \zeta^* Y_{lm}(\mathbf{p}_j)\zeta^* Y_{l'm'}(\mathbf{p}_j)D_{S^2}(\zeta(\mathbf{p}_j))$$

$$= \sum_{u_j \in \mathcal{V}(S^2)} Y_{lm}(u_j)Y_{l'm'}(u_j)D_{S^2}(u_j)$$

$$= \langle Y_{lm}, Y_{l'm'}\rangle_{S^2}$$

Since this is tautology, the order of the numerical accuracy in Z_{lm} is identical to that of spherical harmonics given in the previous section. There is no need for additional validation other than given in the previous section. Hence we conclude that our basis is in fact orthonormal within two decimal accuracy.

We have also constructed an orthonormal basis on a cortical surface with more than 40000 mesh vertices (Figure 8.19). The diagonal elements in the inner product matrix are 0.9999 ± 0.0001 indicating that our basis is orthonormal within three decimal accuracy. As the mesh resolution increases, we expect to have increased accuracy. The proposed orthonormal basis construction methods avoids inverting matrix of size larger than 40000×40000 associated with the eigenfunction approach and the Gram-Smidth orthogonalization process. Although the pattern of tiling in the eigenfunction approach and the pullback based method looks different (Figure 8.18), it can be shown that they are actually linearly dependent.

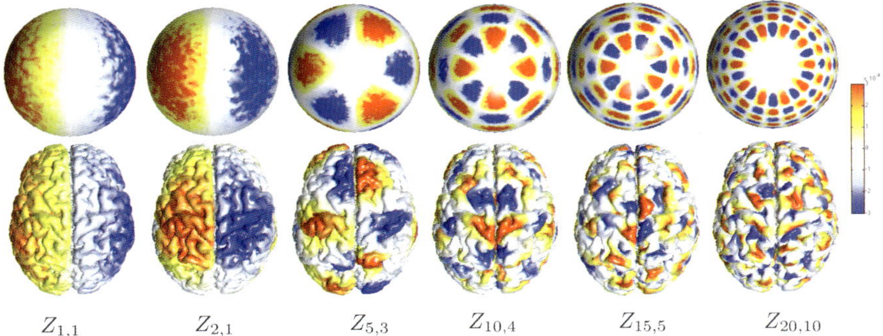

Fig. 8.19 Orthonormal basis Z_{lm} on a cortical surface. The basis is projected on a sphere to show how the nonuniformity of the Jacobian determinant is effecting the spherical harmonics Y_{lm}. The color scale is thresholded at ± 0.003 for better visualization.

8.8.4 *Pullback Representation*

As an application of the proposed basis construction technique, we present the novel *pullback representation* for parameterizing anatomical boundaries that outperforms the traditional spherical harmonic (SPHARM) representation (Brechbuhler *et al.*, 1995; Chung *et al.*, 2007; Gu *et al.*, 2004; Shen *et al.*, 2004; Styner *et al.*, 2006). The proposed representation has far less intersubject variability in the estimated parameters than SPHARM and converges faster to the true boundary with less number of basis.

The spherical harmonic (SPHARM) representation models the surface coordinates with respect to a unit sphere as

$$\mathbf{p}(\theta, \varphi) = \sum_{l=0}^{k} \sum_{m=-l}^{l} \mathbf{p}_{lm}^{0} Y_{lm}(\theta, \varphi) \tag{8.45}$$

where $\mathbf{p}_{lm}^{0} = \langle \mathbf{p}, Y_{lm} \rangle_{S^2}$ are spherical harmonic coefficients, which can be viewed as random variables. The coefficients are estimated using the iterative residual fitting algorithm that breaks a larger least squares problem into smaller ones in an iterative fashion (Chung *et al.*, 2007). The MATLAB code for performing the iterative residual fitting algorithm for arbitrary surface mesh is given in `http://www.stat.wisc.edu/~mchung/softwares/weighted-SPHARM/weighted-SPHARM.hmtl`. Note that all MRIs were reoriented to the pathological plane guaranteeing an approximate global alignment before the surface flattening to increase the robustness of the coefficient estimation.

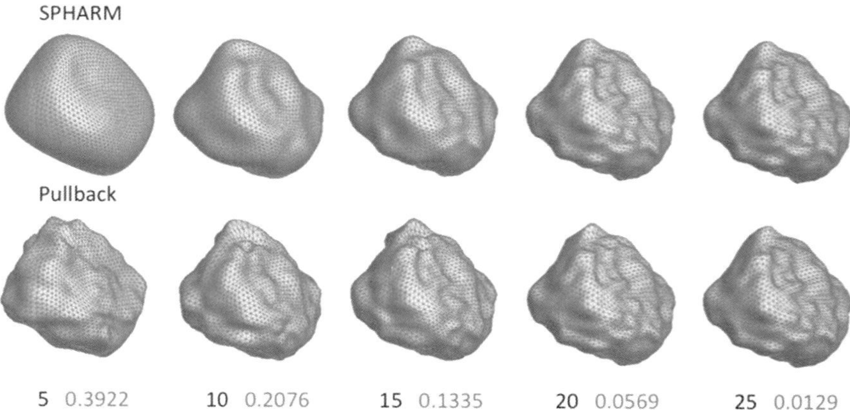

Fig. 8.20   Comparison of SPHARM and the pullback representations for degree 5 to 25. Red colored numbers are the average Euclidean distance between two representations in mm.

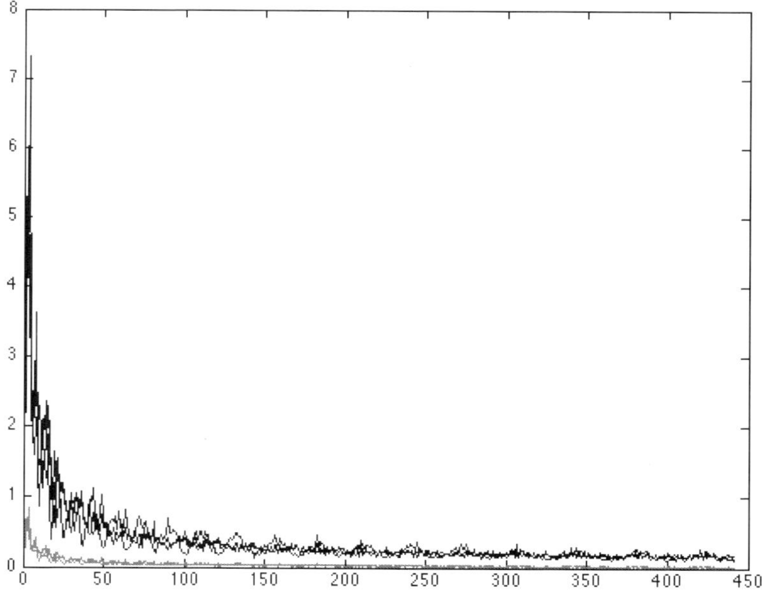

Fig. 8.21   Sample standard deviation of Fourier coefficients of for 47 subjects plotted over the index of basis. In average, the traditional SPHARM representation (black) has 88% more variability than the pull back method (gray).

The shortcoming of the spherical harmonic representation is that the reconstruction is respect to a unit sphere that is not geometrically related to the original anatomical surface. On the other hand, the pullback representation will reconstruct the surface with respect to the average template surface reducing substantial amount of variability compared to SPHARM.

In the pullback representation, we represent the surface coordinates with respect to the template surface $\mathcal{M}$ as

$$\mathbf{p}(\theta, \varphi) = \sum_{l=0}^{k} \sum_{m=-l}^{l} \mathbf{p}_{lm}^{1} Z_{lm}(\theta, \varphi) \tag{8.46}$$

with $\mathbf{p}_{lm}^{1} = \langle \mathbf{p}, Z_{lm} \rangle_{\mathcal{M}}$. Then it can be shown that the pullback representation has smaller variance in the estimated coefficients so that

$$\mathrm{Var}(\mathbf{p}_{lm}^{1}) \leq \mathrm{Var}(\mathbf{p}_{lm}^{0}). \tag{8.47}$$

The equality in (8.47) is obtained when the template $\mathcal{M}$ becomes the unit sphere, in which case the spherical mapping ζ collapses to the identity, and the inner products coincide. We have computed the sample standard deviation of Fourier coefficients for 47 subjects using the both representations. In average, the SPHARM contains 88% more intersubject variability compared to the pullback representation. This implies that SPHARM is an inefficient representation and requires more number of basis to represent surfaces compared to the pullback method.

Although the pullback method is more efficient, the both representations (8.45) and (8.46) converge to each other as k goes to infinity. We have computed the squared Euclidean distance between two representations numerically (Figure 8.20). In average, the difference is 0.0569 mm for 20 degree representation negligible for 1mm resolution MRI. Figure 8.20 also visually demonstrates that the pullback representation converges to the true manifold faster than SPHARM again showing the inefficiency of the SPHARM representation.

8.9 Basis Function Expansion on Multiple Shells

Various cortical measures such as cortical thickness are routinely computed along the vertices of cortical surface meshes. These metrics are used in surface-based morphometric studies. If one wishes to compare the surface-based morphometric studies to 3D volume-based studies at a voxel level, 3D interpolation of the sparsely sampled 2D cortical data is needed. In this section, we present a new framework for explicitly representing sparsely sampled cortical data as a linear combination of eigenfunctions of the 3D Laplacian. The eigenfunctions are expressed as the product of spherical Bessel functions and spherical harmonics. The coefficients of the expansion are estimated in the least squares fashion iteratively by breaking the problem into smaller subproblems to reduce a computational bottleneck. This section summarizes the method first published in Chung *et al.* (2009c) and later applied to the multi-shell reconstruction problem in diffusion weighted imaging (Hosseinbor *et al.*, 2011).

Cortical surfaces have been characterized by various geometric measures such as cortical thickness (Chung *et al.*, 2007; Fischl and Dale, 2000), curvatures (Cachia *et al.*, 2003a; Luders *et al.*, 2006b) and area elements (Chung *et al.*, 2003c). These measures are computed along the vertices of cortical surface meshes. After surface normalization, these measures are feed into statistical analysis pipelines. Surface specific analysis tend to sensitize surface specific tissue change and has been used frequently in quantifying the amount of gray matter change. The limitation of surface based approaches is the additional computational burden of segmenting gray matters accurately and obtaining cortical surfaces meshes.

On the other hand, the volume-based morphometric techniques such as the deformation-based morphometry (Ashburner *et al.*, 1998; Chung *et al.*, 2003c) or voxel-based morphometry (Ashburner and Friston, 2000) do not require the additional step of obtaining cortical surface meshes. If one tries to compare or combine both surface- and volume-based measures, one has to transform the measurements into a common space. Since the voxel space is more densely defined than mesh vertices, it is easier to warp volume measures to a surface. In Chung *et al.* (2007), the computation intensive nearest neighbor search algorithm (Friedman *et al.*, 1997) on an optimized k-D tree is used to compute the distance map and warp volume measures to a cortical surface mesh. If one wishes to warp surface measures such as cortical thickness to the 3D volume space, one has to interpolate voxels that the mesh vertices do not pass through.

In this section, we present a new explicit functional representation technique to address the problem of resampling sparsely sampled cortical data to a densely defined volume space. The cortical data is represented as the linear combination of basis functions, which are the eigenfunctions of the 3D Laplacian. The eigenfunctions are the product of spherical harmonics and spherical Bessel functions. Our approach should offer more unified modeling flexibility than widely used radial basis approaches (Carr *et al.*,

1997; Fornefett *et al.*, 1999) since each basis has the identical mathematical form. On the other hand, the radial basis method represent data as the linear combination of low degree polynomials and radically symmetric functions.

The eigenfunction expansion of cortical data is not a computationally easy problem due to the large number of mesh vertices upward of 700000. If one tries the traditional least squares estimation (Gerig *et al.*, 2001; Shen *et al.*, 2004), one encounters a serious computational bottleneck of solving 700000 linear equations simultaneously. Using the recently developed iterative residual fitting algorithm (Chung *et al.*, 2007), we reduce the computational burden to solving few equations at a time. Our framework is very general that it can be directly applicable to constructing the probability density function that describes water diffusion from multiple shell data without much modification in the framework (Tuch, 2004; Wu and Alexander, 2007).

8.9.1 *Eigenfunction Expansion in a Solid Ball*

Suppose the Cartesian coordinates (p_1, p_2, p_3) are given by the spherical coordinates (r, θ, φ) as

$$(p_1, p_2, p_3) = (r \sin \theta \cos \varphi, r \sin \theta \sin \varphi, r \cos \theta), \tag{8.48}$$

where $(\theta, \varphi) \in [0, \pi] \otimes [0, 2\pi)$. Define the spherical Laplacian on the unit sphere S^2 as

$$\Delta_{S^2} = \frac{1}{\sin \theta} \frac{\partial}{\partial \theta} \left(\sin \theta \frac{\partial}{\partial \theta} \right) + \frac{1}{\sin^2 \theta} \frac{\partial^2}{\partial \varphi^2}.$$

The Laplacian in the solid ball $\mathcal{M}$ of radius 1 is then defined as

$$\Delta_{\mathcal{M}} = \frac{\partial^2}{\partial r^2} + \frac{2}{r} \frac{\partial}{\partial r} + \frac{1}{r^2} \Delta_{S^2}$$

using the spherical coordinates (r, θ, φ). Consider the eigenvalue problem

$$\Delta_{\mathcal{M}} f + \lambda f = 0 \tag{8.49}$$

in the solid ball of radius 1. We may assume the additional Dirichlet boundary condition

$$f(r = 1, \theta, \varphi) = 0 \tag{8.50}$$

Substituting the separable solution of the form

$$f(r, \theta, \varphi) = g(r)h(\theta, \varphi).$$

in (8.49), we obtain

$$r^2 \frac{g''}{g} + 2r\frac{g'}{g} + r^2\lambda = -\frac{\Delta_{S^2} h}{h} = \mu$$

for some constant μ.

Spherical Harmonics. We first solve for the second equation

$$\Delta_{S^2} h + \mu h = 0. \tag{8.51}$$

The solutions to (8.51) are the spherical harmonics Y_{lm}, where l and m are called the degree and the order respectively. The explicit form for spherical harmonics is given in (Chung *et al.*, 2007). The eigenvalues are $\mu_{lm} = l(l+1)$ for $l = 0, 1, 2, \cdots$.

Bessel Functions. The first equation can be written as

$$r^2 g'' + 2rg' + [r^2\lambda - l(l+1)]g = 0. \tag{8.52}$$

If we define a new variable $g = r^{-1/2}G$, we can transform the equation to

$$r^2 G'' + rG' + \left[r^2\lambda - \left(l + \frac{1}{2}\right)^2\right]G = 0.$$

This is the scaled version of the Bessel equation and the only bounded solution at the origin is given in terms of the Bessel function of the first kind as $G(r) = J_{l+\frac{1}{2}}(\sqrt{\lambda}r)$. The solution to (8.52) is given by

$$g(r) = r^{-1/2}J_{l+\frac{1}{2}}(\sqrt{\lambda}r) \propto S_l(\sqrt{\lambda}r), \tag{8.53}$$

where $J_{l+\frac{1}{2}}$ is the Bessel function of the first. The solution is proportional to the spherical Bessel function S_l defined as

$$S_l(x) = \sqrt{\frac{\pi}{2x}}J_{l+1/2}(x).$$

The first term of the spherical Bessel function is

$$S_0(x) = \frac{\sin x}{x}.$$

Other terms are obtained recursively from

$$S_{l+1}(x) = -S'_l(x) + \frac{l}{x}S_l(x).$$

Few other terms are

$$S_1(x) = -\frac{\cos x}{x} + \frac{\sin x}{x^2},$$

$$S_2(x) = \frac{\sin x}{x} - \frac{3\cos x}{x^2} + \frac{3\sin x}{x^3}.$$

In the computer implementation of the spherical Bessel function, one may need to define $S_l(0)$. However, the built-in spherical Bessel functions in most computer programs such as `MATLAB` cause the singularity at $x = 0$. Hence we need to define $S_l(0)$ explicitly. Using the l'Hospital's rule, we have $S_0(0) = 1$ and $S_1(0) = 0$. Then using the l'Hospital's rule iteratively, we have

$$\lim_{x \to 0} S_{l+1}(x) = -\lim_{x \to 0} S'_l(x) + l \lim_{x \to 0} S'_l(x) = 0 \text{ for } l \geq 1.$$

Since the solution should satisfy the boundary condition (8.50), we should have $S_l(\sqrt{\lambda}) = 0$. We order the roots of the spherical Bessel function as

$$0 < \sqrt{\lambda_{l,1}} < \sqrt{\lambda_{l,2}} < \sqrt{\lambda_{l,3}} < \cdots .$$

For the 0-th degree, the roots are trivially given as $\sqrt{\lambda_{0,n}} = n\pi$. All higher roots are numerically estimated.

Eigenfunctions in a Sold Ball. Multiplying the spherical Bessel functions and the spherical harmonics together, the eigenfunctions to (8.49) are then given by

$$Z_{lmn}(r,\theta,\varphi) = S_l(\sqrt{\lambda_{ln}}r)Y_{lm}(\theta,\varphi).$$

Figure 8.22 shows the representative basis sampled in the cube $[-1,1]^3$ at the cross section $p_2 = 0$. These eigenfunctions from a basis within a solid sphere of radius 1. Then any function $f \in L^2(\mathcal{M})$, the space of square integrable functions, can be expanded as

$$f(r,\theta,\varphi) \approx \sum_{l=0}^{k} \sum_{m=-l}^{l} \sum_{n=1}^{j} \beta_{lmn} Z_{lmn}(r,\theta,\varphi).$$

The expansion is truncated at the degree $l = k$ and with $n = j$ roots.

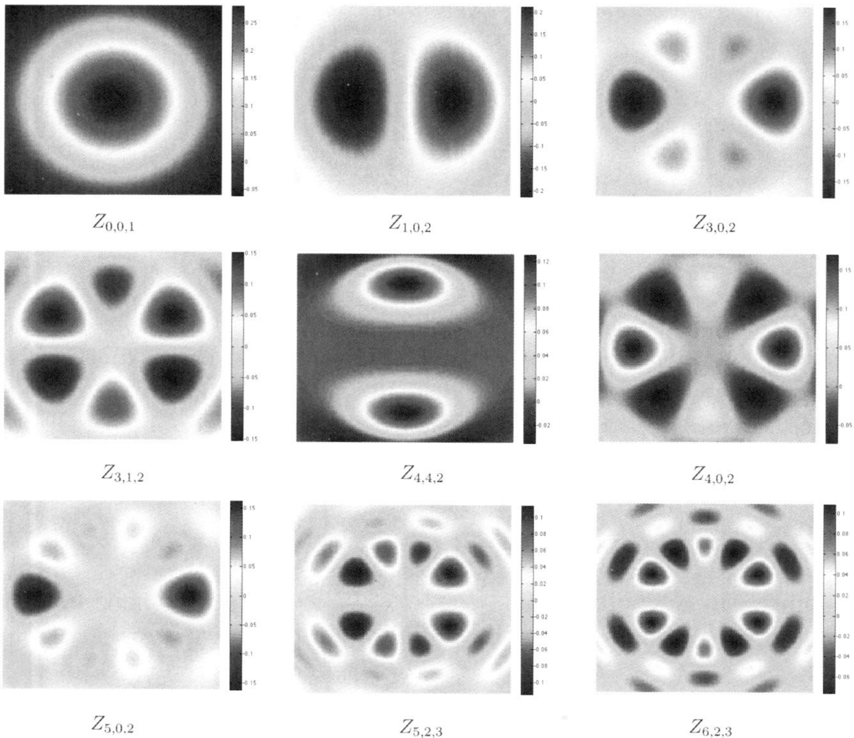

Fig. 8.22 Few Basis functions Z_{lmn} are visualized in the cube $[-1, 1]^3$. The images are the cross sections at $p_2 = 0$ The expansion is only valid within the ball of radius 1. The indices of Z_{lmn} corresponds to the spherical harmonic Y_{lm} and the n-th root of the spherical Bessel function S_l. The index n basically relates to the scale of the pattern Y_{lm} in the radial direction.

8.9.2 *Iterative Residual Fitting*

Previously the coefficients of spherical harmonic series expansion have been estimated using the least squares method by solving the system of linear equations (Chung *et al.*, 2007; Gerig *et al.*, 2001; Shen *et al.*, 2004). For a cortical surface mesh with N vertices, we need to simultaneously solve N linear equations and, in turn, invert an $N \times N$ matrix. For cortical surface meshes, N can easily reach up more than 700000 and it will not fit most computer memories. To address this computational bottleneck, we have developed the iterative residual fitting algorithm (Chung *et al.*, 2007) that divide the extremely large linear problem into manageable small subset of linear problems.

Let $p_i = (r_i, \theta_i, \varphi_i)$ be the mesh vertices where the cortical measurements f are given. We vectorize the measurement as

$$\mathbf{f} = (f(p_1), \cdots, f(p_N)).'$$

Let $\mathbf{Z}_{l,\cdot,n}$ be the $N \times (2l + 1)$ submatrix of basis given by

$$\mathbf{Z}_{l,\cdot,n} = \begin{bmatrix} Z_{l,-l,n}(p_1) & \cdots & Z_{l,l,n}(p_1) \\ \vdots & \ddots & \vdots \\ Z_{l,-l,n}(p_N) & \cdots & Z_{l,l,n}(p_N) \end{bmatrix}.$$

Denote the matrix of all basis corresponding to the l-th degree as

$$\mathbf{Z}_l = [\mathbf{Z}_{l,\cdot,1}, \cdots, \mathbf{Z}_{l,\cdot,j}].$$

Define the vector of coefficients corresponding to $\mathbf{Z}_l$ as

$$\beta_l = (\beta_{l,-l,1}, \cdots, \beta_{l,l,j})'.$$

Then we iteratively estimate the coefficients of low degrees to high degrees using the iterative algorithm.

Algorithm 8.1. Iterative Residual Fitting.

1. $l \leftarrow 0$.
2. $\mathbf{r} \leftarrow \mathbf{f}$.
3. $\beta_0 \leftarrow (\mathbf{Z}_0\mathbf{Z}_0)^{-1}\mathbf{Z}_0'\mathbf{f}$.
4. $l \leftarrow l + 1$.
5. $\mathbf{r} \leftarrow \mathbf{r} - \mathbf{Z}_{l-1}\beta_{l-1}$.
6. $\beta_l \leftarrow (\mathbf{Z}_l\mathbf{Z}_l)^{-1}\mathbf{Z}_l'\mathbf{r}$.
7. If $l \leq k$, go to Step 4.

8.9.3 *3D Resampling of 2D Surface Data*

Among various cortical measures, we have used the cortical thickness to demonstrate the proposed method. High resolution magnetic resonance images were obtained using a 3-Tesla GE SIGNA scanner. The collected images went through intensity nonuniformity correction (Sled *et al.*, 1988) and spatially normalized into the MNI stereotaxic space via a global affine transformation (Collins *et al.*, 1994). A supervised neural network classifier was used for tissue segmentation (Kollakian, 1996). Subsequently a deformable surface algorithm was used to obtain both the inner and the outer cortical surfaces that bound gray matter (MacDonald *et al.*, 2000). The cortical thickness is then defined as the distance between the two surfaces along the vertices of the cortical mesh.

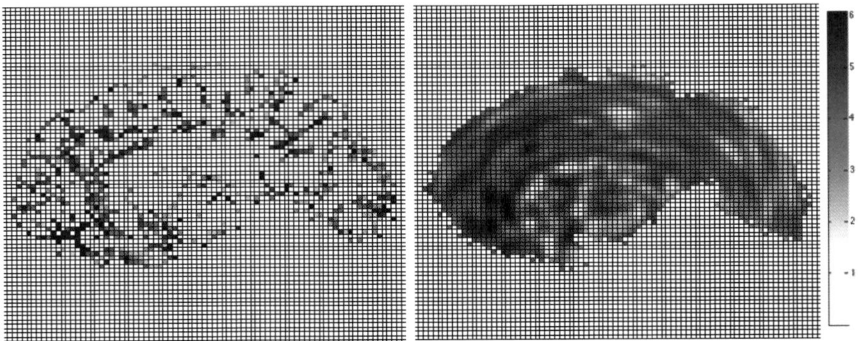

Fig. 8.23   Left: The cortical thickness defined on mesh vertices are rounded to the closest voxel. Thickness is sparsely defined. Right: Eigenfunction expansion with degree 22 and 22 roots. Only the masked brain region is shown. The representation can fill out voxels where cortical thickness is not defined.

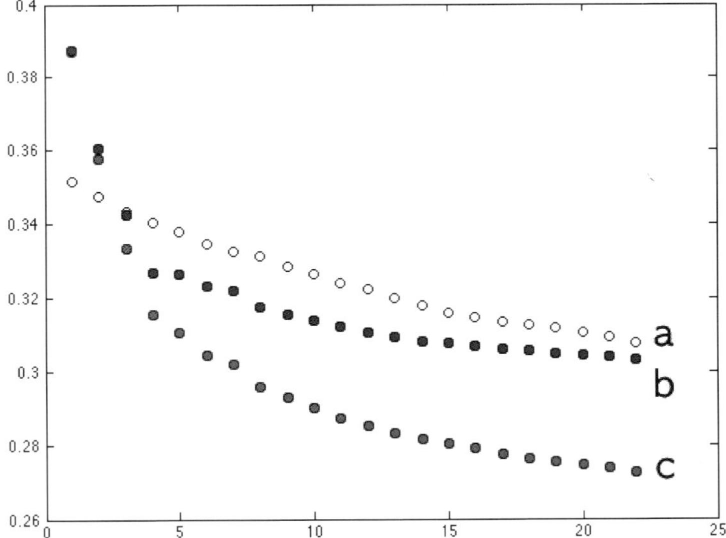

Fig. 8.24   Relative error plot of eigenfunction expansion for various number of degrees and roots. Dots are the errors for varying number of (a) degrees for the fixed number of roots $j = 5$, (b) roots at the fixed degree $k = 20$, (c) roots at the fixed degree $k = 10$. As expected, the error plots show the increasing the number of degrees and roots increases the accuracy.

Since the brain surfaces can not be contained in a ball of radius 1, we have scaled the mesh coordinates to be contained in the ball. Then we have performed the eigenfunction expansion. As the degree and the number of roots increases, the expansion should be able to represent more detailed cortical pattern. Taking the given cortical thickness as the ground truth, we have computed the average relative error between the ground truth and the representation (Figure 8.24). Increasing the number of roots and degrees decreases the discrepancy between the representation and the ground truth. Since there are so many empty voxels where cortical thickness is not defined (Figure 8.23), the effect of the eigenfunction expansion is more like low-pass filtering.

Chapter 9

Structural Brain Connectivity

The cerebral cortex is composed of many functionally and structurally distinct areas, each receiving and sending various neuronal projections from and to each other. Thus the brain forms a very complex network of connections (Young, 1992). Neuroanatomical connectivity places structural constraints on the functional connectivity of the cerebral cortex (Sporns *et al.*, 2000). Therefore, it is crucial to understand functional connectivity in relation to the underlying structural connectivity.

In the usual fMRI connectivity studies, we usually have to either manually or automatically define regions of interest (ROI) first. For instance, Anatomical Automatic Labeling (AAL) can be used to automatically identify multiple ROI in a template (Tzourio-Mazoyer *et al.*, 2002). AAL parcellation provides 45 labels for each hemisphere resulting in total 90 ROI. We then superimpose functional activation on top of ROI and set up a model of how activation in one region is related to other regions. For instance, we can set up a general linear model (GLM) of how fMRI in a ROI is dependent on all other ROI. For 90 ROI, we need to set up 90 linear models and solve them simultaneously while accounting for various covariates. From the model fit, we can obtain correlation measures which can be used to build a connectivity matrix that characterize the whole brain network. Unlike other static imaging modalities such as FDG-PET and DTI, fMRI has the temporal component so it is possible to code the cause and effect as directional information in the connectivity matrix.

Structural connectivity studies have been fairly popular in recent years due to the advancement of diffusion tensor imaging (DTI). DTI is a new imaging technique that has been used to characterize the macrostructure of biological tissues using magnitude, anisotropy and aniotropic orientation associated with water diffusion in the brain (Basser *et al.*, 1994). DTI provides directional and connectivity information that MRI usually does not provide. The white matter fibers poses a physical constrain on the movement of water molecules along the direction of fibers. It is assumed that the direction of greatest diffusivity is most likely aligned to the local orientation of the white matter fibers. White matter fibers consist mostly of myelinated axons which connect grey matter regions of the brain to each other. The axons are filled with neuronal filaments running along its longitudinal axis, which contributes to the anisotropy of water diffusion (Mori and van Zijl, 2002).

9.1 White Matter Fiber Tractography

White matter tractography offers the unique opportunity to characterize the trajectories of white matter fiber bundles noninvasively in the brain. Whole brain tractography studies routinely generate up to half million tracts per brain. Various deterministic tractography have been used to visualize and map out major white matter pathways in individuals and brain atlases (Basser *et al.*, 2000; Catani *et al.*, 2002; Conturo *et al.*, 1999; Lazar *et al.*, 2003; Mori *et al.*, 1999, 2002; Thottakara *et al.*, 2006; Yushkevich *et al.*, 2007); however, tractography data can be challenging to interpret and quantify. Recent efforts have attempted to cluster (O'Donnell *et al.*, 2006) and automatically segment white matter tracts (O'Donnell and Westin, 2007) as well as characterize tract shape parameters (Batchelor *et al.*, 2006). Many of these techniques can be quite computationally demanding. Efficient methods for extracting tracts, representing tract shape, regional tract segmentation and clustering, tract registration and quantification would be of tremendous value to researchers.

The DTI has been widely used to estimate the patterns of white matter connectivity. The white matter connectivity is mainly obtained by the streamline based tractography, in which a continuous path of connection between two brain regions is estimated as a streamline whose tangential velocity field is given by the principal eigenvectors. Most of current white matter tractography is based on streamlines (Conturo *et al.*, 1999; Mori *et al.*, 1999; Basser *et al.*, 2000) or its variations such as tensor deflection (TEND) method (Lazar *et al.*, 2003).

9.1.1 *Diffusion Tensors*

The directional information of water diffusion is usually represented as a symmetric positive definite 3×3 matrix $D = (d_{ij})$ which is usually termed as the *diffusion tensor* or *diffusion coefficients* (m^2/s). The diffusion tensors are usually normalized by its transpose, i.e. $D/\mathrm{tr}D$. This normalization guarantees that the sum of eigenvalues of D equals 1. The eigenvectors and eigenvalues of D are obtained by solving

$$D\mathbf{v} = \lambda\mathbf{v},$$

which results in 3 eigenvalues $\lambda_1 \geq \lambda_2 \geq \lambda_3$ and the corresponding eigenvectors $\mathbf{v}_1, \mathbf{v}_2, \mathbf{v}_3$. We may assume that the eigenvectors are normalized as $\|\mathbf{v}_j\| = 1$. The principal eigenvector $\mathbf{v}_1$ usually determines the direction of the water diffusion, and mainly used in streamline based tractography.

9.1.2 *Streamlines*

For the given principal vector fields $\mathbf{v}_1$, the corresponding streamline $p = \psi(t)$ satisfies the ordinary differential equation

$$\frac{d\psi}{dt} = \mathbf{v}_1(\psi(t)) \tag{9.1}$$

This ordinary differential equation gives a family of integral curves whose tangent vector is $\mathbf{v}_1$ (Betounes, 1998). By integrating (9.1) with respect to the parameter t, we obtain the equivalent integral version

$$\psi(t) = \int_0^t \mathbf{v}_1(\psi(t))\, dt + \psi(0). \tag{9.2}$$

The most common numerical methods for solving (9.1) are Euler's method and the Runge-Kutta algorithm (Basser *et al.*, 2000).

The streamline-based techniques for obtaining fiber tracts have three main steps: defining seed points, performing integration (9.2) and determining stopping criteria (Vilanova *et al.*, 2004). The stopping criteria avoids the area where the principal vector fields are not robustly defined. Note that streamlines have been encountered in the context of estimating cortical thickness using the Laplace equation (Jones *et al.*, 2000). See Section 7.2 for details.

9.1.3 *Probabilistic Methods*

There are various probabilistic and stochastic models for tracing fibers (Basser and Pierpaoli, 1996; Batchelor *et al.*, 2001; Behrens *et al.*, 2007; Hagmann *et al.*, 2000). Tench *et al.* (2002) introduced a hybrid streamline-based tractography where the direction of principal eigenvector is modeled stochastically to overcome the shortcomings of DTI. Koch *et al.* (2002) introduced a Monte-Carlo random walk simulation that uses a different transition probability than our own. Their algorithm has a certain restrictions built in the random walk so that it was only allowed to jump in a direction within 90 degrees from the previous jump direction, which restricts the jump to a very small number of voxels in the neighborhood. Furthermore they considered the voxels with the FA-values (Basser and Pierpaoli, 1996) and sum of the eigenvectors bigger than certain thresholds. Then based on the Monte-Carlo simulation of 4000 random walks, they computed the probabilistic connectivity measure.

Hagmann *et al.* (2000) used a hybrid approach combining Monte-Carlo random walk simulation with information about the white fiber track curvature function in the corpus callosum. Then assuming bivariate normal distribution of the random walk hitting a vertical plane at some distance apart, they estimated the covariance matrix and performed a statistical hypothesis testing of the homogeneity of covariance matrix in the different regions of the corpus callosum.

Batchelor et al. (2001) solved an anisotropic heat equation where the diffusion coefficients of the heat equation are the diffusion coefficients of DTI (Batchelor *et al.*, 2001). To get the probabilistic measure of the connectivity, the diffusion equation is solved with the initial condition where every vertex is zero except a seed region where it is given the value one:

$$\frac{\partial f}{\partial t}(p, t) = \nabla \cdot D\nabla f(p, t) \tag{9.3}$$

$$f(p, t = 0) = 1 \text{ at } p = p_0 \text{ and } 0 \text{ elsewhere.} \tag{9.4}$$

The value 1 is diffused though the white matter and the numerical values between 0 and 1 is taken as a probability of white matter connectivity. Mathematically it is equivalent as the Monte-Carlo random walk simulation without restriction. The boundary condition $D\nabla f \cdot \mathbf{n} = 0$, i.e. the boundary is insulated and no heat diffuses out of the boundary, can be also enforced. A Crank-Nicholson scheme with Galerkin finite element discretization in space, and finite difference in time was then used to solve (9.4) (Babuška *et al.*, 2004). Instead of solving the diffusion equation (9.4) directly, we can perform an equivalent iterative anisotropic kernel smoothing scheme (Chung *et al.*, 2003a; Yoruk *et al.*, 2005). Recently, fast marching based tratography has been popularized (Parker *et al.*, 2002; Jbabdi *et al.*, 2008; Staempfli *et al.*, 2006). Unlike probabilistic tractography, the fast marching methods do not present a computational burden.

The white fiber tracking is prone to cumulative acquisition noise and partial volume effect so the estimated white fiber tracks might possibly be erroneous in some cases (Basser *et al.*, 2000; Tench *et al.*, 2002). So it is crucial to develop a connectivity metric that is robust under the effect of acquisition noise and partial voluming. Such a robust connectivity metric can be used in VBM type of voxelwise inference on connectivity difference between two populations (Ashburner and Friston, 2000). In the classical VBM, the gray and white matter densities are computed and used for inference on tissue concentration at each voxel. In DTI, instead of the tissue densities, we can use the connectivity metric that measures the strength of how two regions of the brain are connected via the white fiber tracts.

9.2 Probabilistic Connectivity

In this section, a probabilistic connectivity based on the transition probability of diffusion is presented in detail (Chung *et al.*, 2003a; Yoruk *et al.*, 2005). Let $P_t(p, q)$ be the *transition density* of a particle going from p to q under diffusion. This is the conditional probability density of the particle hitting q at time t when the particle is at p at time 0. Similarly the *transition probability* of going from point p to another region of interest Q is given by

$$P_t(p, Q) = \int_Q P_t(p, x) \, dx.$$

Note that

$$P_t(p, \mathbb{R}^n) = \int_{\mathbb{R}^n} P_t(p, x) \, dx = 1.$$

The region Q can be a collection of voxels and it may possibly be consisting of a single voxel p. So we will interchangeably use $P_t(p, q)$ as either transition probability density or transition probability if there is no ambiguity. The transition probability is the most natural probabilistic measure associated with diffusion process and the connectivity measure based on the transition probability will be presented in this section.

If the diffusion coefficient D is constant in $\mathbb{R}^n$, it can be shown that

$$P_t(p, q) = K_t(q - p),$$

the Gaussian kernel of the form (4.14) (Stevens, 1995). Since D is varying over the brain regions, it is only valid when p and q are short distance apar_ and we may take $D(x)$ to be constant in the neighborhood of voxel position x.

The transition probability of a particle going from p to any arbitrary q is the total sum of the probabilities of going from p to q through all possible intermediate points $x \in \mathbb{R}^n$. Therefore,

$$P_t(p, q) = \int_{\mathbb{R}^n} P_s(p, x) P_{t-s}(x, q) \, dx \tag{9.5}$$

for any $0 < s < t$. It is traditionally called the Chapman-Kolmogorov equation (Paul and Baschnagel, 1999). The equation still hold in the case when s is either 0 or t, since in that case one of the probability in the integral becomes the Dirac-delta function and, in turn, the integral collapses to the probability on the left side.

Note that the probability $P(p, x)$ decreases exponentially as the distance between p and x increases so we approximate (9.5) in a small region B_p centered around p. For any point $x \in B_p$,

$$P_s(p, x) \doteq K_s(p - x).$$

Then for any arbitrary points p and q,

$$P_t(p, q) \doteq \frac{\int_{B_p} K_s(p - x) P_{t-s}(x, q) \, dx}{\int_{B_p} K_s(p - x) \, dx}. \tag{9.6}$$

When $s \to 0$, the approximation becomes exact since all the weights of the kernel will be in B_p. The denominator is a correction term for compensating the underestimation in the numerator. Note that this is the integral version of Gaussian kernel smoothing of data $P_{t-s}(x, q)$ for given q. Comparing with the formulation of Gaussian kernel smoothing, we rewrite (9.6) as

$$P_t(p, q) \doteq \tilde{K}_s * P_{t-s}(p, q), \tag{9.7}$$

where the convolution is with respect to the first argument p and $\tilde{K}_s$ is the truncated Gaussian kernel normalized by $\int_{B_p} K_s(p - x) \, dx$. Note that when $s \to 0$, the equation becomes exact.

The kernel smoothing formulation (9.7) is mainly valid when s is small. For large s, we borrow the iterative smoothing framework developed in Section 6.3. We discretize t into N equal time intervals $t = N\Delta t$ and let $s = \Delta t$. Then (9.7) can be written as

$$F_j(q) = \tilde{K}_{\Delta t} * F_{j-1}(q), \tag{9.8}$$

where $F_j(q) = P_{j\Delta t}(p, q)$ for a given p and the initial condition

$$F_0(q) = P_0(p, q) = \delta(p - q).$$

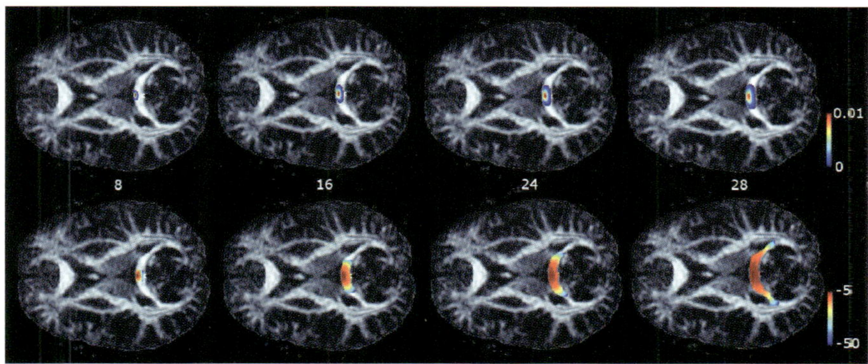

Fig. 9.1 The dispersion of transition probability from the seed at the splneium of in the corpus callosum with $\Delta t = 0.1$ and $N = 8$, 16, 24, 28 iterations. The scale in the top images is 10^{-3} while the natural log is taken for the bottom image.

The reason we get the Dirac-delta function is that the transition probability of a particle at p hitting any point q instantaneously is zero except when $q = p$.

One important property of our iterative procedure is the conservation of the total probability at each iteration. From (9.8), we have

$$\int_{\mathbb{R}^n} F_{j+1}(x)\,dx = \int_{B_x} \tilde{K}_{\Delta t}(x - y)\,dy \int_{\mathbb{R}^n} F_j(x)\,dx$$

$$= \int_{\mathbb{R}^n} F_j(x)\,dx.$$

Since

$$F_1(\mathbf{q}) = \tilde{K}_{\Delta t} * \delta(q) = \tilde{K}_{\Delta t}(q),$$

F_1 is a probability function and it will integrate to one so

$$\int_{\mathbb{R}^n} F_j(x)\,dx = 1.$$

Hence F_j is also a probability function at each iteration. As the number of iteration increases, the total probability will be dispersed over all region of white matter from the seed (Figure 9.1).

If there are one million voxels within the brain, in average, each voxel will have the connection probability of one over a million, which is extremely small. So even though the connectivity measure based on the transition probability is a mathematically sound one, it may not be a good one fcr visualization. So what need is the log-scale of the transition probability, i.e.

$\rho = \ln P_t(p, q)$ and we propose this as a probabilistic metric for measuring the strength of the anatomical connectivity. We will refer this metric as the *log-transition probability*. For simplicity we may let $p = 0$ and let $\rho(q) = \ln P_t(0, q)$ for fixed t. If the diffusion coefficient is constant, the log-transition probability can be represented in a simple formula

$$\rho(x) = -x'D^{-1}x - \sum_{i=1}^{n} \ln \lambda_i - \frac{n}{2} \log(4\pi t),$$

where λ_i are the eigenvalues of D. When $D = I$,

$$\rho(x) = -x'x - \frac{n}{2} \log(4\pi t).$$

For a region of interest Q, the log-transition probability of reaching Q would be

$$\rho(q) = \ln \int_Q P_t(\mathbf{0}, x) \, dx.$$

See Figure 9.1 for log-transition probability obtained by taking the splenium as the seed.

9.3 Cosine Series Representation of Fiber Tracts

Unlike the nonparametric way of representing white matter fiber connectivity probabilistically, parametric methods can be used to model white matter fibers explicitly. In this section, we show how to represent white matter fiber tracts suing cosine basis functions.

Splines have also been often used for modeling and matching 3D curves (Clayden *et al.*, 2007; Gruen and Akca, 2005; Kishon *et al.*, 1990). Unfortunately, splines are not easy to model and to manipulate explicitly compared to Fourier descriptors, due to the introduction of internal knots. In Clayden *et al.* (2007), the cubic-B spline is used to parameterize the median of a set of tracts for tract dispersion modeling. Matching two splines with different numbers of knots is not computationally trivial and has been solved using a sequence of ad-hoc approaches. In Gruen and Akca (2005), the optimal displacement of two cubic spline curves are obtained by minimizing the sum of squared Euclidean distances. The minimization is nonlinear so an iterative updating scheme is used. On the other hand, there is no need for any numerical optimization in curve matching in Fourier descriptors due to the nature of the Hilbert space framework. Instead of using the squared distance of coordinates, others have used the curvature and torsion as features to be minimized to match curves (Corouge *et al.*, 2004; Gueziec *et al.*, 1997; Kishon *et al.*, 1990; Leemans *et al.*, 2006).

9.3.1 *Cosine Basis in a Unit Interval*

We are interested in encoding a smooth curve $\mathcal{M}$ consisting of n noisy ordered control points $p_1, \cdots, p_n$. Consider a mapping ζ^{-1} that maps the control point p_j onto the unit interval $[0, 1]$ as

$$\zeta^{-1} : p_j \to \frac{\sum_{i=1}^{j} \|p_i - p_{i-1}\|}{\sum_{i=1}^{n} \|p_i - p_{i-1}\|} = t_j. \tag{9.9}$$

This is the ratio of the arc-length from the point p_1 to p_j, to p_1 to p_n. We let this ratio to be t_j. We assume $\zeta^{-1}(p_1) = 0$. The ordering of the control points is also required in obtaining smooth one-to-one mapping. Then we parameterize the smooth inverse map

$$\zeta : [0, 1] \to \mathcal{M}$$

as a linear combination of continuous basis functions.

Consider the space of square integrable functions in $[0, 1]$ denoted by $\mathcal{L}^2[0, 1]$. The orthonormal basis $\psi_0, \psi_1, \cdots$ in $\mathcal{L}^2[0, 1]$ is obtained by solving the eigenequation

$$\Delta \psi + \lambda \psi = 0 \tag{9.10}$$

in $\mathcal{L}^2[0, 1]$ with 1D Laplacian $\Delta = \frac{d^2}{dt^2}$. Instead of solving (9.10) in the domain $[0, 1]$, we solve it in the larger domain $\mathbb{R}$ with the periodic constraint

$$\psi(t + 2) = \psi(t). \tag{9.11}$$

The eigenfunctions are then Fourier sine and cosine basis

$$\psi_l = \sin(l\pi t), \cos(l\pi t)$$

with the corresponding eigenvalues $\lambda_l = l^2 \pi^2$. The period 2 constraint forces the basis function expansion to be only valid in the intervals $\cdots, [-2, -1], [0, 1], [2, 3], \cdots$ while there are gaps in $\cdots, (-1, 0), (1, 2), (3, 4), \cdots$. We can fill the gap by padding with zeros but this will result in the Gibbs phenomenon (ringing artifacts) at the points of jump discontinuities (Chung *et al.*, 2007).

One way of filling the gap automatically while making the function continuous across the whole intervals is by putting the constraint of evenness, i.e.

$$\psi(t) = \psi(-t) \tag{9.12}$$

Then the only eigenfunctions satisfying two constraints (9.11) and (9.12) are the cosine basis of the form

$$\psi_0(t) = 1, \psi_l(t) = \sqrt{2} \cos(l\pi t) \tag{9.13}$$

with the corresponding eigenvalues $\lambda_l = l^2\pi^2$ for integers $l > 0$. The constant $\sqrt{2}$ is introduced to make the eigenfunctions orthonormal in $[0, 1]$ with respect to the inner product

$$\langle \psi_l, \psi_m \rangle = \int_0^1 \psi_l(t)\psi_m(t)\,dt = \delta_{lm}, \tag{9.14}$$

where δ_{lm} is the Dirac-delta function. With respect to the inner product, the norm $\|\cdot\|$ is then defined as

$$\|\psi\| = \langle \psi, \psi \rangle^{1/2}.$$

9.3.2 *Cosine Series Representation of 3D Curves*

Denote the coordinates of $\boldsymbol{\zeta}$ as $(\zeta_1, \zeta_2, \zeta_3)$. Then each coordinate is modeled as

$$\zeta_i(t) = \mu_i(t) + \epsilon_i(t), \tag{9.15}$$

where μ_i is an unknown smooth function to be estimated and ϵ_i is a zero mean random field, possibly Gaussian. Instead of estimating μ_i in $\mathcal{L}^2[0, 1]$, we estimate in a smaller subspace $\mathcal{H}_k$, which is spanned by up to the k-th degree eigenfunctions:

$$\mathcal{H}_k = \left\{ \sum_{l=0}^k c_l \psi_l(t) : c_l \in \mathbb{R} \right\} \subset \mathcal{L}^2[0, 1].$$

Then the least squares estimation of μ_i in $\mathcal{H}_k$ is given by

$$\widehat{\mu}_i = \arg \min_{f \in \mathcal{H}_k} \|f - \zeta_i(t)\|^2.$$

Obviously, the minimization is simply given as the k-th degree expansion:

$$\widehat{\mu}_i = \sum_{l=0}^k \langle \zeta_i, \psi_l \rangle \psi_l. \tag{9.16}$$

With this motivation in mind, we have the following k-th degree *cosine series representation* for a 3D curve:

$$\zeta_i(t) = \sum_{l=0}^k c_{li}\psi_l + \epsilon_i(t), \tag{9.17}$$

where ϵ_i is a zero mean random field. It is also possible to have slightly different but equivalent model that will be used for statistical inference.

Assuming Gaussian random field, ϵ_i can be expanded using the given basis ψ_l as follows.

$$\epsilon_i(t) = \sum_{l=0}^{k} Z_l \psi_l(t) + e_i(t),$$

where $Z_l \sim N(0, \tau_l^2)$ are possibly *correlated* Gaussian and e_i is the residual error field that cab be neglected in practice. This is the direct consequence of the Karhunen-Loeve expansion (Adler, 1990; Dougherty, 1999; Kwapien and Woyczynski, 1992; Yaglom, 1987). Therefore we can equivalently model (9.17) as

$$\zeta_i(t) = \sum_{l=0}^{k} X_l \psi_l(t) + e_i(t), \tag{9.18}$$

where $X_l \sim N(c_{li}, \tau_l^2)$.

We only observe the curve $\mathcal{M}$ in finite number of control points $\zeta_j(t_1), \cdots, \zeta_j(t_n)$ so we further need to estimate the Fourier coefficient $c_{li} = \langle \zeta_i, \psi_l \rangle$ as follows. At control points we have normal equations

$$
\underbrace{\begin{pmatrix} \zeta_1(t_1) & \zeta_2(t_1) & \zeta_3(t_1) \\ \zeta_1(t_2) & \zeta_2(t_2) & \zeta_3(t_2) \\ \vdots & \vdots & \vdots \\ \zeta_1(t_n) & \zeta_2(t_n) & \zeta_3(t_n) \end{pmatrix}}_{Y}
=
\underbrace{\begin{pmatrix} \psi_0(t_1) & \psi_1(t_1) & \cdots & \psi_k(t_1) \\ \psi_0(t_2) & \psi_1(t_2) & \cdots & \psi_k(t_2) \\ \vdots & \vdots & \ddots & \vdots \\ \psi_0(t_n) & \psi_1(t_n) & \cdots & \psi_k(t_n) \end{pmatrix}}_{\Psi}
\underbrace{\begin{pmatrix} c_{01} & c_{02} & c_{03} \\ c_{11} & c_{12} & c_{13} \\ \vdots & \vdots & \vdots \\ c_{k1} & c_{k2} & c_{k3} \end{pmatrix}}_{C}.
$$

The coefficients are simultaneously estimated in the least squares fashion as

$$\widehat{C} = (\Psi'\Psi)^{-1}\Psi'Y.$$

The least squares estimation technique avoids using the Fourier transform (FT) (Batchelor *et al.*, 2006; Bulow, 2004; Gu *et al.*, 2004). The drawback of the FT is the need for a predefined regular grid system so some sort of interpolation is needed. The advantage of the cosine representation is that, instead of recording the coordinates of all control points, we only need to record $3 \cdot (k+1)$ number of parameters for all possible tract shape. This is a substantial data reduction considering that the average number of control points is 105 (315 parameters). We recommend readers to use $10 \le k \le 30$ degrees for modeling white matter fiber tracts. The degree $k = 19$ representation given in Figure 9.2 has the average absolute error of 0.26mm along the tract. The `MATLAB` code for performing the least squares estimation can be obtained from `brainimaging.waisman.wisc.edu/~chung/tracts`

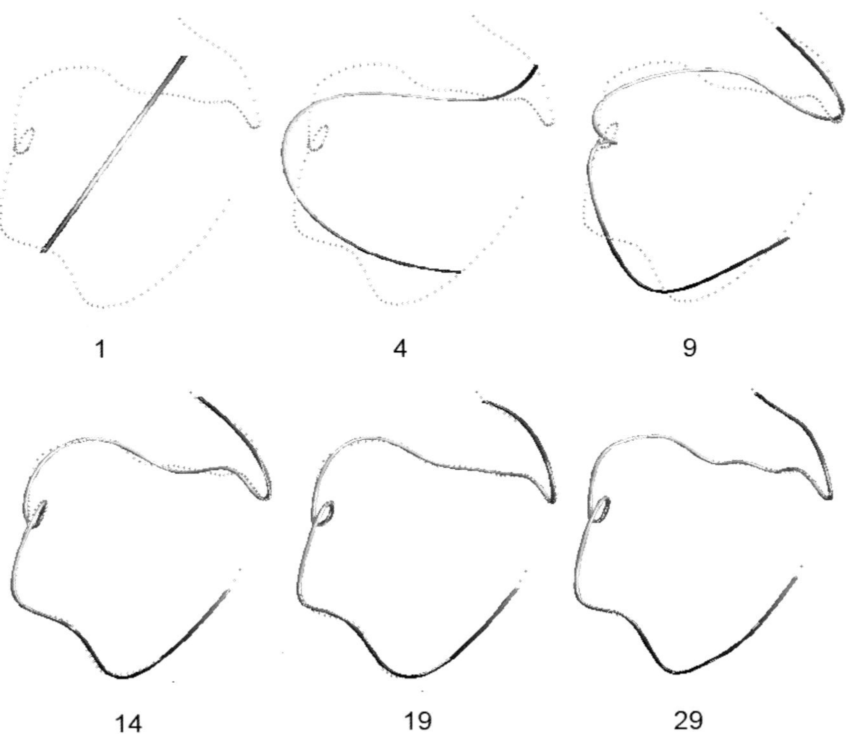

Fig. 9.2 Cosine representation of a tract at various degrees. Dots are control points obtained from a streamline based tractography. The degree 1 representation is a straight line that fits all the control points in a least squares fashion. The degree 19 representation is used through the paper.

9.3.3 *Optimal Degree Selection*

The optimal degree is determined by using a stepwise model selection framework. This framework for Fourier descriptors was first presented in Chung *et al.* (2007) and Chung *et al.* (2008b) for cortical surfaces. Although increasing the degree of the representation increases the goodness-of-fit, it also increases the number of estimated coefficients linearly. So it is necessary to stop the series expansion at the degree where the goodness-of-fit and the number of coefficients balance out.

Assuming up to the $(k-1)$-degree representation is proper in (9.17), we determine if adding the k-degree term is statistically significant by testing

$$H_0 : c_{ki} = 0.$$

The k-th degree *sum of squared errors* (SSE) for the i-th coordinate is

$$\mathrm{SSE}_k = \sum_{j=1}^{n} \left[\zeta_i(t_j) - \sum_{l=0}^{k} \widehat{c_{li}}\psi_l(t_j) \right]^2 ,$$

where $\widehat{c_{li}}$ are the least squares estimation. As the degree k increases, SSE decreases until it flattens out. So it is reasonable to stop the series expansion when the decrease in SSE is no longer significant. Under H_0, the test statistic F follows

$$F = \frac{\mathrm{SSE}_{k-1} - \mathrm{SSE}_k}{\mathrm{SSE}_{k-1}/(n-k-2)} \sim F_{1,n-k-2},$$

the F-distribution with 1 and $n - k - 2$ degrees of freedom. We compute the F statistic at each degree and stop increasing the degree of expansion if the corresponding p-value first becomes bigger than the pre-specified significance $\alpha = 0.01$. The forward model selection framework hierarchically builds the cosine series representation from lower to higher degree.

In many Fourier descriptor and spherical harmonic representation literature, the issue of the optimal degree has not been addressed properly and the degree is simply selected based on a pre-specified error bound (Bulow, 2004; Gerig *et al.*, 2001; Gu *et al.*, 2004; Shen and Chung, 2006; Shen *et al.*, 2004). Since the stepwise model selection framework chooses the optimal degree for each coordinate separately, the maximum of optimal degrees for all coordinates can be chosen as optimal. The optimal degree changes if a different tract is chosen. For instance, the optimal degrees for 4987 randomly chosen whole brain white matter tracts longer than 30mm are 13.94 ± 7.02 and the upper 80 percentile is approximately 19. For simplicity in numerical implementation and inference, it is crucial to choose the same fixed degree for all tracts. We may not want to choose the degree 14 as optimal since then about 50% of tracts will not be represented optimally. Therefore, we may choose the degree corresponding to the upper 80 percentile. Figure 9.4 shows the 19 degree representation of parts of tracts from the brain stem.

The optimal degree is not related to the length of tracts. The correlation between the length of tracts and the optimal degree is 0.06, which is statistically insignificant. The increased degree should correspond to the increased curvature and bending rather than the the length of tracts.

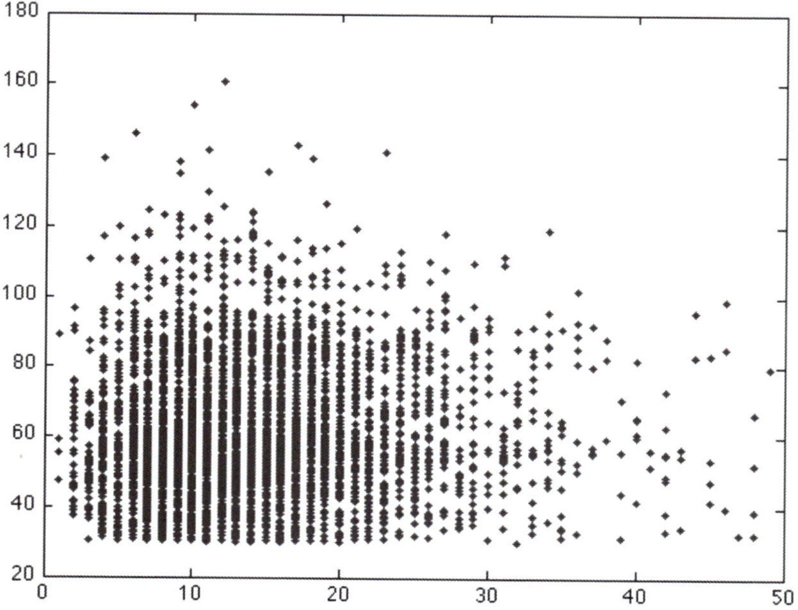

Fig. 9.3 The lengths of tracts (vertical) is not related to the optimal degrees (horizontal). The optimal degree should be related to the bending and curvedness of tracts, which are further related to the spatial frequency of the tract shapes.

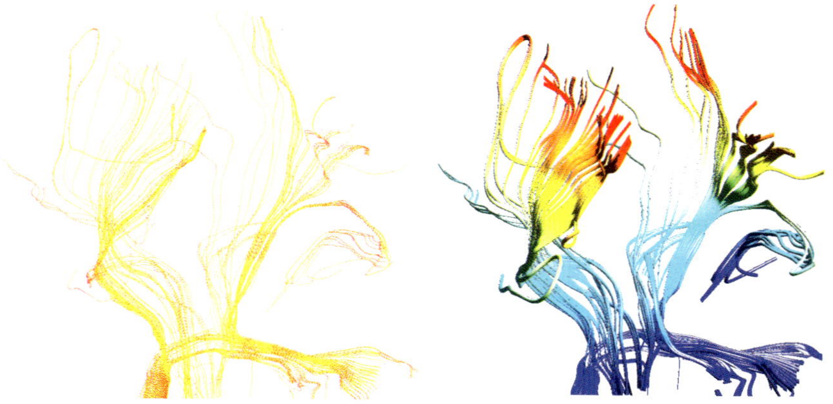

Fig. 9.4 Left: control points (red) are obtained from the second order Runge-Kutta streamline algorithm. Subsampled 500 tracts with length larger than 50mm are only shown here. Yellow lines are line segments connecting connecting the control points. Right: 19 degree cosine series representation of tracts.

9.3.4 *Distance Between Tracts*

The cosine series representation can be used to analyze a collection of fiber bundles consisting of similarly shaped curves. The ability to register one tract to another tract is necessary to establish anatomical correspondence for a subsequent population study. Since curves are represented as combinations of cosine functions, the registration will be formulated as a minimization problem in the subspace $\mathcal{H}_k$ which avoids brute-force style numerical optimization schemes (Gruen and Akca, 2005; Gueziec *et al.*, 1997; Kishon *et al.*, 1990; Leemans *et al.*, 2006; Ramsay and Silverman, 1997). This simplicity makes the cosine series representation more well suited than the usual spline representation of curves in subsequent statistical analysis (Gruen and Akca, 2005).

With the abuse of notations, we will interchangeably use curves to be estimated and their estimation with the same notations when the meaning is clear. Let the cosine series representation of two curves $\boldsymbol{\eta}$ and $\boldsymbol{\zeta}$ be

$$\boldsymbol{\eta}(t) = \sum_{l=0}^{k} \boldsymbol{\eta}_l \psi_l(t), \tag{9.19}$$

$$\boldsymbol{\zeta}(t) = \sum_{l=0}^{k} \boldsymbol{\zeta}_l \psi_l(t) \tag{9.20}$$

where $\boldsymbol{\eta}_l$ and $\boldsymbol{\zeta}_l$ are the Fourier coefficient vectors.

Consider the displacement vector field $\mathbf{u} = (u_1, u_2, u_3)$ that is required to register $\boldsymbol{\zeta}$ to $\boldsymbol{\eta}$ (Figure 9.5). We will determine an optimal displacement $\mathbf{u}$ such that the discrepancy between the deformed curve $\boldsymbol{\zeta} + \mathbf{u}$ and $\boldsymbol{\eta}$ is minimized with respect to a certain discrepancy measure ρ. The discrepancy measure ρ between $\boldsymbol{\eta}$ and $\boldsymbol{\zeta}$ are defined as the integral of the sum of squared distance:

$$\rho(\boldsymbol{\zeta}, \boldsymbol{\eta}) = \int_0^1 \|\boldsymbol{\zeta}(t) - \boldsymbol{\eta}(t)\|^2 \, dt. \tag{9.21}$$

The discrepancy ρ can be further simplified as

$$\rho(\boldsymbol{\zeta}, \boldsymbol{\eta}) = \int_0^1 \sum_{j=1}^{3} \left[\sum_{l=0}^{k} (\zeta_{lj} - \eta_{lj}) \psi_l(t) \right]^2 dt$$

$$= \sum_{j=1}^{3} \sum_{l=0}^{k} (\zeta_{lj} - \eta_{lj})^2.$$

We have used the orthogonality condition (9.14) to simplify the expression. The discrepancy measure ρ can be used in clustering tracts (Figure 9.6).

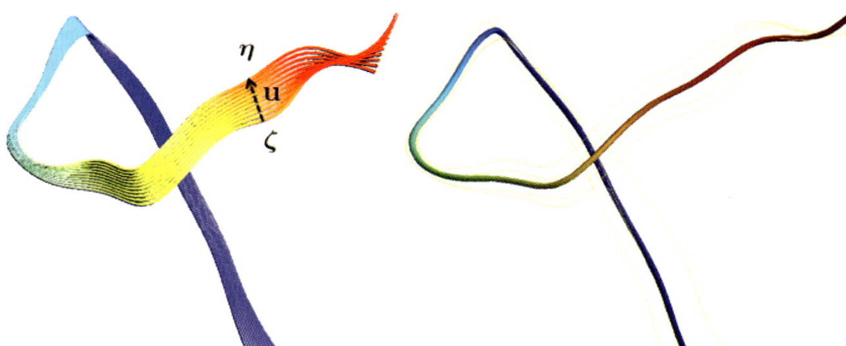

Fig. 9.5   Left: the curve ζ is registered to η by the displacement vector field $\mathbf{u}$. The other intermediate curves are generated by plotting $\zeta + \alpha\mathbf{u}$ with $\alpha \in [0,1]$ to show how the different amount of displacement deforms the curve ζ. Right: the average of a fiber bundle consisting of 5 tracts.

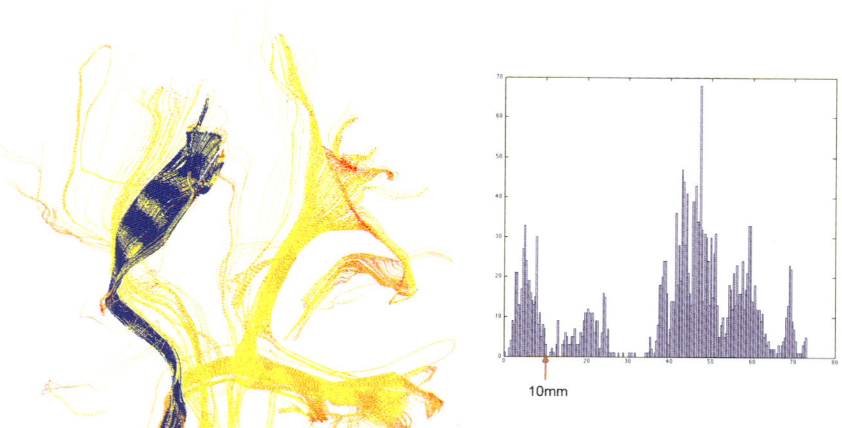

Fig. 9.6   Left: histogram of discrepancy measure from a single tract (one of blue tracts). By thresholding the histogram at 10mm gives the clustered blue colored tracts. The discrepancy measure can be used in clustering fibers in the whole brain automatically.

9.3.5 *Tract Registration*

The algebraic manipulation then shows that the optimal displacement $\mathbf{u}^*$, which minimizes the discrepancy between $\boldsymbol{\zeta} + \mathbf{u}$ and $\boldsymbol{\eta}$, is given by

$$\mathbf{u}^*(t) = \arg \min_{u_1, u_2, u_3 \in \mathcal{H}_k} \rho(\boldsymbol{\zeta} + \mathbf{u}, \boldsymbol{\eta}) \tag{9.22}$$

$$= \sum_{l=0}^{k} (\boldsymbol{\eta}_l - \boldsymbol{\zeta}_l) \psi_l(t). \tag{9.23}$$

The proof requires substituting

$$\mathbf{u}(t) = \sum_{l=0}^{k} \mathbf{u}_l \psi_l(t)$$

in the expression (9.22), which becomes the unconstrained positive definite quadratic program with respect to variables $\mathbf{u}_l = (u_{l1}, u_{l2}, u_{l3})$. So the global minimum always exists and obtained when $\rho(\boldsymbol{\zeta} + \mathbf{u}^*, \boldsymbol{\eta}) = 0$. Figure 9.5 shows the schematic view of registration.

The simplicity of the above approach is that curve registration is done by simply matching the corresponding Fourier coefficients without any sort of numerical optimization as in spline curve matching. Based on the idea of registering tracts by matching coefficients, we construct the average of a white fiber bundle consisting of m curves $\boldsymbol{\zeta}^1, \cdots, \boldsymbol{\zeta}^m$ by finding the optimal curve that minimizes the sum of all discrepancy in $\mathcal{H}_k$:

$$\overline{\boldsymbol{\zeta}}(t) = \arg \min_{\zeta_1, \zeta_2, \zeta_3 \in \mathcal{H}_k} \sum_{j=1}^{m} \rho(\boldsymbol{\zeta}^j, \boldsymbol{\zeta}).$$

Again the algebraic manipulation will show that the optimum curve is obtained by the average of representation:

$$\overline{\boldsymbol{\zeta}}(t) = \frac{1}{m} \sum_{j=1}^{m} \sum_{l=0}^{k} \boldsymbol{\zeta}_l^j \psi_l(t) = \sum_{l=0}^{k} \overline{\boldsymbol{\zeta}}_l \psi_l(t), \tag{9.24}$$

where $\overline{\boldsymbol{\zeta}}_l$ is the average coefficient vector

$$\overline{\boldsymbol{\zeta}}_l = \frac{1}{m} \sum_{j=1}^{m} \boldsymbol{\zeta}_l^j.$$

This simplicity is the consequence of Fourier series having the best representation in the Hilbert space. So any optimization involving our quadratic discrepancy will simplify the expression as the sum of squared Fourier coefficients making the problem a fairly simple quadratic problem. Similarly we can define the sample variance of m curves and it will turn out to be the cosine representation with the coefficient vector consisting of the sample variance of m coefficients. The construction of the sample variance of m curves should be fairly straightforward and we will not go into the detail.

Given another population of curves $\eta^1, \cdots, \eta^n$, we are interested in performing statistical inference on the equality of curve shape in the two populations. The null hypothesis of interest is then

$$H_0 : \overline{\zeta} = \overline{\eta}. \tag{9.25}$$

Here we again abused the notation so we are testing the equality of mean representations of populations. From the very property of Fourier series in Hilbert space, the uniqueness of the cosine series representation is guaranteed so the two representations are equal if and only if the coefficients vectors match. Therefore, the equivalent hypothesis to (9.25) is given by

$$H_0' : \overline{\zeta}_1 = \overline{\eta}_1, \cdots, \overline{\zeta}_k = \overline{\eta}_k.$$

Obviously this is a multiple comparisons problem. Under the Gaussian assumption in (9.18), testing the equality of the mean coefficient vector can be done using the Hotelling's T-square statistic. For correcting for the multiple comparisons, the Bonferroni correction can be used.

9.3.6 *Limitation of Cosine Series Representation*

Although the cosine representation is efficient for normalizing and averaging tracts, unfortunately it is not translation, rotation and scale invariant. One simple way of obtaining translation, rotation and scale invariant representation is to project white matter fiber tracts onto a unit sphere. Given the control points p_i that defines a tract, consider directional vectors $v_i = p_i - p_{i-1}$ with the convention $v_1 = p_1$. The vectors v_i contain all the necessary information to reconstruct the original tract.

The advantage of using the spherical projection method is that it offers a translation, rotation and scale invariant tract representation. Two tracts with the identical shape but at different positions will be identically represented as the same spherical curve. The translation information is stored in v_1 value, which should be stored separately.

Since v_i are represented as a unit vectors (except v_1) in some of tractography algorithm such as Lazar *et al.* (2003), they are all in S^2. For a general case, which will likely happen for other tractography algorithms, we project v_i onto S^2 via the spherical projection P:

$$P : v_i \rightarrow w_i = \frac{v_i}{\|v_i\|}.$$

w_j defines control points for a spherical curve. The spherical curves can be parameterized using the cosine representation

$$\zeta_o(t_j) = \sum_{l=0}^{k} c_{lo} \psi_l(t_j). \tag{9.26}$$

However, directly solving for each coordinate ζ_o will violate the quadratic constraint that the spherical curve has to be embedded on S^2, i.e.

$$\sum_{o=1}^{3} \left[\sum_{l=0}^{k} c_{lo} \psi_l(t_j) \right]^2 = 1. \tag{9.27}$$

This is easily seen from Figure 9.7, in which the degree 10 representation is visibly not embedded in S^2. The average absolute error for reconstruction is relatively large for low degree due to the fact that the representation is no longer embedded in S^2 (Figure 9.8). Note that at degree 30, the average absolute error is small enough, i.e. 0.0153mm, to be used for subsequent modeling.

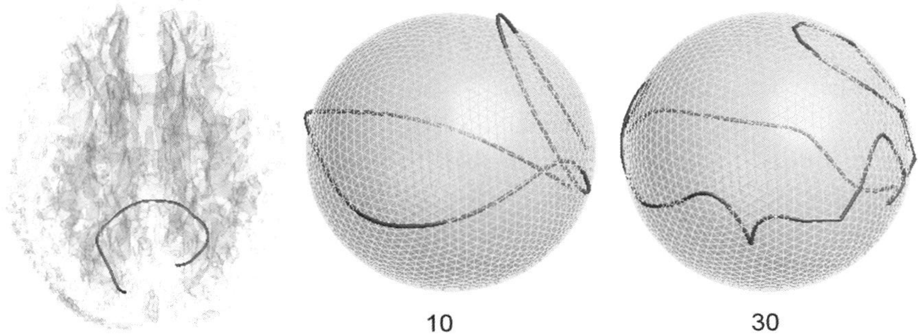

Fig. 9.7   Left: a single white matter fiber tract passing through the splenium of the corpus callosum. Middle and right: the cosine representation of the spherical projection of the tract at degree 10 and 30.

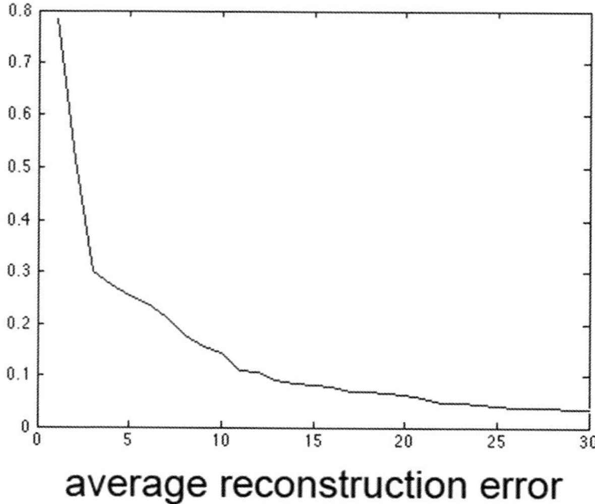

Fig. 9.8   The error plot displays the average reconstruction error in millimeter (vertical) vs. degree (horizontal) in the spherical projection method.

The spherical projection based representation can not be obtained in a straightforward fashion and requires solving three least squares problem simultaneously with the quadratic constraint (9.27) that relates the three equations (9.26). We will not consider this issue in this paper and leave it for a future study.

9.4   Parcellation-Free Brain Networks

Structural brain connectivity can be modeled as a network graph using white matter fiber bundles obtained from DTI tractography algorithms. Whole brain tractography studies routinely generate up to half million tracts per brain, which serves as edges in an extremely large 3D graph.

The whole gray matter has been traditionally parcellated into n disjoint regions. White matter fibers provide information of how one gray matter region is connected to another via a n-by-n connectivity matrix. The connectivity matrix is then thresholded to produce a binarized adjacency matrix, which is further used for a graph with n nodes (Fornito *et al.*,

2010; Gong *et al.*, 2009; Hagmann *et al.*, 2007; Zalesky *et al.*, 2010). However, there is no gold standard for gray matter parcellation which makes the identification of node depends on the choice of parcellation. Depending on the scale of parcellation, the parameters of graph, which characterize graph topology, varies considerably up to 95% (Fornito *et al.*, 2010; Zalesky *et al.*, 2010). Another major problem of traditional parcellation based network construction is the arbitrariness of thresholding connectivity matrix. The topological parameters such as sparsity and clustering coefficients change substantially depending on the level of threshold (Gong *et al.*, 2009).

The problems of parcellation and the subsequent arbitrary thresholding can be avoided if we do not use any parcellation. So the question is whether if it is possible to construct a network graph without the usual parcellation scheme. In this section, we present a parcellation-free, scalable and iterative connectivity network construction technique.

9.4.1 *Why Parcellation Free?*

This section presents a novel network graph modeling technique called the ϵ-*neighbor construction* that avoids parcellation and the subsequent connectivity matrix thresholding (Chung *et al.*, 2011a,b). Instead of using the pre-specified parcellation, we propose to use the two end points of fibers as network nodes while the fibers themselves serve as the edges connecting nodes.

Rips Complex. The ϵ-neighbor construction is motivated by the Rips complex of point cloud data (Ghrist, 2008), which is used to characterize the topology of the point cloud data. The Rips complex is a graph constructed by connecting two data points if they are within specific distance. The problem of the Rips complex is that given n data points, it exactly produce a graph with n nodes so the resulting graph becomes very complicated when n becomes large. Unlike the Rips complex, the ϵ-neighbor method does not use every data points in constructing a graph so it significantly reduce the complexity of data. Further, while the point cloud data does not have any hidden topological constraint, the two end points of white matter fibers are connected so we are actually dealing with paired point cloud data. So the ϵ-neighbor construction is different than building the Rips complex while offer substantial computational advantage.

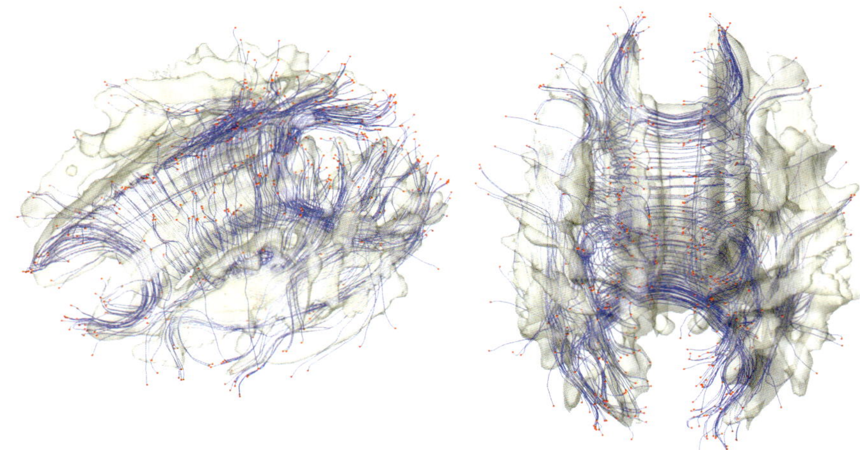

Fig. 9.9   White matter fiber bundles obtained from TEND (Cook *et al.*, 2006; Lazar *et al.*, 2003).   The tracts are sparsely subsampled for better visualization.   The end points are colored as red.   The surface is the isosurface of the template FA map so some tracts are expected to be outside of the surface.   The ϵ-neighbor method will use the proximity of the ends points in constructing the network graph.

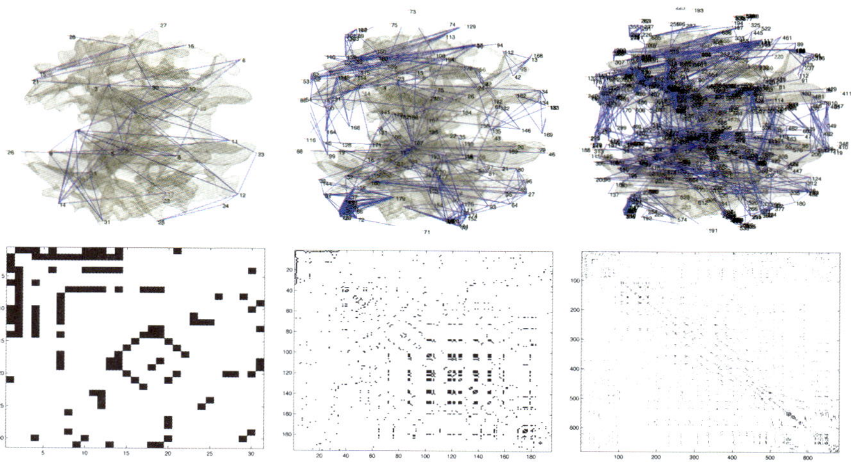

Fig. 9.10   The ϵ-neighbor graph construction on white matter fibers with 20, 10 and 6mm radius.   The corresponding adjacency matrices are also shown.

DTI Registration. Spatial normalization of DTI plays a key role in constructing brain network graphs that are spatially compatible across different subjects. The quality of spatial normalization determines the extent to which white matter tracts are aligned. It has direct impacts on the successful removal of shape confounds and consequently on the validity, specificity, and sensitivity of the subsequent statistical inferences of group differences. Inadequate normalization with coarse registration algorithms can result in insufficient removal of shape differences that is necessary for obtaining topologically invariant network graph. For instance, we can use nonlinear tensor image registration algorithm implemented in DTI-TK for spatial normalization (Zhang *et al.*, 2007b). This approach combines full tensor co-registration and high-dimensional diffeomorphic spatial normalization. The registration is based on an iterative strategy (Joshi *et al.*, 2004; Zhang *et al.*, 2007b) where the initial template was computed as the average of original DTI. Then DTI were first affinely aligned to the template. The tensor images after the affine alignment were provided as the input to the registration algorithm. The algorithm leverages full tensor-based similarity metrics while optimizing tensor orientation explicitly. The metric is based on the L_2-distance between the anisotropic parts of diffusion profiles associated with the diffusion tensors (Zhang *et al.*, 2006). The algorithm then approximates smooth transformations using a dense piecewise affine parameterization which is sufficient when the required deformations are not large. Now compute a refined template as an average of the normalized images. If the change between templates from consecutive iterations is sufficiently small, we stop the iteration otherwise we continue the iterative process of getting a new template and refitting.

From now on, we will assume the ϵ-neighbor network construction is done in the normalized space. After DTI were alined to a template space, we can perform streamline based tractography using TENsor Deflection (TEND) in the normalized space (Cook *et al.*, 2006; Lazar *et al.*, 2003). Figure 9.9 shows the subsampled tractography result for a single subject. Then the ϵ-neighbor method is applied in obtaining the binary network (Figure 9.10). The overall pipeline for the ϵ-neighbor brain network construction is illustrated in Figure 9.11.

9.4.2 *Epsilon Neighbor Networks*

A graph G consists of a vertex set V and an edge set E, i.e. $G = \{V, E\}$. A point p is the ϵ-neighbor of G if the shortest distance between p and some point q in V is smaller than given ϵ. Then we identify the point p and q as the same point. Formally, we define distance $d(p, G)$ of a point p to the graph G to be shortest Euclidean distance between p and points in V, i.e.

$$d(p, G) = \min_{q \in V} \|p - q\|.$$

We say point p is the ϵ-*neighbor* of graph G if $d(p, G) \leq \epsilon$.

With these definitions, we construct a connectivity graph iteratively. In constructing the brain network, only two end points of the tract were considered since all other points along the tract are connected to these two points. Figure 9.11 shows the extracted end points in subsampled tracts. We now construct the graph in an iterative fashion by adding one tract at a time to an existing graph. Initially graph G_1 consists of a single tract consisting of two end points e_{11} and e_{12}, and an edge $e_{11}e_{12}$ connecting the end points. Consider a tract with two end points . The algorithm then starts with the graph $G_1 = \{V_1, E_1\}$, where

$$V_1 = \{e_{11}, e_{12}\}, E_1 = \{e_{11}e_{12}\}.$$

In the next iteration, we consider how to add the second tract to the existing graph G_1 and obtain a new graph G_2. Consider the second tract with two end points e_{21}, e_{22} to the existing graph G_1. There are four possibilities in adding the two end points to G_1 depending if the end points are the ϵ-neighbors of G_1:

(1) e_{21} and e_{22} are all ϵ-neighbors of G_1. Since the end points e_{21} and e_{22} are close to the already existing graph G_1, we do not change the vertex set. i.e. $V_2 = V_1$. Now check if the edge $e_{21}e_{22}$ is in the edge set E_1 and add them if it is not found in the edge set. In this case we have

$$E_2 = E_1 \cup \{e_{21}e_{22}\}.$$

(2) Only e_{21} is an ϵ-neighbor. We only to add e_{22} to VV_1 and let

$$V_2 = V_1 \cup \{e_{21}\}, \ E_2 = E_1 \cup \{e_{21}e_{22}\}.$$

(3) Only e_{22} is an ϵ-neighbor. We add e_{21} to V_1 and let

$$V_2 = V_1 \cup \{e_{22}\}, \ E_2 = E_1 \cup \{e_{21}e_{22}\}.$$

(4) e_{21} and e_{22} are not ϵ-neighbors. We add the end points to the vertex set and add the edge to the edge set. In this case, $e_{21}e_{22}$ forms a disjoint edge and we have

$$V_2 = V_1 \cup \{e_{21}, e_{22}\}, \ E_2 = E_1 \cup \{e_{21}e_{22}\}.$$

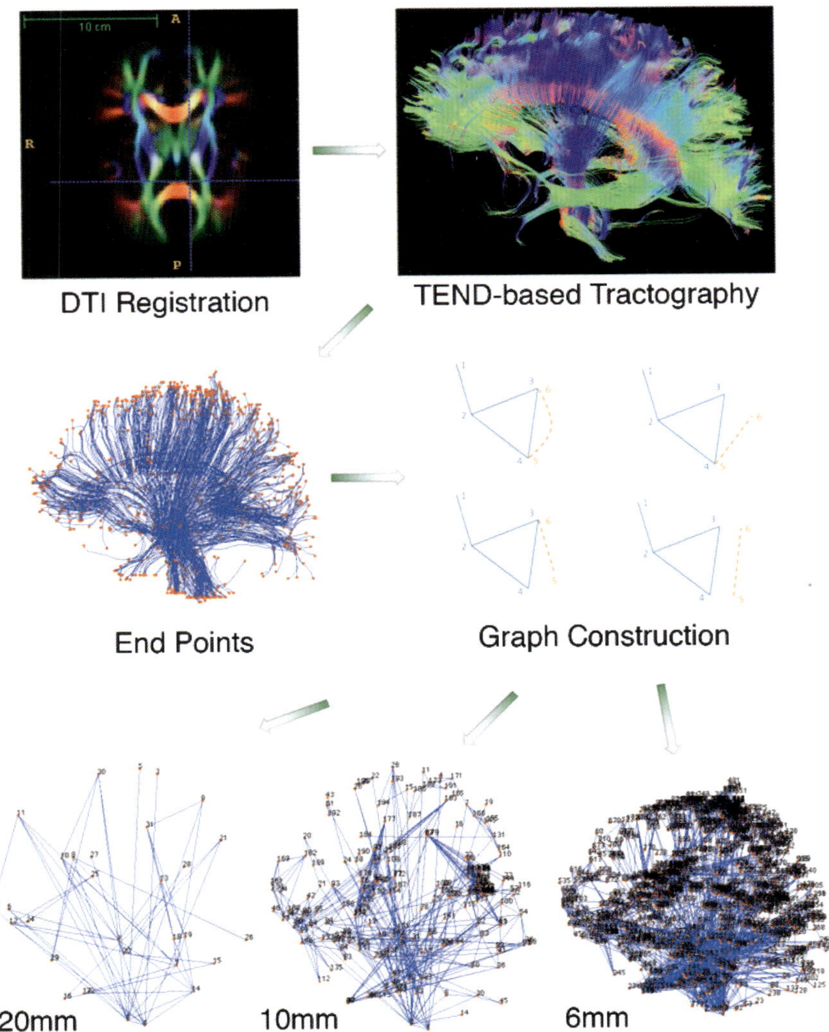

Fig. 9.11 Pipeline for building structural network in DTI. DTI needs to be aligned to a template and tractography is done in the standard space. End points of tracts are identified and used as possible nodes of the network. The networks are constructed using the ϵ-neighbor method (Chung *et al.*, 2010a).

The procedure is iteratively performed to every tracts until we exhaust all the tracts. The `MATLAB` code for performing ϵ-neighbor construction is given in `http://brainimaging.waisman.wisc.edu/~chung/graph`.

The constructed 3D networks graph can be uniquely parameterized by transforming the graph into adjacent matrices. The adjacency matrix $A = (a_{ij})$ of a graph is constructed on the fly at each iteration by checking if we are adding a new edge to the existing edge set. If nodes i and j are connected, we let $a_{ij} = 1$ and $a_{ij} = 0$ otherwise. The diagonal terms a_{ii} are assumed to be zero. The adjacency matrix is symmetric. The adjacency matrix of a graph can be constructed on the fly at each iteration by checking if we are adding a new edge to the existing edge set. The adjacency matrix contains sufficient information to construct a graph. Statistical analysis can be done on the ensemble of adjacency matrices and we can determine if two groups significantly differ in connectivity. The graph construction pipeline is illustrated in Figure 9.11. For the subsequent discussions on the graph complexity, 6mm-neighbor graph was used. This particular resolution is chosen since it is the largest integer resolution that produces nodes below 1000.

9.4.3 *Connected Components*

Identifying connected components in a network is important to understand in decomposing the network into disjoint subnetworks. The number of connected components of a graph is a topological invariant that measures the number of structurally independent or disjoint subnetworks. It can be interpreted as the zeroth Betti number β_0 in algebraic topology (Edelsbrunner *et al.*, 2002). The connected components can be identified using the Dulmage-Mendelsohn decomposition (Pothen and Fan, 1990), which has been widely used for decomposing sparse matrices into block triangular forms in speeding up matrix operations.

Figure 9.12 shows connected components in 4 brain networks. All nodes in the same connected component are colored identically. Surprisingly, most of nodes belong to the largest connected component indicating the brain network is highly connected. There are only 4% of nodes that are not connected to the largest connected component while the remaining 96% are all connected. We have plotted those 4% of nodes that are not part of the largest connected component for all subjects (Figure 9.12).

We tested if the size of the largest connected components differ between the groups. At 6mm resolution, control subjects have 642.86 ± 68.60 nodes

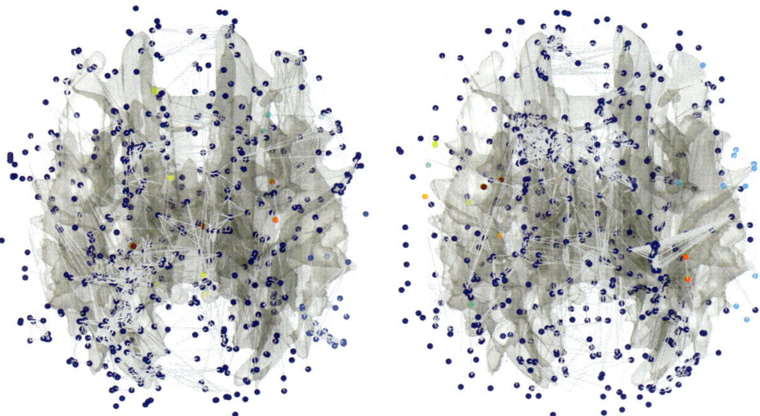

Fig. 9.12 Top: DTI networks constructed by the ϵ-neighbor method for two control subjects. All nodes in the same connected component are colored identically. DTI-based brain network is characterized by giant component that connects almost all regions of brain. In average 4% of nodes do not belong to the giant components in 30 controls subjects.

in the largest component while autistic subjects have 607.12 ± 39.39 nodes. Note that we do not need to account for brain size difference since networks constructed in the normalized space. The cluster size difference is significant (p-value $= 0.079$). We expect a larger sample size would increase the statistical significance.

9.4.4 *Epsilon Filtration*

The previous analysis about the size of largest component is at the last iteration of the ϵ-neighbor construction. Here, we present the idea of quantifying the network over all iterations *via* ϵ-filtration, which is motivated by the Rips filtration in persistent homology. We will cover the Rips filtration in detail in the last chapter.

For each given ϵ, we have Rips complex $\mathcal{G}_\epsilon$. By increasing the ϵ value, we have the Rips filtration (Edelsbrunner and Harer, 2008; Ghrist, 2008; Horak *et al.*, 2009; Zomorodian and Carlsson, 2005), a sequence of larger Rips complexes:

$$\mathcal{G}_{\epsilon_1} \subset \mathcal{G}_{\epsilon_2} \subset \mathcal{G}_{\epsilon_3} \subset \cdots$$

for

$$\epsilon_1 \leq \epsilon_2 \leq \epsilon_3 \leq \cdots .$$

During the Rips filtration, the topological features such as the Betti numbers change. The topological change over the filtration can be visualized by using the barcode. In the barcode, we plot the zeroth Betti number β_0 over the changing ϵ value. The resulting barcode is a decreasing function of ϵ and its decreasing pattern can be used to discriminate groups (Lee et al., 2011a). Although the Rips filtration completely characterizes the topological change of a network, it is difficult to biologically interpret what it really means to have changing network over scale ϵ.

Similar to the Rips filtration, the ϵ-filtration is a sequence of networks obtained from the ϵ-neighbor method. At the k-th iteration, we have a network $\mathcal{G}_k$. As the number of iteration increases, we are generating a sequence of larger networks

$$\mathcal{G}_1 \subset \mathcal{G}_2 \subset \mathcal{G}_3 \subset \cdots,$$

which we will call the ϵ-filtration. On the other hand, the ϵ-filtration is much easier to interpret since it shows the actual process of network construction.

We computed the size of the largest component in each iteration in the ϵ-filtration (Figure 9.13). It is always an increasing function and at about 6000 iterations, we begin to see the significant group difference in the increasing pattern. For instance, at 6000, 7000 and 8000 iterations, we have the p-values of 0.058, 0.038, 0.04 respectively. The control network (blue) is integrating into the largest component much faster than the autistic

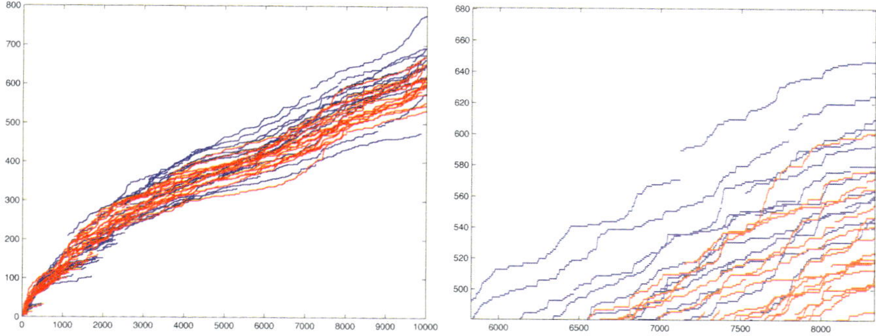

Fig. 9.13 The size of largest connected component (vertical) over the number of iterations in the ϵ-filtration showing group difference (control = blue, autism= red). At about 10000 iterations, we have 642.86 ± 68.60 and 607.12 ± 39.39 nodes in the control and autistic subjects respectively. Sudden jumps in the plot is caused by the introduction of hub nodes that connect all the disjointed components.

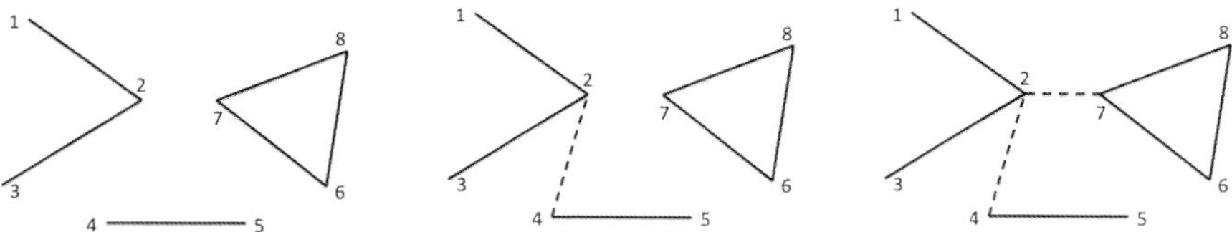

Fig. 9.14 An example of how the size of connected component changes in the ϵ-filtration. Originally a network consists of three disjoint components $\{1, 2, 3\}, \{4, 5\}, \{6, 7, 8\}$. The size of the largest components is 3. In the next iteration, we connect the nodes 2 and 4 and obtain two components $\{1, 2, 3, 4, 5\}, \{6, 7, 8\}$. The size of the largest component is 5. In the 2nd iteration, we connect the nodes 2 and 7 and eventually obtain a giant component of size 8. The node 2 is more than a hub and connects all disjoint components together. By removing the node 2, the giant components disintegrate into three disjoint components. The sudden jumps in Figure 9.13 are showing the introduction of such nodes in the network.

network (red). The growth of the size of the largest component is higher in controls. A schematic understanding of the underlying process is given in Figure 9.14. The control subjects are expected to have hub nodes that speed up the integration of disjoint components into the largest component.

9.4.5 *Electrical Circuit Model for Fiber Tracts*

Diffusion tensor imaging (DTI) is a non-invasive imaging modality often used in mapping macroscopic brain connectivity through the tractography. The strength of connection from one gray matter region to another is often measured by counting the number of fiber tracts connecting the two regions in predefined parcellations. However, the problems with this approach are the use of arbitrary parcellation and the negligence of the distance between the regions (Zalesky *et al.*, 2010).

Motivated by these limitations, we present another parcellation-free data driven network model, which is related to the ϵ-neighbor network construction. We model white matter fiber tracts as wires in an electrical circuit. The strength of connection corresponds to the resistance of the wire. Any complex circuit can be replaced by a simpler circuit with the equivalent resistance. Similarly we can simplify whole brain tractography result into smaller number of tracts.

Electronic Circuits. The brain network can be modeled as an electrical system consisting of series and parallel circuits. Each fiber tract is viewed

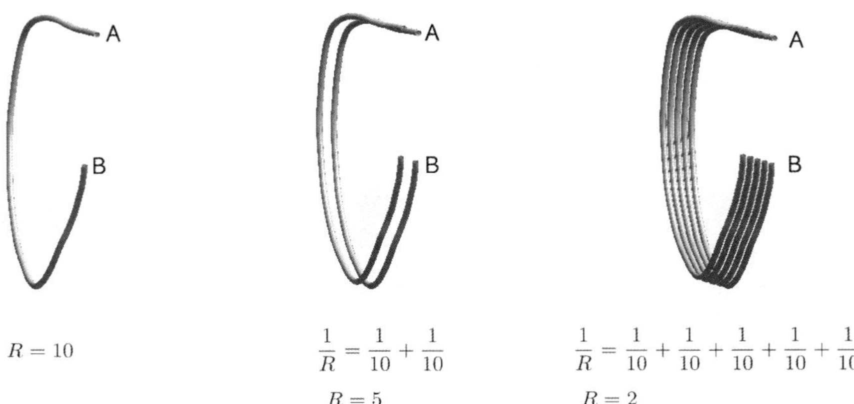

$$R = 10$$

$$\frac{1}{R} = \frac{1}{10} + \frac{1}{10}$$

$$R = 5$$

$$\frac{1}{R} = \frac{1}{10} + \frac{1}{10} + \frac{1}{10} + \frac{1}{10} + \frac{1}{10}$$

$$R = 2$$

Fig. 9.15   Multiple fiber tracts connectiong the regions A and B are modeled as a parallel circuit. The resistance in a wire is proportional to the length of the wire. As more tracts connect the regions in parallel, the strength of connection increases and the resistance decreases. In this example, we let the resistance of each tract be equal to the length of the tract. If all the tracts are 10 cm in length, the total resistance becomes 10, 5 and 2 as the number of tracts increases to 1, 2 and 5.

as a wire with resistance R proportional to the length of the wire. If two regions are connected through an intermediate region, it forms a series circuit. In the series circuit, the total resistance is addictive so we have

$$R = R_1 + \cdots + R_k,$$

where R_k is the resistance of the k-th tract. If multiple fiber tracts connect two regions, it forms a parallel circuit, where the total resistance is

$$\frac{1}{R} = \frac{1}{R_1} + \cdots + \frac{1}{R_k}.$$

Figure 9.15 shows examples of parallel circuits. Any parallel circuits in an electrical system can be simplified using a single wire with the equivalent resistance. This idea is used in simplifying the whole brain fiber tracts into a small number of tracts.

Equivalent Circuits. The proposed electronic circuit model is used in constructing the brain network without a predefined parcellation. All the tracts are sorted in terms of length and the two end points are identified. Every tract whose end points are within the ball of ϵ-radius is considered as

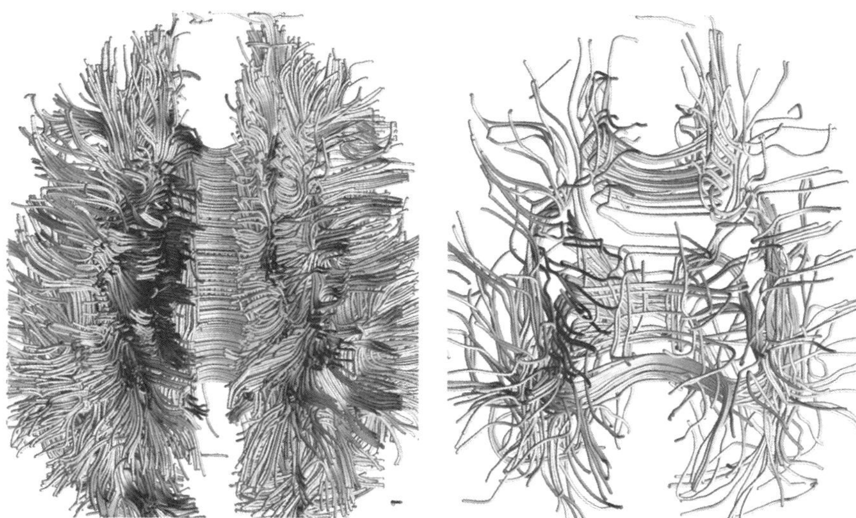

Fig. 9.16 Left: The end points of tracts are identified. Tracts whose end points are within the ball of epsilon radius are considered as connected. The fiber tracts and the balls constitute a complex electronic circuit. Right: All the parallel circuits present in the system (a) are shown. Each parallel circuit is replaced by a single tract with equivalent resistance. (c) The simplified circuit then forms a graph where the edge weights are given by the resistance.

connected. The method is similar to the proposed ϵ-neighbor method in the previous section except that we assign the edge weights using resistance. $\epsilon = 10$ mm is used for the study. The collection of tracts and ϵ-radius balls form a complex circuit, which is iteratively simplified by replacing a parallel circuit with a single equivalent tract (Figure 9.16). Initially we start with the longest tract and go on to the second longest tract in the next iteration. This process completely removes all the parallel circuits. So for any two ϵ-radius balls, there is only one tract connecting them . Hence, the simplified circuit forms a graph with the resistances as the edge weights. The graph has uniformly distributed nodes and no two nodes will be within ϵ-distance. So the nodes sufficiently cover all the brain regions.

Autistic Brain Network. DTI were acquired on a 3-Tesla scanner. The imaging parameters are given in Chung *et al.* (2010b). Spatial normalization of DTI data was done using via a diffeomorphic registration strategy (Zhang *et al.*, 2007a). A population specific tensor template was

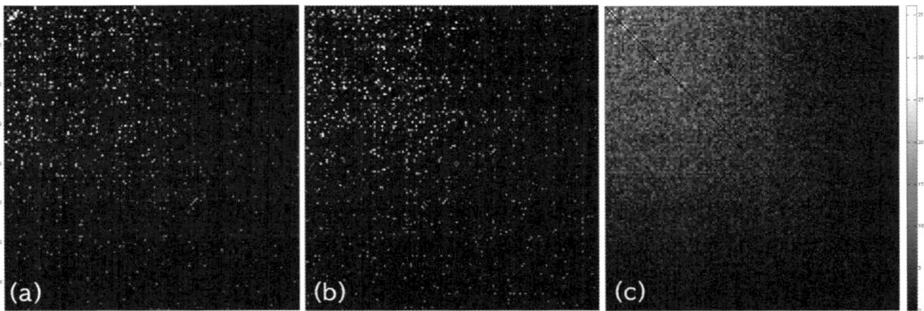

Fig. 9.17	Connectivity matrix for subject 1 (a) and subject 2 (b). (c) The average connectivity matrix of all 36 control subject.

constructed. Tractography was done in the normalized space using the TEND algorithm (Lazar *et al.*, 2003). As an application, we applied the proposed technique in constructing the structural network of 26 autistic and 41 normal control (NC) subjects.

The connectivity matrix is determined using resistance for each subject (Figure 9.17). Smaller resistance corresponds to stronger connection. The nodes are indexed in such a way that long tracts have smaller indexing. Long tracts tend to have higher resistance. Entries are sparser at the bottom right. The connectivity matrix is normalized by the maximum resistance. The total resistance is computed by summing all the entries of the connectivity matrix. The average resistance is 225 for NC and 212 for autistic subjects. The difference is found to be statistically significant using the rank-sum test (p=0.07). Higher resistance implies that NC must have more longer tracts and less redundant parallel circuits.

## 9.5	Structural Brain Connectivity without DTI

So far brain networks were constructed using DTI. However, it is also possible to construct structural brain connectivity exclusively using T1-weighted MRI without DTI. It is based on the idea of correlating local morphological features obtained from MRI in constructing a structural brain network (Lerch *et al.*, 2006; Worsley *et al.*, 2005b; Chung *et al.*, 2010c; Kim *et al.*, 2011, 2012b). The previous works mainly focused on the cortico-cortical connectivity using cortical thickness, which is defined along the gray matter.

Using the cross-correlation of cortical thickness, we then determine when the anatomy of one region changes, if there are corresponding morphological changes in other regions (Lerch *et al.*, 2006; Worsley *et al.*, 2005b,a). Cortical thickness was mainly chosen because it reflects the size, density and arrangement of neurons (He *et al.*, 2007). However, cortical thickness cannot be used in directly characterizing the connectivity within the white matter. To overcome the limitation of the previous studies, we correlate the Jacobian determinant obtained from the tensor-based morphometry (TBM) over different white matter voxels in determining association within the white matter. The detailed construction is given in [Chung *et al.* (2010c); Kim *et al.* (2011, 2012b)].

9.5.1 *Correlating Jacobian Determinants*

TBM has been often used in characterizing tissue volume difference between populations at voxel level (Chung *et al.*, 2001a; Thompson *et al.*, 2001). So far most TBM studies have performed massive univariate tests in every voxels mainly using the Jacobian determinant. Such massive univariate approaches are ill suited for addressing more complex hypotheses about brain network connectivity. Most of structural brain network models involve diffusion tensor images (DTI) in establishing edges in connectivity graphs (Bullmore and Sporns, 2009; Hagmann *et al.*, 2007; Li *et al.*, 2009; Zalesky and Fornito, 2009). Here we present a new framework for structural connectivity analysis. Instead of using cortical thickness for constructing structural connectivity maps (He *et al.*, 2007; Lerch *et al.*, 2006; Worsley *et al.*, 2005b,a), we use voxel-wise morphometric measures such as tissue density or the Jacobian determinant in building whole brain 3D connectivity maps. The main innovation is then the proposed framework does not utilize DTI but still able to construct the population specific connectivity maps only using T1-weighted MRI.

TBM usually produces the displacement $u = (u_1, u_2, u_3)'$ of warping a template image to an individual subject image. With respect to the spatial coordinates $x = (x_1, x_2, x_3)'$, the Jacobian matrix $J = (J_{ij})$ is given by

$$J = I + \frac{\partial u}{\partial x'}.$$

The Jacobian determinant is then linearly approximated using the volume dilatation (3.1) (Chung *et al.*, 2001a):

$$\det J \approx 1 + \frac{\partial u_1}{\partial x_1} + \frac{\partial u_2}{\partial x_2} + \frac{\partial u_3}{\partial x_3}. \tag{9.28}$$

We will compute the cross-correlation ρ of the Jacobian determinants between different voxel positions as a way to establish structural connectivity. Since correlation is invariant under translation, the number 1 in (9.28) does not contribute to the cross-correlation. Therefore, if $K = (K_{ij})$ is another Jacobian matrix at a different voxel position, the cross-correlation ρ between the Jacobian determinants is approximated by

$$\rho(\operatorname{tr} J, \ \operatorname{tr} K) = \sum_{i,j} \rho(J_{ii}, K_{jj}).$$

By fixing one region to be a seed, we can construct a correlation map which looks similar to seed based probabilistic connectivity maps in DTI (Batchelor *et al.*, 2001; Koch *et al.*, 2002). The resulting correlation map measures the strength of connection from the seed to other white matter regions. Statistical analysis on connectivity map difference can be done using the Fisher transform. Given two connectivity maps ρ_1 and ρ_2, we can construct the Z-statistic using the Fisher transform:

$$Z = c(\tanh^{-1} \rho_1 - \tanh^{-1} \rho_2)$$

with some normalizing constant c.

9.5.2 *Seed-Based Connectivity*

We can correlate the Jacobian determinants over the whole brain by fixing one voxel. Figure 9.18 shows the pipeline for the proposed seed-based connectivity analysis. We illustrate the method with MRI of post-institutionalized children.

T1-weighted MRIs were collected using a 3T GE SIGNA scanner for 32 maltreated children who have been post-institutionalized (PI) in orphanages in East Europe and China but later adopted to the families in US and age matched 33 normal control (NC) subjects. The mean age for PI is 11.19 ± 1.73 years while that of NC is 11.48 ± 1.62 years. There are 13 boys and 19 girls in PI, and 20 boys and 13 girls in NC.

A study-specific template construction and non-linear normalization of individual images were done by Advanced Normalization Tools (ANTS) (Avants *et al.*, 2008). A seed voxel is identified at the genu of the corpus callosum in the template (Figure 9.18 b). The connectivity maps were computed for normal controls and PI. The overlay of the connectivity maps over the template.

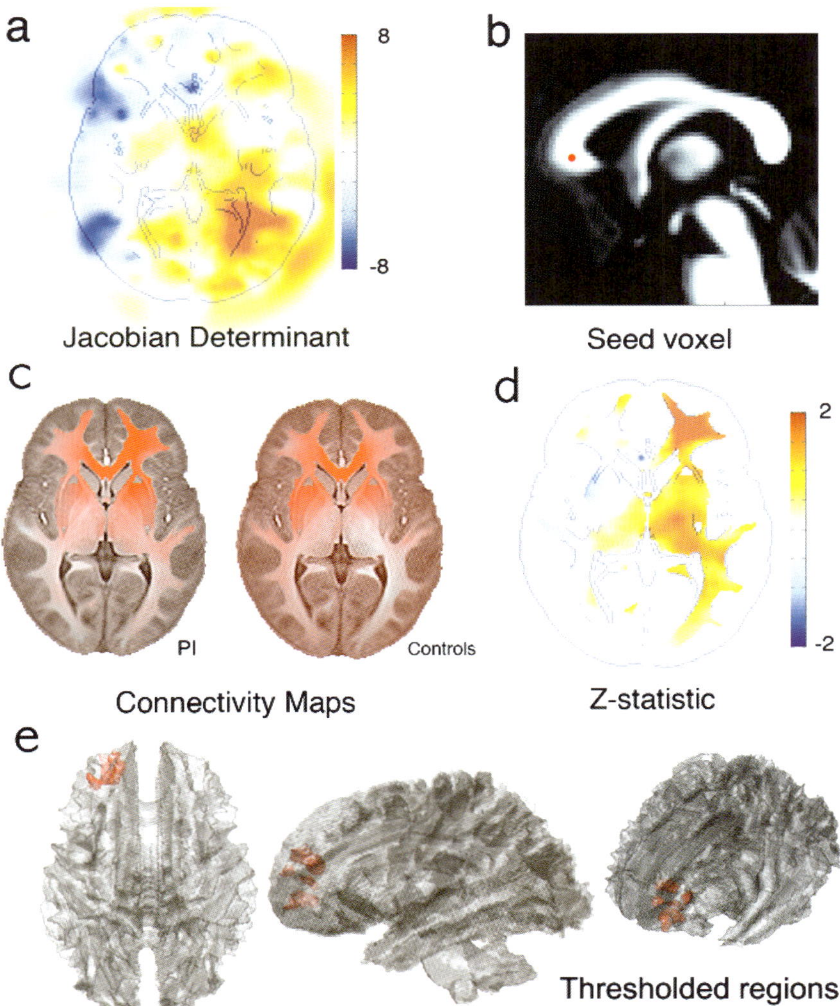

Fig. 9.18   Structural connectivity pipeline: (a) Jacobian determinant map from a subject to a template. (b) Seed voxel is chosen at the genu of the corpus callosum. (c) connectivity maps computed from the seed for post-institutionalized (PI) in orphanages and controls. (d) Z-statistic showing the connectivity difference (e). Region of significant connectivity difference thresholded at $p = 0.01$.

The regions of high connectivity are shown in darker red while the regions of low connectivity is shown in lighter red (Figure 9.18 c). Since the seed is taken at the genu, white matter regions near the genu should have higher connectivity as expected. It is remarkable that the connectivity maps look exactly like probabilistic connectivity maps often obtained in DTI. One can actually trace the gradient of connectivity maps by solving the streamline equation and obtain tracts that should behave like white matter fiber tracts.

From the connectivity maps, Z-statistic is constructed by the Fisher transform (Figure 9.18 d). The regions of the most significant connectivity difference are localized by thresholding the p-values of the Z-statistic (PI - controls) at p=0.01 and overlaid on the white matter boundary. The effected regions are white matter regions connecting the anterior prefrontal cortex. We mainly observe the highly clustered regions of positive correlation difference only. Increase in the white matter volume in the genu corresponds to increase of white matter in the anterior prefrontal cortex indicating the abnormal corpus callosum connectivity in PI. However, this does not imply that PI has more white matter volume in these regions.

9.5.3 *Parcellation-Based Connectivity*

Instead of correlating the Jacobian determinants while fixing one voxel, we can correlate them across different voxels using a parcellation. Using the publicly available DTI-based white matter atlas (ICBM-DTI-81) (Mori *et al.*, 2008), we can determine the the regions of abnormal white matter connectivity in PI in the whole brain. The method does not rely on identifying seed voxels. The framework can be further used in showing the agreement between the TBM-based connectivity and the white matter parcellation.

Once we obtain the deformation field from the individual MRI to the template, we compute the Jacobian determinant. The Jacobian determinant maps were smoothed with a Gaussian kernel with 2mm FWHM. Then we correlate Jacobian determinant across different voxels. The details on constructing Jacobian determinant-based correlation maps is given in Kim *et al.* (2011). Among the 336363 voxels with white matter density larger than 0.8, 12484 voxels were subsampled at every 3mm as possible network nodes. For the nodes i and j, we computed partial correlations $\widehat{\rho_{ij}}$ of Jacobian determinant while factoring out the confounding effect of age and gender. This is done as follows:

(1) Fit the general linear model (GLM) of the form
$$\texttt{Jacobian} = \lambda_0 + \lambda_1 \cdot \texttt{age} + \lambda_2 \cdot \texttt{gender}$$
at each node independently using the least squares method.
(2) Compute the residual between the observation and the model fit at each node.
(3) Compute the Pearson correlation between the residuals on the nodes i and j. This Pearson correlation is the partial correlation.

We will only considered positive correlations as conventionally investigated in the many structural brain network studies (He *et al.*, 2008). The constructed partial correlation maps were superimposed on top of the DTI-based white matter atlas (ICBM-DTI-81) (Mori *et al.*, 2008). In the atlas, 50 anatomical subregions in white matter were manually parcellated by radiologists guided by the fractional anisotropy (FA) map and the orientation map based on DTI. The atlas does not segment all the white matter voxels into partitions, but only labels reliably identifiable voxels that correspond to the major fiber bundles such as corpus callosum, corona radiata and longitudinal fasiculus.

9.5.4 *Validation*

In this section, we validate the TBM-based connectivity framework to ICBM-DTI-81 parcellation. See Kim *et al.* (2012b) for details. The ICBM-DTI-81 white matter parcellations are given in the MNI-152 template space. In order to normalize the white matter parcellations into our study-specific template, we first warped the MNI-152 T1-weighted template into our template, then applied the warping field to the parcellations.

We assume that, if the white matter connectivity obtained from TBM follows that of DTI, the connectivity within a parcellation will be greater than the connectivity between different parcellations. Note that we should not expect any connectivity between different white matter parcellations.

Connectivity Matrix. Let C_k be the region containing a collection of nodes that belongs to the k-th parcellation. The connectivity matrix $X = (X_{mn})$ between the parcellations is then given by averaging partial correlations $\widehat{\rho_{ij}}$ over all possible connections:

$$X_{mn} = \frac{1}{N} \sum_{i \in C_m, j \in C_n} \widehat{\rho_{ij}}, \tag{9.29}$$

where N is the total number of correlations.

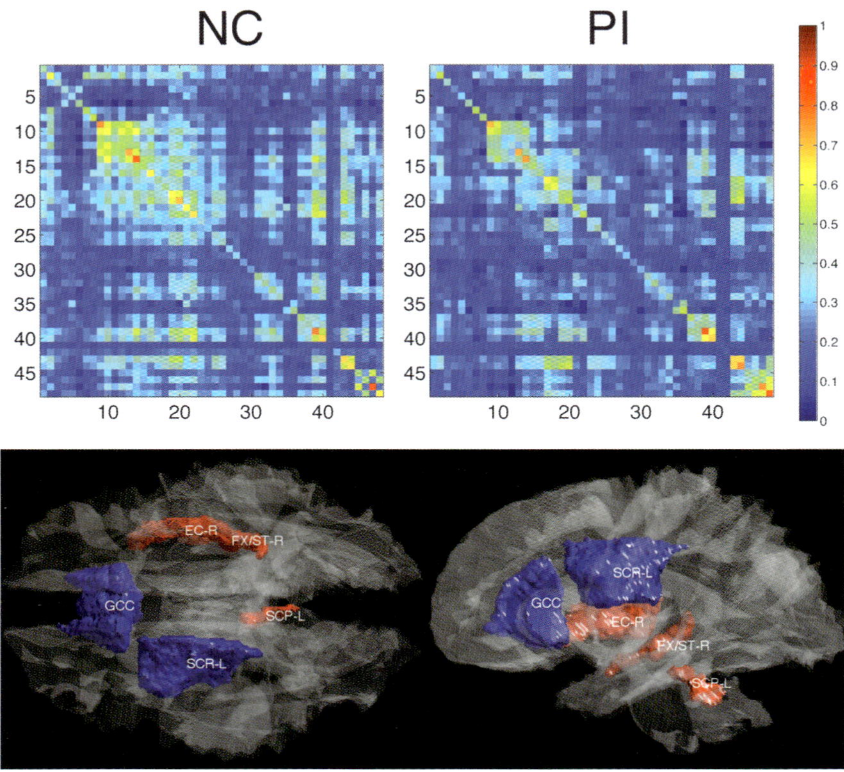

Fig. 9.19 Estimated connectivity matrices X_{mn} for NC and PI. The white matter parcellations show significant group differences in the connectivity between NC and PI. The mean correlation is greater in the PI than the NC (red) at the right external capsule (EC-R), the right fornix and stria terminalis (FX/ST-R) and the left superior cerebellar peduncle (SCP-L). The mean correlation is smaller in the PI than the NC (blue) at the genu of corpus callosum (GCC) and the left superior corona radiata (SCR-L). See Kim *et al.* (2012b) for details. Figure is generated by Seung-Goo Kim of Seoul National University.

The diagonal elements in X measure connectivity within each parcellation. We will call the diagonal term as *within-connectivity*. The off-diagonal elements measure connectivity between two different parcellations, and will be called as *between-connectivity*. The resulting connectivity maps are given in Figure 9.19. It is expected that there is no or minimal connectivity between distinct white matter parcellations. If the TBM-based connectivity map really follows the underlying white matter fibers, the within-connectivity should be relatively larger than the between-connectivity.

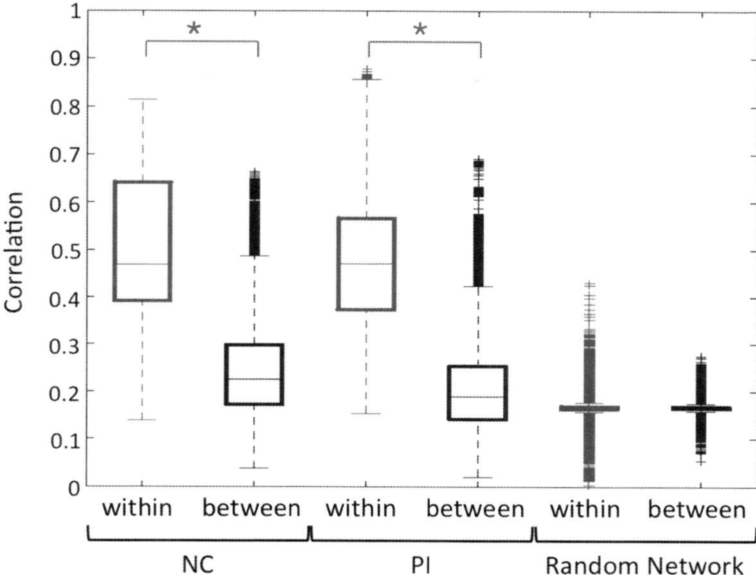

Fig. 9.20 The Wilcoxon rank sum test was applied to testing the between- and within-connectivity difference in the NC-, PI- and random networks. Significant differences are indicated with asterisks at $\alpha = 0.001$ level. See Kim *et al.* (2012b) for details.

Jackknife Resampling Technique. To test our hypothesis, we constructed 500 random networks as a null model having no meaningful connections. The random networks are generated by simulating ρ_{ij} as uniformly distributed in $[-1, 1]$. Then the corresponding connectivity matrix is also computed following (9.29). Then we tested if the median of the within-connectivity is different to the median of the between-connectivity using Wilcoxon rank sum test. Since we have only one connectivity matrix for a group, we used the jackknife resampling for inferences. In jackknifing on k subjects, one subject is removed and the remaining $k - 1$ subjects are used to generate a single network. This process is repeated for each subject to produce k networks.

Validation Results. The median of the within-connectivity is significantly greater than that of the between-connectivity both in the NC- and PI-networks $(p < 0.001)$ whereas the difference is not significant in the random networks $(p = 0.42)$ (Figure 9.20). The within-connectivity is significantly greater than the between-connectivity in the human brain. The result suggests that the connectivity maps obtained in TBM is in agreement with the existing white matter fiber bundles. However, an analysis that factors out the high correlation in ROI due to spatial regularity of registration is needed as well as a further study that directly compares the TBM to DTI tractography in the same subject.

We also tested if the connectivity is locally different between PI and NC. We only tested on the significance of diagonal elements X_{mm} since the off-diagonal elements are fairly noise and close to zero. The resulting p-values were corrected for multiple comparisons using the Bonferroni procedure. We found significant differences in the within-connectivity between the NC and the PI ($p < 0.01$). The regions of significant network differences are shown in Figure 9.19. We found smaller connectivity at the genu of corpus callosum (GCC) connecting anterior regions of hemispheres, and at the left superior corona radiata (SCR-L) connecting hypothalamic projection to the superior regions of neocortex (blue). We also found greater connectivities at three fiber bundles at the right external capsule (EC-R), the right fornix and stria terminalis (FX/ST-R) and the left superior cerebellar peduncle (SCP-L) (red).

Severe stress during the early developmental stage is found to related to atrophy in brain structures including the corpus callosum (Jackowski *et al.*, 2009). Our result shows an altered integrity of white matter connectivity due to stressful early maltreatment.

9.5.5 *RV-Coefficient*

The problem of using the Jacobian determinant in constructing the connectivity map is that it summarize a 3×3 multivariate measures into a single scalar value so we are not utilizing the full Jacobian matrix information. We need a more general approach in correlating matrices using a multivariate extension of correlation. Instead of correlating Jacobian determinants, we can correlate Riemmanian metric tensors induced by the Jacobian determinants (Chung *et al.*, 2008a). The Jacobian matrix J induces the Riemannian metric tensor

$$g = (g_{ij}) = J'J.$$

Then we can use the induced metric tensor instead of the Jacobian determinant in the log-Euclidean framework Arsigny *et al.* (2005); Lepore *et al.* (2006). Note that the volume element $\sqrt{\det g}$ is identical to the Jacobian determinant $\det J$.

Since the metric tensor g is symmetric and positive definite, we can use the *RV coefficient* (Abdi, 2007; Robert and Escoufier, 1976; Shinkareva *et al.*, 2006). If $h = K'K$, RV-coefficient ρ between g and h is defined as

$$\rho(g, h) = \frac{\text{tr}(gh)}{\sqrt{\text{tr}(g^2)\,\text{tr}(h^2)}}.$$

tr is equivalent to the vector product if we vectorize the entries of matrices and $\text{tr}(g^2)$ is the square of the Frobenius norm of g. The numerator represents a generalized covariance between J and K while the denominator normalized the numerator to have values between 0 and 1. Unfortunately, the statistical distribution of the RV-coefficient is unknown analytically but the exact permutation distribution can be obtained so that the exact mean and variance can be computed (Abdi, 2007; Kazi-Aoual *et al.*, 1995). We define a sphericity index of tensor g to be

$$\beta_g = \frac{\text{tr}^2 g}{\text{tr}(g^2)}.$$

Note that the sphericity index was mainly used in estimating the degrees of freedom for multivariate tests (Worlsey *et al.*, 1995). Then the mean of RV-coefficient between tensors g and h is

$$\mathbb{E}(\rho) = \frac{\beta_g \beta_h}{n-1},$$

where n is the dimension of matrices. The mean is taken over all possible permutations between g and h. The computation for the variance of RV-coefficient is more complicated.

$$\mathbb{V}(\rho) = \frac{2(n-1-\beta_g)(n-1-\beta_h)}{(n+1)(n-1)^2(n-2)}\left[1 + \frac{n-3}{2n(n-1)}\gamma\right]$$

for some γ. For $n = 3$, we do not need to know the value of γ since the term vanishes in the expression.

The Z statistic for testing the significance of correlation map difference between two RV-coefficients ρ_1 and ρ_2 is then given by

$$Z = \frac{\rho_1 - \mathbb{E}\rho_1 - (\rho_2 - \mathbb{E}\rho_2)}{\sqrt{\mathbb{V}\rho_1 + \mathbb{V}\rho_2}}$$

which follows the standard normal distribution.

9.6　Network Complexity Measures

So far we have discussed various brain network construction methods. Here, we discuss often used network complexity measures. Recent developments in graph theoretic analysis of complex networks have lead to deeper understanding of brain networks. Many complex networks show similar macroscopic behaviors despite differences in the microscopic details (Bullmore and Sporns, 2009). Probably two most often observed characteristics of complex networks are scale-free and small-world properties (Song *et al.*, 2005). In this section, we will explore if structural brain networks also follow scale-free and small-worldness.

9.6.1　*Degree Distribution*

Probably the most important and simplistic graph complexity measure is node degree. The *degree of a node* is the number of edges connected to a given node. It measures the local complexity of network at the node. Once we have the adjacency matrix of a network, various network connectivity measures including the node degree can be computed. The node degree is obtained by summing up the corresponding rows in the adjacency matrix. It is the most fundamental complexity measure and many other measures are related to node degree (Bullmore and Sporns, 2009). Figure 9.21 shows the node degree obtained form the DTI connectivity network using the ϵ-neighbor technique (Chung *et al.*, 2011a). For undirected network, the average degree is

$$\mathbb{E}k = \frac{2e}{n},$$

where n is the number of nodes and e is the number of links in the graph.

The *degree distribution $P(k)$*, probability distribution of the number of connecting edges in each node, can be represented by a power-law with a degree exponent γ usually in the range $2 < \gamma < 3$ for diverse networks (Bullmore and Sporns, 2009; Song *et al.*, 2005):

$$P(k) \sim k^{-\gamma}.$$

Such networks exhibits gradual decay of tail regions (heavy tail) and are said to be *scale-free.* In a scale-free network, a few hub nodes hold together many nodes while in a random network, there are no highly connected hub nodes. The smaller the value of γ, the more important the contribution of the hubs in the network.

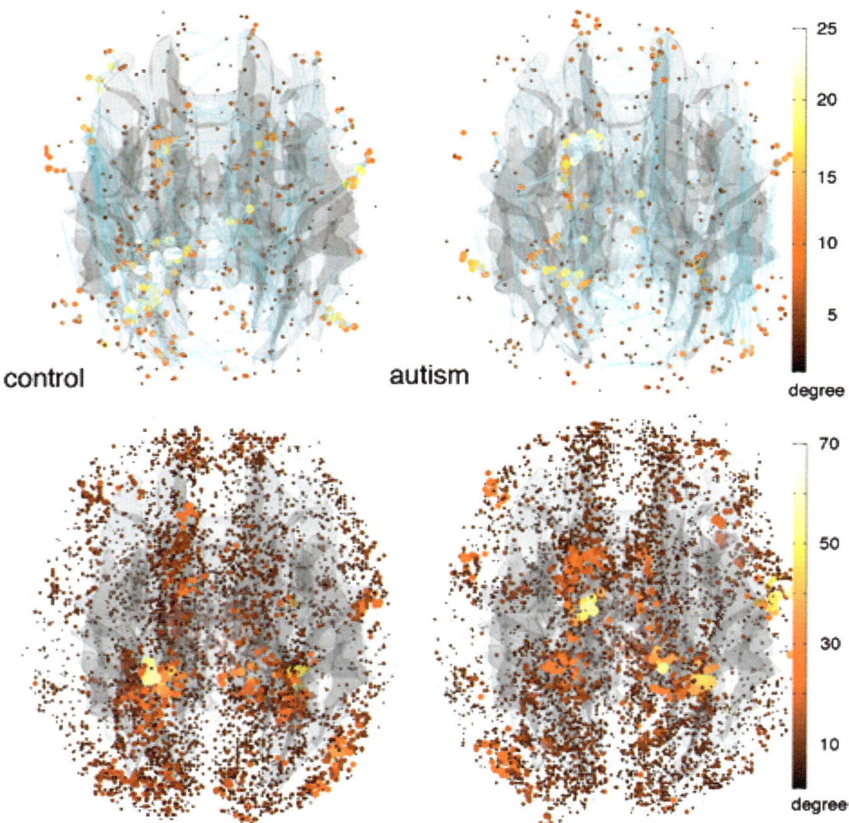

Fig. 9.21 Top: node degrees are shown as colored spheres superimposed on top of the white matter surface for a control and an autistic subject. The size of a sphere at a node is proportional to the degree. Bottom: the superimposition of node degrees for all subject in each group showing clear group discriminant.

Figure 9.22 shows the degree distributions for autistic and control subjects. The degree distributions clearly demonstrate the small-worldness of the brain network such as sparse connectivity and local clustering (Sporns and Zwi, 2004). The autistic brain network has more nodes with low degree of connectivity, which implies that there are more regions in the brain that are not connected to other regions of brain compared to the control subjects. In this example, we have thresholded at degree 25 since there are not many nodes with degree larger than 25 so the tail regions are fairly noisy.

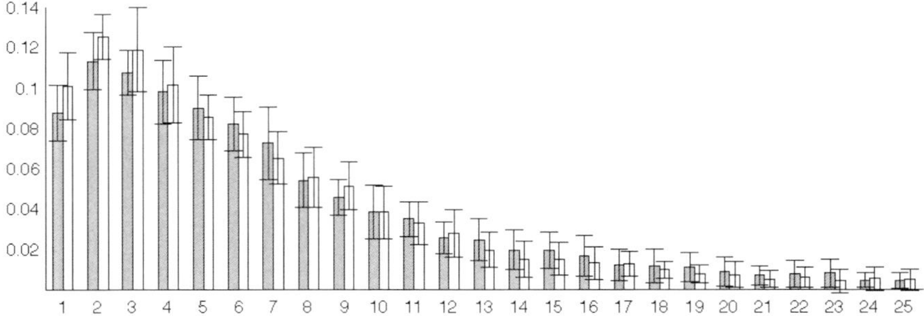

Fig. 9.22 Degree distribution for autistic (white) and control (gray) subjects. Autistic network is more stratified showing higher concentration of low degree nodes (degree 1 to 3) compared to the control subjects (pvalues = 0.024, 0.015, 0.080 respectively) (Chung *et al.*, 2010a).

The usual two-sample t-test will not work in the tail regions since the variance is too large due to small sample size. Inference on tail regions requires the extreme value theory which deals with modeling extreme events and has seen applications in environmental studies (Smith, 1989) and insurance (Embrechts *et al.*, 1999). One main tool in the extreme value theory is that for wide variety of distributions, they follow the generalized Pareto distribution at high thresholds. A standard technique is to estimate tail regions with parametric models and perform inferences on the parameters of the model fit. For low degrees, since the sample size is usually large, two-sample t-test is sufficient.

9.6.2 *Small-Worldness*

The *distance (path length)* between two nodes in a network is the number of edges in a shortest path connecting them. If most nodes can be connected in a very small number of steps, the network is said to be *small-world*. Small world networks have dense short range connections with relatively small number of long range connections (Watts and Strogatz, 1998). Let l be the shortest distance between two nodes and n is the number of nodes in a graph. If we take the average of l for every pairs of vertices and over all realizations of the randomness in the model, we have the mean path length $\mathbb{E}l$. The mean path length $\mathbb{E}l$ measures the overall navigability of a network. $\mathbb{E}l$ is sometime called the diameter of the network. However, in general, the *diameter* of a network usually means the maximum l (longest geodesic path) (Newman, 2003).

For regular lattices, $\mathbb{E}l$ scales linearly with the number of nodes n while for random graphs, $\mathbb{E}l$ is proportional to $\ln n$ (Newman and Watts, 1999; Watts and Strogatz, 1998). The small-world model is somewhere between them so the small-worldness is mathematically expressed as (Song *et al.*, 2005):

$$\mathbb{E}l \sim \ln n. \tag{9.30}$$

The relation (9.30) links the over all size of the graph to the number of nodes and implies that as n increases, the average path length is bounded by the logarithm of n. (9.30) can be rewritten as

$$n \sim e^{\mathbb{E}l}.$$

(9.30) implies that the small-world networks are not self-similar, since self-similarity requires a power-law relation between l and n. However, Song *et al.* (2005) was able to show that the model (9.30) might be biased for inhomogenous networks. Using a scale-invariant renormalization procedure through the box counting method, Song *et al.* (2005) was able to show diverse complex networks are in fact self-similar. Here we briefly go over the technique for computing the fractal dimension for networks. The explained method is simpler than Song *et al.* (2005).

9.6.3 *Fractal Dimension*

Benoit B. Mandelbrot termed *fractal* in 1960 Mandelbrot (1982). Mathematically, a fractal is a set with non-integral Hausdorff dimension (Hutchinson, 1981). While classical geometry deals with objects with integer dimension, fractals have non-integral dimension. Fractals have infinite details at every points of the object, and have self-similarity between parts and overall features of the object. The smaller scale structure of fractals are similar to the larger scale structure. Hence, fractals do not have a single characteristic scale. Many anatomical objects such as cortical surfaces and cardiovasular system are self-similar. The complexity of such objects can be quantified using the fractal dimension (FD). The main question is if the brain networks exhibit the characteristic of self-similarity. To answer this question, we need to compute FD.

Let ϵ be the scale and N_ϵ be the number of self-similar parts that can cover the whole structure. Then FD is defined as

$$\text{FD} = \lim_{\epsilon \to 0} \frac{\ln N_\epsilon}{\ln \frac{1}{\epsilon}}.$$

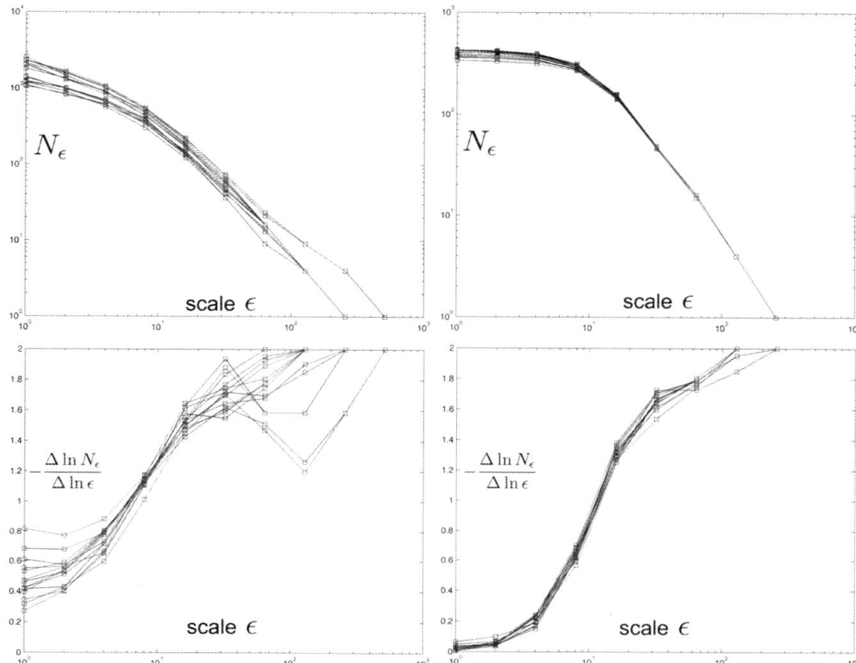

Fig. 9.23   The plots of $\ln N_\epsilon$ and $-\frac{\Delta \ln N_\epsilon}{\Delta \ln \epsilon}$ over scale $\ln \epsilon$. The first column is for 14 normal control subjects and the second column is for 14 Erdös-Rényi random graphs $G(200, 0.01)$. The FD characteristic of the random graph is different from the brain networks.

In practice, we cannot compute the limit as ϵ goes to zero for real anatomical objects so we resort to the box-counting method (Hutchinson, 1981; Mandelbrot, 1982). For k different scales $\epsilon_1, \cdots, \epsilon_k$, we have corresponding number of covers $N_{\epsilon_1}, \cdots, N_{\epsilon_k}$. Then we draw the log-log plot of $(N_{\epsilon_i}, 1/\epsilon_i)$ and fit a linear line in a least squares fashion. The slope of the fitted line is the estimated FD. We can also estimate the FD locally using the finite difference using neighboring measurements as

$$FD = -\frac{\Delta \ln N_\epsilon}{\Delta \ln \epsilon},$$

where Δ is the second order finite difference (Figure 9.23).

For networks, we have avoided using the box-counting method to the space where the network is embedded or the graph itself (Song *et al.*, 2005). Rather we have applied the method to the structure that defines link connections, i.e. adjacency matrix. The use of adjacency matrix simplifies a lot of computation. The method is applied to the ϵ-neighbor graph obtained in Section 9.4. Figure 9.23 shows the log-lot plot of N_ϵ over ϵ for 14 normal control subjects and Erdös-Rényi random graphs $G(200, 0.01)$. The Erdös-Rényi random graph $G(n, p)$ is defined as a random graph generated with n nodes where two nodes are connected with probability p (Erdös and Rényi, 1961). The FD characteristic of the brain networks is different from that of random graphs.

9.6.4 *Clustering Coefficient*

The clustering coefficient of a node measures the propensity of pair of nodes to be connected to each other if they are connected to another node in common (Newman *et al.*, 2001; Watts and Strogatz, 1998). There are two different definitions of the clustering coefficients but we will use the one originally given in Watts and Strogatz (1998). Let k_p be the number of neighbors of a node p. At most $k_p(k_p - 1)/2$ edges can exists among k_p neighbors if they are all connected to each other. The clustering coefficient $c(p)$ of the node p is the fraction of allowable edges that actually exists over $k_p(k_p - 1)/2$. Then the clustering coefficient of a graph G, $c(G)$, is simply the average of the clustering coefficient $c(p)$ over all nodes, i.e.

$$c(G) = \frac{2}{\#V} \sum_{p \in V} \frac{\text{number of edges among neighboring nodes}}{k_p(k_p - 1)}, \quad (9.31)$$

where $\#V$ is the total number of nodes in V. Note that $0 \le c(G) \le 1$.

Random graphs are expected to have smaller clustering coefficient compared to more structured one (Sporns and Zwi, 2004). For a complete graph, where all nodes are connected to each other, $c(G)$ obtains the maximum 1 and tends to zero for a random graph as the graph becomes large (Newman *et al.*, 2006). Unfortunately, the definition (9.31) is biased for a graph with low degree nodes due to the factor $k_p(k_p-1)$ in the denominator. Further, the definition (9.31) is not the mean probability of if two nodes with a common connected node are connected. The correct probability is computed by counting the total number of paired nodes and dividing it by the total number of such pairs that are also connected.

Compared to random networks, the brain network is known to have higher clustering coefficient and shorter path length. These are the characterization of *small-world networks* (Sporns and Zwi, 2004). Figure 9.24 (c) shows clustering coefficents for a control and a autistic subject, and (d) shows the superimposition of clustering coefficents for all subjects.

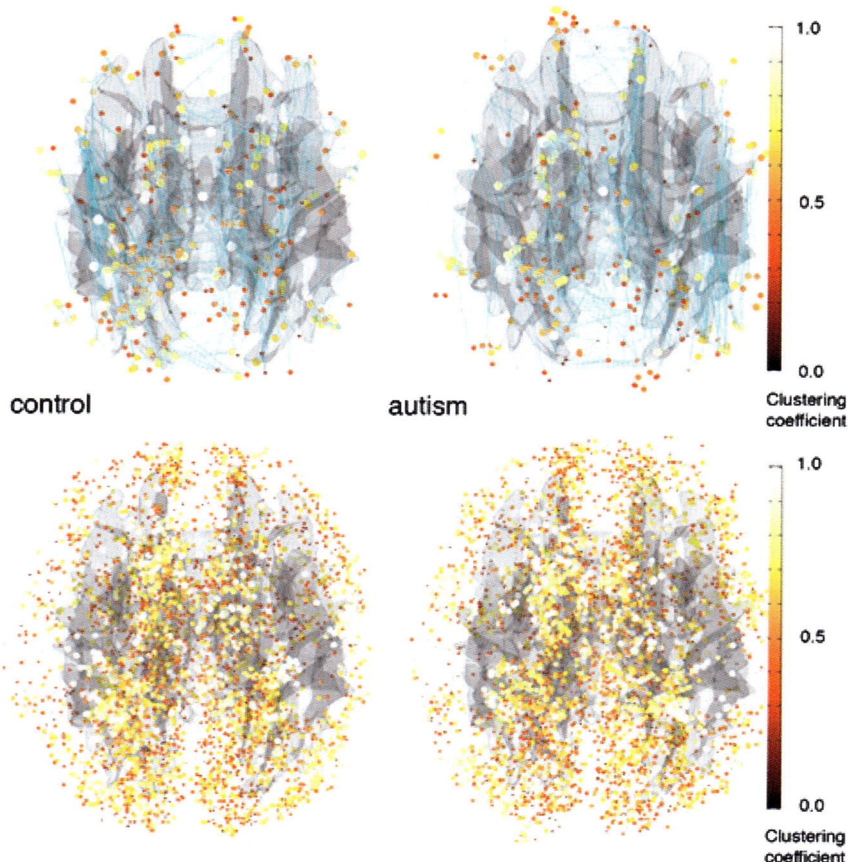

Fig. 9.24   Top: clustering coefficients are shown as colored spheres superimposed on top of the white matter surface for a control and an autistic subject. The size of a sphere at a node is proportional to the degree. Bottom: Superimposition of clustering coefficients for all subject. There are no significant group differences in the distributions of the clustering coefficients.

Although we do not observe clear group discrimination, it clearly demonstrate the small-worldness of the structural brain network.

Although we do not discuss them in detail here, other various popular graph theoretic measures are also proposed: entropy (Sporns *et al.*, 2000), path length, hub centrality (Freeman, 1977) and modularity. A review on various graph measures can be found in (Bullmore and Sporns, 2009). The path length is the minimum number of edges that need to be traversed to go from one node to another (Bullmore and Sporns, 2009). Random and complete networks have shorter mean path lengths. The centrality of a node measures the number of shortest paths between all other nodes that pass through the given node, and motivated in part by modeling social network (Freeman, 1977). Nodes with high centrality, which are likely to be with high degree, are called hubs. The modularity of a network measures the number of components or modules possibly using hierarchical clustering (Girvan and Newman, 2002).

9.7 Sparse Brain Network Models

The brain network connectivity analysis has its roots in modeling effective connectivity in fMRI, where they looked at the causal influence of one neuronal system exerts over another (Friston *et al.*, 1993a; Friston 1994; Marrelec *et al.*, 2009). Traditionally the effective connectivity has been modeled using structural equation modeling (SEM) (McIntosh and Gonzalez-Lima, 1994) and dynamic causal modeling (DCM) (Friston *et al.*, 2003). Recently partial correlation based effective connectivity modeling has been also popularized (Marrelec *et al.*, 2006, 2009).

Multivariate approaches can be used to characterize inter-dependency of morphometric measures across voxels and to produce the representational of structural networks (Brickman *et al.*, 2007). For example, the subprofile scaling model has been used to quantify the covarying patterns of tissue density at a voxel with age as well as with other voxels (Brickman *et al.*, 2007). Subtle changes in tissue density in aging may not be detected at each voxel using standard univariate analyses but the subprofile scaling model may detect subtle age-related changes in interregional dependency.

9.7.1 *Correlation Thresholding*

The majority of functional and structural connectivity studies in brain imaging are usually performed following the standard analysis framework (Gong *et al.*, 2009; Hagmann *et al.*, 2007; Fornito *et al.*, 2010; Zalesky *et al.*, 2010). From 3D whole brain images, n regions of interest (ROI) are identified and serve as the nodes of the brain network. Measurements at ROIs are then correlated in a pair-wise fashion to produce the connectivity matrix of size $n \times n$. The connectivity matrix is then thresholded to produce the adjacency matrix consisting of zeros and ones that define the link between two nodes. The binarized adjacency matrix is then used to construct the brain network. However, for a large number of nodes, this brute force approach has a serious computational bottleneck of manipulating huge number of connections and storing them. Even if we solve the computational problem, biomedical interpretation of network will be difficult with the huge number of links. For example, for 3×10^5 voxels in an image, we can possibly have a total of 9×10^{10} links in the graph. For this reason there is a strong need for a sparse regression framework in obtaining a far smaller number of significant links.

The majority of connectivity analyses have been based on thresholding correlation in detecting focal regions of correlated voxels (Cao and Worsley, 1999a; Koch *et al.*, 2002). On the other hand, Worsley *et al.* (2005b) used the singular value decomposition (SVD) in showing that SVD is better at detecting extensive regions of correlated voxels compared to the traditional method of simple correlation thresholding. Let $X_{n \times p} = (x_{ij})$ be the matrix of p regions and n subjects. Unless it is large sample size studies, we expect the *large p small n problem*. We assume X to be centered by subtracting their mean value. We further assume that each column of X is normalized by dividing by its root sum of squares, so that the diagonal elements of the cross-correlation matrix $\Sigma_{p \times p} = X'X$ is 1. The SVD of Σ is:

$$\Sigma = UWU',$$

where U is an orthonormal matrix and W is a diagonal matrix of component weights.Worsley *et al.* (2005b) proposed to estimate Σ by setting the smaller weights in W to be zero. This is exactly the principal component analysis or partial least squares (PLS) (McIntosh *et al.*, 1996; McIntosh and Lobaugh, 2004). PSL is similar to PCA but the solutions of PSL are constrained to be the part of the covariance structure. Since p can possibly reach upward of few million voxels, the computational burden of finding SVD of Σ can be prohibitive in small computers. (Worsley *et al.*, 2005b) proposed to bypass the problem by matrix decompositions. Afterward, the statistical inference is done either using permutation tests (Nichols and Holmes, 2002) or the random field theory (Cao and Worsley, 1999a; Worsley *et al.*, 1998). Since the brain networks are known to be sparse and highly clustered (Achard and Bullmore, 2007; He *et al.*, 2007), it is reasonable to incorporate the sparsity of network structures into PCA further. There have been various attempts in incorporating spasticity in PCA using LASSO (least absolute shrinkage and selection operator) in statistics (Jolliffe *et al.*, 2003; Zou *et al.*, 2006). LASSO is a widely used variable selection technique that produces sparse models (Tibshirani, 1996). It is based on the observation that PCA can be reformulated as the optimal solution of a regression so that LASSO can be integrated into the regression.

The main limitation of connectivity analyses based on correlation or covariance matrices is that it fails to explicitly factor out the confounding effect of other regions. To remedy this limitation, partial correlation has been naturally introduced in factoring out the dependencies of other regions (He *et al.*, 2007; Marrelec *et al.*, 2006) or eliminating the effect of the experimental design (McIntosh *et al.*, 1996). Since the partial correlation corresponds to the off-diagonal entries of the inverse covariance matrix, sparse PCA can be used to the inverse covariance matrix. A similar frameworks found applications in image classification (Berge *et al.*, 2007), gene expression (Dobra *et al.*, 2004), flow cytometry data (Friedman *et al.*, 2008) and functional brain network model (Huang *et al.*, 2009, 2010).

9.7.2 *Sparse Partial Correlation*

In many real-world applications, the number of nodes p are expected to be larger than the number of observations n, which gives an underdetermined system. Consider measurement matrix $X_{n \times p} = (x_{ij})$ of n subjects and p regions. At node j, we have the random variable x_j, which is realized by the random sample $x_{1j}, \cdots, x_{nj}$. We will denote this realization as

$$\mathbf{x}_j = (x_{1j}, \cdots, x_{nj})'.$$

So at the node j, the i-th measurement is given by x_{ij}. The collection of random variables x_j are assumed to be distributed with mean zero and covariance $\Sigma = (\sigma_{jj'})$ i.e.

$$\mathbb{E}x_j = 0, \ \mathbb{E}(x_j x_{j'}) = \sigma_{jj'}.$$

If $\mathbb{E}x_j \neq 0$, we can always center the data by translation. The correlation $\gamma_{jj'}$ between the two nodes j and j' is given by

$$\gamma_{jj'} = \frac{\sigma_{jj'}}{\sqrt{\sigma_{jj}\sigma_{j'j'}}}.$$

By thresholding the correlation, we can establish a link between two nodes. However, there is a problem with this simplistic approach in that it fails to explicitly factor out the confounding effect of other nodes. To remedy the problem, partial correlations have be used in factoring out the dependency of other nodes (He *et al.*, 2007; Marrelec *et al.*, 2006; Huang *et al.*, 2009, 2010; Peng *et al.*, 2009).

If we denote the inverse covariance matrix as $\Sigma^{-1} = (\sigma^{jj'})$, the *partial correlation* between the nodes j and j' while factoring out the effect of all other nodes is given by

$$\rho_{jj'} = -\frac{\sigma^{jj'}}{\sqrt{\sigma^{jj}\sigma^{j'j'}}}. \tag{9.32}$$

Equivalently, we can compute the partial correlation *via* a linear model as follows. Consider a linear model of correlating measurement at node j to all other nodes:

$$x_j = \sum_{k \neq j} \beta_{jk} x_k + \epsilon_k. \tag{9.33}$$

The parameters β_{jk} are estimated by minimizing the sum of squared residual of (9.33)

$$L(\beta) = \sum_{j=1}^{p} \left\| \mathbf{x}_j - \sum_{k \neq j} \beta_{jk} \mathbf{x}_k \right\|^2 \tag{9.34}$$

in a least squares fashion. If we denote the least squares estimator by $\widehat{\beta}_{jk}$, the residuals are given by

$$r_j = x_j - \sum_{k \neq j} \widehat{\beta}_{jk} x_k. \tag{9.35}$$

The partial correlation is then obtained by computing the correlation between the residuals of the model fit (9.33) (He *et al.*, 2007; Lerch *et al.*, 2006; Peng *et al.*, 2009):

$$\rho_{jj'} = \mathrm{corr}\,(r_j, r_{j'}).$$

The minimization of (9.34) is exactly given by solving the normal equation:

$$\mathbf{x}_j = \sum_{k \neq j} \beta_{jk} \mathbf{x}_k, \tag{9.36}$$

which can be turned into standard linear form $y = A\beta$ (Chung *et al.*, 2011c). A slightly different linearization is given in Lee *et al.* (2011d). Note that (9.36) can be written as

$$\mathbf{x}_j = \underbrace{[\mathbf{x}_1, \cdots, \mathbf{x}_{j-1}, \mathbf{0}, \mathbf{x}_{j+1}, \cdots, \mathbf{x}_p]}_{\mathbf{X}_{-j}} \underbrace{\begin{pmatrix} \beta_{j1} \\ \beta_{j2} \\ \vdots \\ \beta_{jp} \end{pmatrix}}_{\beta_j},$$

where $\mathbf{0}_{n\times 1}$ is a column vector of all zero entries. Then we have

$$\underbrace{\begin{pmatrix} \mathbf{x}_1 \\ \mathbf{x}_2 \\ \vdots \\ \mathbf{x}_p \end{pmatrix}}_{y_{np\times 1}} = \underbrace{\begin{pmatrix} \mathbf{X}_{-1} & \mathbf{0} & \cdots & \mathbf{0} \\ \mathbf{0} & \mathbf{X}_{-2} & \cdots & \mathbf{0} \\ \vdots & \vdots & \ddots & \vdots \\ \mathbf{0} & \mathbf{0} & \cdots & \mathbf{X}_{-p} \end{pmatrix}}_{A_{np\times p^2}} \underbrace{\begin{pmatrix} \beta_1 \\ \beta_2 \\ \vdots \\ \beta_p \end{pmatrix}}_{\beta_{p^2\times 1}}, \tag{9.37}$$

where A is a block diagonal matrix and $\mathbf{0}_{n\times p}$ is a matrix of all zero entries.

9.7.3 *Sparse Network Recovery*

There is a serious problem with the least squares estimation framework. Since $n \ll p$, this is a significantly underdetermined system. This is also related to the covariance matrix Σ being singular so we cannot just invert the covariance matrix in (9.32). So we need to regularize (9.37) by incorporating l_1 LASSO-penalty J (Tibshirani, 1996; Peng *et al.*, 2009; Lee *et al.*, 2011d):

$$J = \sum_{j,j'} |\beta_{jj'}|.$$

The sparse estimation of $\beta = (\beta_{jj'})$ is then given by minimizing

$$L(\beta) + \lambda J(\beta). \tag{9.38}$$

The larger the value of λ, more sparsity constraint we are enforcing. Note that (9.38) can be equivalently formulated as

$$\min_{\beta} L(\beta) \ \text{ subject to } \ J(\beta) \le \epsilon$$

for some $\epsilon \ge 0$ (Figueiredo *et al.*, 2008). This formulation is often used in compressed sensing (Candes and Wakin, 2008; Haupt *et al.*, 2008).

Since there is dependency between y and A, (9.37) is not exactly a standard compressed sensing problem. Nevertheless, as a first order exploratory analysis, we can undergo the investigation as if they are independent as has been done in others (Peng *et al.*, 2009; Lee *et al.*, 2011d).

It should be intuitively understood that sparsity makes the linear equation (9.36) less underdetermined. The larger the value of λ, the more sparse the underlying topological structure gets. Since

$$\rho_{jj'} = \beta_{jj'} \sqrt{\frac{\sigma^{jj}}{\sigma^{j'j'}}}, \tag{9.39}$$

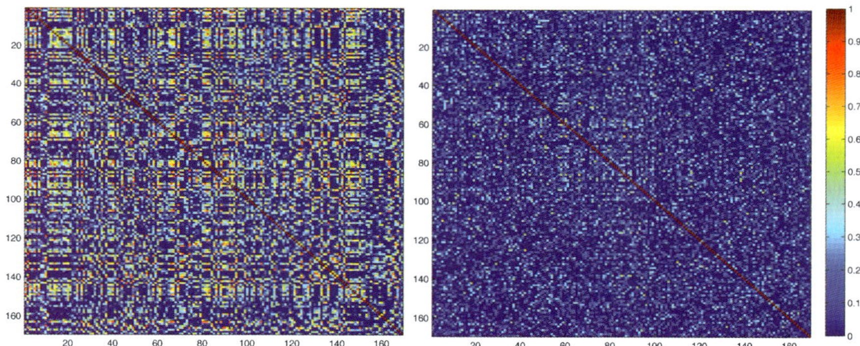

Fig. 9.25 Partial correlation estimation using the least squares estimation (left) and LASSO with $\lambda = 100$ (right). Only positive correlations are shown. The LASSO penalty reduces the number of links in the network by forcing sparsity on partial correlations.

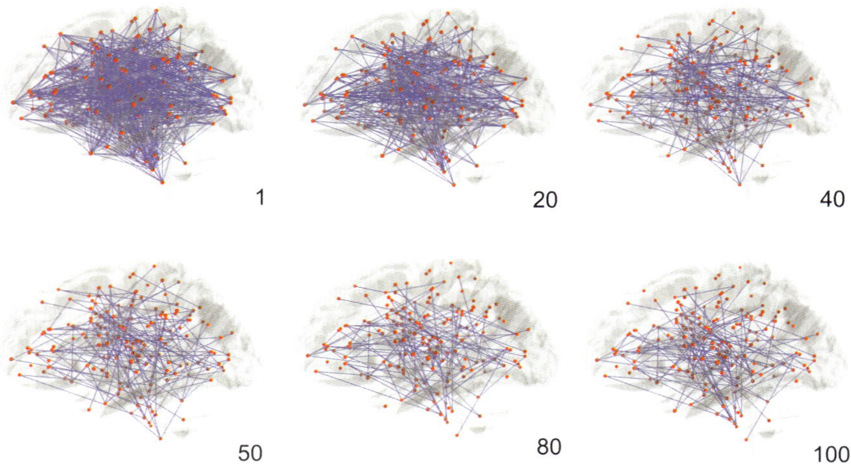

Fig. 9.26 Structural brain network of 33 control subjects. The LASSO-penalty is used for various λ values from 1 to 100. Increasing the λ value increases the sparsity of connections and, in turn, simplifies the topological structure of the network. Persistent topological features such as Betti numbers over increasing λ can be then used in the characterization of brain networks (Lee *et al.*, 2011a)

the sparsity of $\beta_{jj'}$ directly corresponds to the sparsity of $\rho_{jj'}$, which is the strength of the link between nodes j and j' (Peng *et al.*, 2009; Lee *et al.*, 2011d). Once the sparse partial correlation matrix ρ is obtained, we can simply link nodes j and j', if $\rho_{jj'} > 0$ and assign the weight $\rho_{jj'}$ to the edge. This way, we obtain the weighted graph. To simplify the problem, we will only consider positive partial correlations ρ^+ (Figure 9.25). Since the partial correlation matrix is likely to be very sparse, the resulting weighted graph will have an easily interpretable topological structure.

Example. We have applied the method to a group of 33 normal control (NC) subjects. T1-weighted MRIs were collected using a 3T GE SIGNA scanner. Details on the image preprocessing pipelines are explained in Hanson *et al.* (2010). The Jacobian determinant of deformation from individual MRI to a template is computed at each voxel. 169 voxels in the white matter are uniformly selected to form nodes of the network. We have sparsely estimated the partial correlation of the Jacobian determinants across nodes (Figure 9.25). This is a huge l_1-minimization problem and requires to estimate a total of 169^2 parameters. For instance, the matrix A is of size 5577×28561. We have used the interior-point method with various λ values in sparsely estimating the partial correlation matrix (Kim *et al.*, 2008). Then using the positive entries of the matrix as link weights, we can construct the weighted graphs (Figure 9.26).

Limitation of Compressed Sensing. However, the compressed sensing framework has a serious computational bottleneck. For n measurements over p nodes, it is required that we solve a linear system with an extremely large A matrix of size $np \times p^2$, so that the complexity of the problem increases by a factor of p^3! Consequently, for a large number of nodes, the problem immediately becomes almost intractable for a small computer. For example, for 1 million nodes, we have to compute 1 trillion possible pairwise relationships between nodes. One practical solution is to modify (9.33) so that the measurement at node j is represented more sparsely over some possible index set S_j:

$$x_j = \sum_{k \in S_j} \beta_{jk} x_j + \epsilon_i.$$

making the problem substantially smaller.

An alternate approach is to simply follow the *homotopy path*, which enables to add network links one by one with a very limited increase of computational complexity so we do not need to compute β repeatedly from scratch (Donoho and Tsaig, 2006; Plumbley, 2005; Osborne *et al.*, 2000). The trajectory of the optimal solution β in LASSO follows a piecewise linear path as we change λ. By tracing the linear path, we can substantially reduce the computational burden of reestimating β when λ changes.

Beyond sparse regression, others have proposed the likelihood methods. The Gaussian log-likelihood of data X with the covariance matrix Σ is given by

$$L(\Sigma^{-1}) = \log \det \Sigma^{-1} - \operatorname{tr}(S\Sigma^{-1}) - \rho\|\Sigma^{-1}\|_1,$$

where S is the sample covariance, $\|\cdot\|_1$ is the sum of the absolute value of the matrix entries and $\rho > 0$ controls the sparsity of solution (Banerjee *et al.*, 2006, 2008; Friedman *et al.*, 2008). This needs to be maximized over all positive-definite matrices numerically:

$$\widehat{\Sigma^{-1}} = \arg\max_{\Sigma > 0} \ \log \det \Sigma^{-1} - \operatorname{tr}(S\Sigma^{-1}) - \rho\|\Sigma^{-1}\|_1 \qquad (9.40)$$

The relationship of (9.40) to LASSO framework is explored in (Friedman *et al.*, 2008).

9.8 Dynamic Network Modeling

Motivated by the dynamic causal model (DCM) (David *et al.*, 2006; Friston *et al.*, 2003; Penny *et al.*, 2004), we present a *dynamic linear model* that model the dynamic change of anatomical networks. Let us briefly explain DCM, which models the dynamic change of neuronal response in fMRI. Let $z = (z_1, \cdots, z_n)'$ be the neuronal response at n nodes and $u_j = (u_{j1}, \cdots, u_{jm})'$ be the j-th input signal. Then the neuronal activity is modeled as

$$\frac{dz}{dt} = Az + \sum_{j=1}^{m} u_j B^j z + Cu.$$

Friston *et al.* (2003) termed $A = (a_{ik})$ and $B^j = (b^j_{ik})$ as the latent and induced connectivity matrices. A and B^j matrices measure the dependency between nodes. Figure 9.27 shows the schematic of DCM. The temporal change in the neuronal response is basically modeled using the measurements obtained in all other nodes simultaneously. We have already seen a similar statistic network model in Section 9.7, where sparse regression framework is introduced.

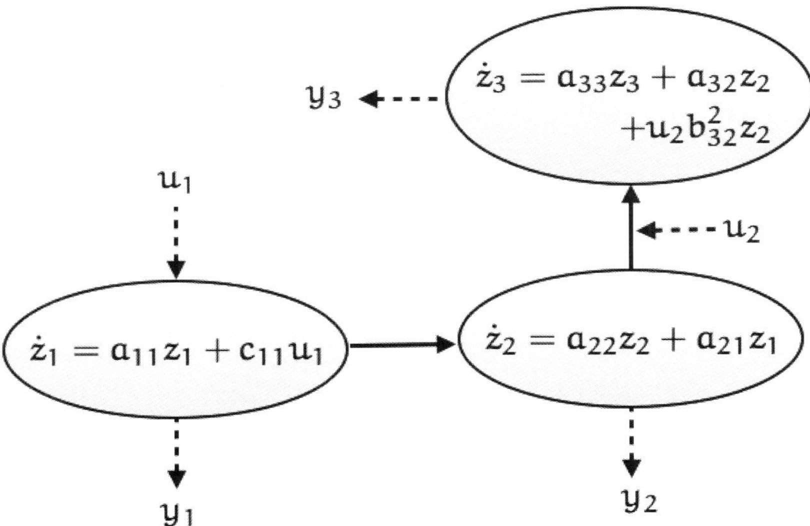

Fig. 9.27   The schematic of dynamic causal model (DCM) on 3 nodes with 2 inputs. The output y_j is somehow obtained from the neuronal response z_j.

Dynamic Linear Model. The sparse regression framework introduced to handle static networks can be adapted to handle temporally changing networks by introducing time dependency in the model. We will not consider rapidly changing functional networks based on functional measurements such as fMRI and EEG.

The system of linear equations (9.33) characterizes the network for a population at specific fixed time point. In the static model, the interest is testing the significance of partial correlations:

$$H_0 : \rho_{jj'} = c \quad \text{vs.} \quad H_1 : \rho_{jj'} \neq c.$$

From (9.39), this is equivalent to testing $\beta_{jj'} = d$ for some d. Hence, the inference on the statistic network can be based on the parameter matrix $\beta = (\beta_{jj'})$ rather than the partial correlations.

For a temporally changing network, the measurements x_{ij} and parameters β are also considered as temporally changing. Thus the change should be characterized by the change of β over time. By differentiating (9.33) with respect to t, we have a dynamic model at node j:

$$\dot{x}_j = \sum_{k \neq j} \beta_{jk}\dot{x}_k + \sum_{k \neq j} \dot{\beta}_{jk}x_k + \dot{\epsilon}_j, \tag{9.41}$$

where $\dot{x}_j = dx_j/dt$. If there is no temporal change in the network, we expect $\dot{\beta}_{jk} = 0$. So the hypothesis of interest in dynamic networks is

$$H_0 : \dot{\beta}_{jk}(t) = 0 \ \ \text{vs.} \ \ H_1 : \dot{\beta}_{jk}(t) \neq 0.$$

Therefore, it is necessary to estimate the derivative $\dot{\beta}_{jk}$ somehow. There are few possible approaches available. Since we already have a LASSO estimate $\widehat{\beta}_{jk}$ for the parameters, (9.42) can be written

$$\dot{x}_j - \sum_{k \neq j} \widehat{\beta}_{jk} \dot{x}_k = \sum_{k \neq j} \dot{\beta}_{jk} x_k + \dot{\epsilon}_j, \tag{9.42}$$

The only unknowns are $\dot{\beta}_{jk}$ which can be further estimated again using LASSO.

Chapter 10

Topological Data Analysis

In this chapter, we present a new framework for characterizing signals in images using techniques borrowed from persistent homology, a branch of computational algebraic topology. This technique is general enough for dealing with noisy multivariate data including geometric noise. This field is usually referred to as topological data analysis. The main aims of the topological data analysis are to (1) infer high dimensional structure from low dimensional representation and (2) assemble discrete points into global structure (Ghrist, 2008).

The main tool is persistent homology is persistence diagrams and barcodes. These diagrams visually show how the topological invariants such as Betti numbers of the sublevel sets of the signal changes. The use of local critical values of a function differs from the usual statistical parametric mapping framework, which mainly uses the mean signal in quantifying imaging data. The method uses all the local critical values in characterizing the signal and by doing so offers a completely new data reduction and analysis framework for quantifying the signal.

Persistent homology is popular in computational algebraic topology with applications in protein structure analysis (Sacan and Wang, 2007), gene expression (Edelsbrunner *et al.*, 2008), activity patterns in visual cortex (Singh *et al.*, 2008), sensor networks (de Silva and Ghrist, 2007) and complex networks (Horak *et al.*, 2009). However, it has not seen any applications in medical image analysis except for Chung *et al.* (2009a) and Chung *et al.* (2009b).

In this chapter, we will offer a basic introduction to topological computations in medical images. For example, we will also show how to generate the persistence diagram without going through the simplex-based topological algorithms (Edelsbrunner *et al.*, 2002; Zomorodian and

Carlsson, 2005). Let us start the chapter with the survey of traditional topological approaches used in brain image analysis.

10.1 Detecting Topological Defect in Images

The topological computation in medical imaging has been traditionally done in connection with correcting for topological defects in anatomical objects (Ségonne *et al.*, 2007; Shattuck and Leahy, 2001). The human cerebral cortex has the topology of a 2D highly convoluted grey matter shell with an average thickness of 3mm. The outer and inner boundaries are assumed to be topologically equivalent to a sphere (Davatzikos and Bryan, 1995; MacDonald *et al.*, 2000). Image acquisition and processing artifacts, and partial voluming will likely produce topological defects such as holes and handles in cortical segmentation. Further since it is needed to remove the brain stem and other parts of the brain in the triangulated mesh representation of the cortex, the resulting cortical surfaces are not likely to have spherical topology. So it is necessary to automatically determine and correct the topological defects using the topological invariants such as the Euler characteristic.

Topological defects are often encountered in image reconstruction. For instance, since the mandible and teeth have relatively low density, unwanted cavities, holes and handles can be introduced in CT image segmentation (Andresen *et al.*, 2000). An example is shown in Figure 10.1 where the tooth cavity forms a bridge over the mandible. In mandibles, these topological noises can appear in thin or cancellous bone, such as in the condylar head and posterior palate (Stratemann *et al.*, 2010). If we apply the isosurface extraction on the topologically defect segmentation results, the resulting surface will have many tiny handles (Wood *et al.*, 2004; Yotter *et al.*, 2009). These handles complicate subsequent mesh operations such as smoothing and parameterization. So it is necessary to correct the topology by filling the holes and removing handles. If we correct such topological defects, it is expected the resulting isosurface is topologically equivalent to a sphere. There have been various topological correction techniques have been proposed in medial image processing. Rather than attempting to repair the topological defects of the already extracted surfaces (Wood *et al.*, 2004; Yotter *et al.*, 2009), we can performe the topological simplification on the volume representation directly using morphological operations (Guskov and Wood, 2001; Yotter *et al.*, 2009). The direct correction on surface meshes can possibly cause surfaces to intersect each other (Wood *et al.*, 2004).

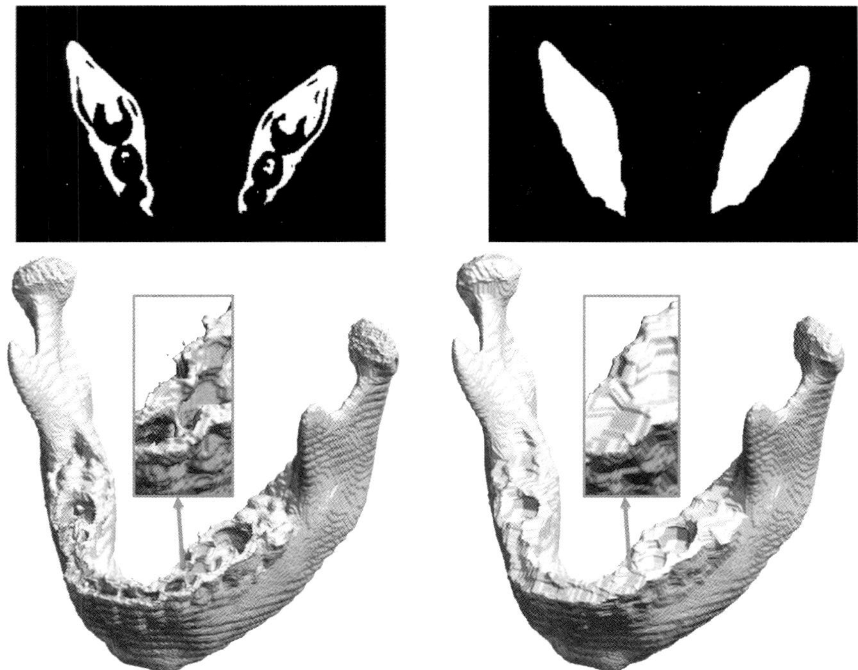

Fig. 10.1   Topological defects occurs in any type of medical image segmentation. Bridges and handles are visible in the teeth regions of the mandible segmentation obtained from CT images. Topological correction on mandible binary segmentation and surface. Disjoint tiny speckles of noisy components are removed by labeling the largest connected component, and holes and handles are removed by the morphological closing operation. Left: A slice shows holes and handles in teeth regions. The isosurface has Euler characteristic $\chi = 50$. Right: After the correction with $\chi = 2$. See Seo *et al.* (2011b) for details. The figure was generated by Seongho Seo of Seoul National University.

Here we briefly present a simplest way to correct topology. We first remove the speckles of noise components by identifying the largest connected component in the binary volume. Then we apply the morphological closing operation in each 2D slice of CT images one by one in all three axises. This basically removes a lot of holes and handles present in each slides (Figure 10.1). Recombining the topology corrected 2D slices results in topologically correct surface meshes.

Euler Characteristic. Determining topological defects on surface can be by checking the topological invariants such as the Betti numbers or Euler characteristic. Let χ be the Euler characteristic of a surface. The sphere has Euler characteristic of 2. If the surface has genus g, the number of handles, the Euler characteristic is given by

$$\chi = 2 - 2g.$$

Each handle in the object reduces χ by 2 while the increase of the disconnected components raise χ by 2. On the surface mesh, the Euler characteristic is given in terms of the number of vertices V, the number of edges E and the number of faces F using the polyhedral formula:

$$\chi = V - E + F.$$

Note that for each triangle, there are three edges. For a closed surface topologically equivalent to a sphere, two adjacent triangles share the same edge. Hence, the total number of edges is $E = 3F/2$. The relationship between the number of vertices and the triangles is $F = 2V - 4$. We simply need to compute the Euler characteristic as $\chi = V - F/2$ and check if it is 2 at the end. All binary volumes produced the topologically correct surfaces without an exception. Figure 10.1 shows an example of before and after the topology correction.

10.2 Expected Euler Characteristic

Other than topological defect corrections in images, topological concepts have been also used in statistical inference. In medical imaging and science in general, it is usually assumed that measurements f to follow the familiar signal plus noise framework

$$f(x) = \mu(x) + \epsilon(x), \ x \in \mathcal{M} \subset \mathbb{R}^d, \tag{10.1}$$

where μ is the unknown mean signal, to be estimated, and ϵ is noise (Kiebel *et al.*, 1999; Worsley *et al.*, 1996b; Miller *et al.*, 1997; Joshi, 1998; Chung *et al.*, 2001a; Friston., 2002). The unknown signal is usually estimated by various spatial smoothing techniques over $\mathcal{M}$. The most widely used smoothing method is kernel smoothing and its variants because of their simplicity, and because they provide the theoretical basis for scale spaces and Gaussian random field theory (Worlsey *et al.*, 1995; Worsley *et al.*, 1996b).

In the usual statistical parametric mapping (SPM) framework (Friston., 2002; Kiebel *et al.*, 1999; Worsley *et al.*, 1996b), inference on the model (10.1) proceeds as follows. If we denote an estimate of the signal by $\widehat{\mu}$, the residual $f - \widehat{\mu}$ gives an estimate of the noise. One then constructs a test statistic $T(x)$, corresponding to a given hypothesis about the signal. As a way to account for spatial correlation of the statistic $T(x)$, the global maximum of the test statistic over the search space $\mathcal{M}$ is taken as the subsequent test statistic. Hence a great deal of the neuroimaging and statistical literature, have been devoted to determining the distribution of $\sup_{x \in \mathcal{M}} T(x)$ using random field theory (Taylor and Worsley, 2008; Worsley *et al.*, 1996b), permutation tests (Nichols and Hayasaka, 2003) and the Hotelling–Weyl volume of tubes calculation (Naiman, 1990).

For the hypothesis of the form

$$H_0 : \mu(x) = 0 \text{ for all } x \text{ vs. } H_1 : \mu(x) > 0 \text{ for some } x,$$

the region of statistically significant signal corresponding to the alternate hypothesis is given by $A_h = \{x \in \mathcal{M} : T(x) > h\}$. Then it is known in the random field theory that

$$P\left(\sup_{x \in \mathcal{M}} T(x) > h \right) \approx \mathbb{E}\chi(A_h),$$

where $\chi(A_h)$ is the Euler characteristic of A_h (Adler, 1981; Taylor and Worsley, 2007; Worsley, 2003). See Section 1.3 for the detailed exposition of the Euler characteristic approach. This indirectly links the problem of statistical inference to that of topology (Figure 10.2).

One the other hand, there has been a parallel development that tried to link topology to statistical analysis via persistence homology (Bubenik and Kim, 2007; Chung *et al.*, 2009a,b). The use of the mean signal is one way of performing data reduction; however, this may not necessarily be the best way to characterize complex multivariate imaging data. Thus instead of using the mean signal, we can to use topological features such as persistent homology, which pairs local critical values (Edelsbrunner and Harer, 2008; Edelsbrunner *et al.*, 2002; Zomorodian and Carlsson, 2005). It is intuitive that local critical values of $\widehat{\mu}$ approximately characterizes the shape of the continuous signal μ using only a finite number of scalar values. By pairing these local critical values in a nonlinear fashion and plotting them, one constructs the persistence diagram (Cohen-Steiner *et al.*, 2007; Edelsbrunner and Harer, 2008; Morozov, 2008; Zomorodian, 2001).

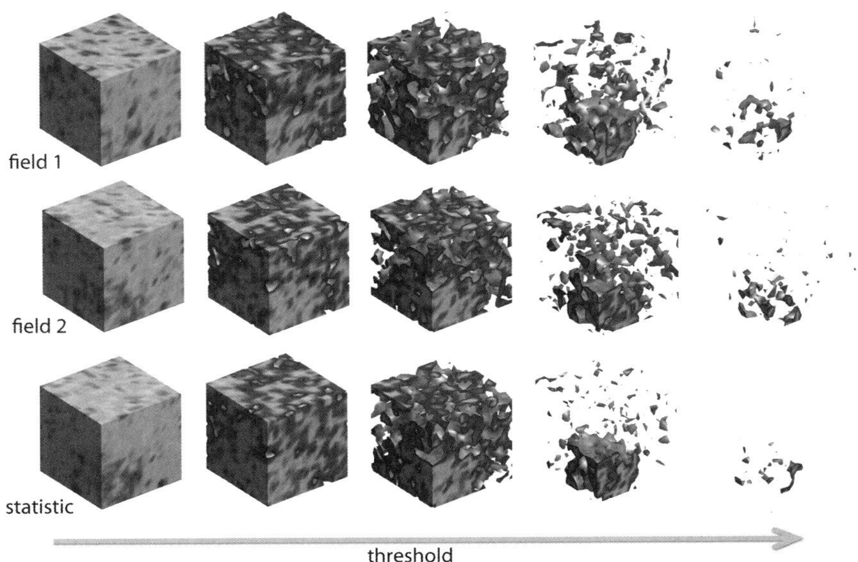

Fig. 10.2   Given fields $f_i = \mu + \epsilon_i$, we are interested in detecting the regions of significant signal $\mu > 0$. In the random field theory (Worsley, 2003), we construct a test statistic T out of the fields f_i and determine the topological change of the excursion set $A_h = \{x \in \mathcal{M} : T(x) > h\}$ as we increase the threshold h. This determine the type-I error associated with the hypothesis testing. On the other hand, what we are advocating is to determine the topological change of the individual excursion sets $B_{i,h} = \{x \in \mathcal{M} : f_i(x) > h\}$ first. Then we construct a statistical test on the topological change of $B_{i,h}$.

10.3   Rips Complex

Cortical surfaces already have surface meshes as the underlying topological representation. So topological computation on cortical surfaces can be easily done. However, for other type of data and images, it is crucial to obtain the most accurate topological representation that approximates them. Often an object can be easily observed and represented as an unordered collection of points in a Euclidean space (Ghrist, 2008). Such the collection of points is often refereed as *point cloud data*. For instance, the point cloud data approximates the underlying gray shaded object in Figure 10.3. Then by connecting the point cloud data somehow, we can obtain higher dimensional topological information.

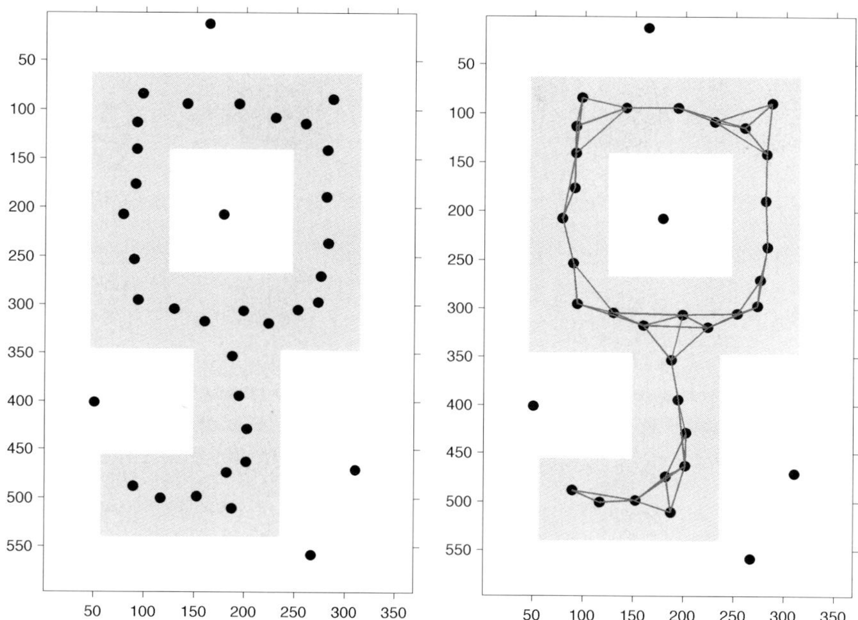

Fig. 10.3 Left: A sparsely sampled point cloud that approximate the underlying object (gray). Right: The rips complex of the point cloud data. $\epsilon = 70$ is used for construction. If two points are within the ϵ radius, we connect them with a link. There are 36 nodes and 56 links. Three outlying data are not connected to the largest connected component.

10.3.1 *Topology*

A high dimensional object can be approximated by the point cloud data X consisting of p number of points. If we connect points of which distance satisfy a given criterion, the connected points start to recover the topology of the object. Hence, we can represent the underlying topology as a collection of the subsets of X that consist of nodes which are connected (Edelsbrunner and Harer, 2009; Hart, 1999). Suppose $U \subset 2^X$, the collection of all possible subsets of X. Then (X, U) is a topological space on X if

(1) $\emptyset, X \subset U$,
(2) $u_1, u_2 \subset U$ implies $u_1 \cup u_2 \subset U$ and
(3) $u_1 \cap u_2 \subset U$.

Note that every metric space is a topological space. In general, given a point cloud data set X with a rule for connections, the topological space is a simplicial complex and its element is a simplex (Zomorodian, 2009). For point cloud data, the Delaunay triangulation is probably the most widely used method for connecting points. The Delaunay triangulation represent the collection of points in space as a graph whose face consists of triangles.

10.3.2   *Simplex*

The k-simplex σ is the convex hull of $(k+1)$ independent points $x_0, \cdots, x_k$. A point is a 0-simplex, an edge is a 1-simplex, and a triangle is a 2-simplex. A complete graph with k nodes is a $(k-1)$-simplex. A *simplicial complex K* is a finite collection of simplices satisfying (Edelsbrunner and Harer, 2009)

(1) any face of $\sigma \in K$ is also in K, and
(2) for $\sigma_1, \sigma_2 \in K$, $\sigma_1 \cap \sigma_2$ is a face of both σ_1 and σ_2.

Hence a graph is a simplicial complex consisting of 0-simplices (nodes) and 1-simplices (edges). There are various simplicial complexes. One of them is the Rips complex.

10.3.3   *Rips complex*

The Rips complex has been also used for triangulation (Ghrist, 2008). The *Rips complex* is a graph constructed by connecting two data points if they are within specific distance ϵ. Figure 10.3 shows an example of the Rips complex that approximates the gray object. Given a point cloud data X, the Rips complex $R(X, \epsilon)$ is a simplicial complex whose k-simplices correspond to unordered $(k+1)$-tuples of points which are pairwise within distance ϵ (Ghrist, 2008).

While a graph has at most 1-simplices, the Rips complex has at most k-simplices. One major problem of the Rips complex is that given n points, it exactly produces a graph with n nodes so the resulting graph becomes very complicated when n becomes large. Figure 10.4 shows an example where the increased sample size increases the complexity of the graph as well as the number of outliers.

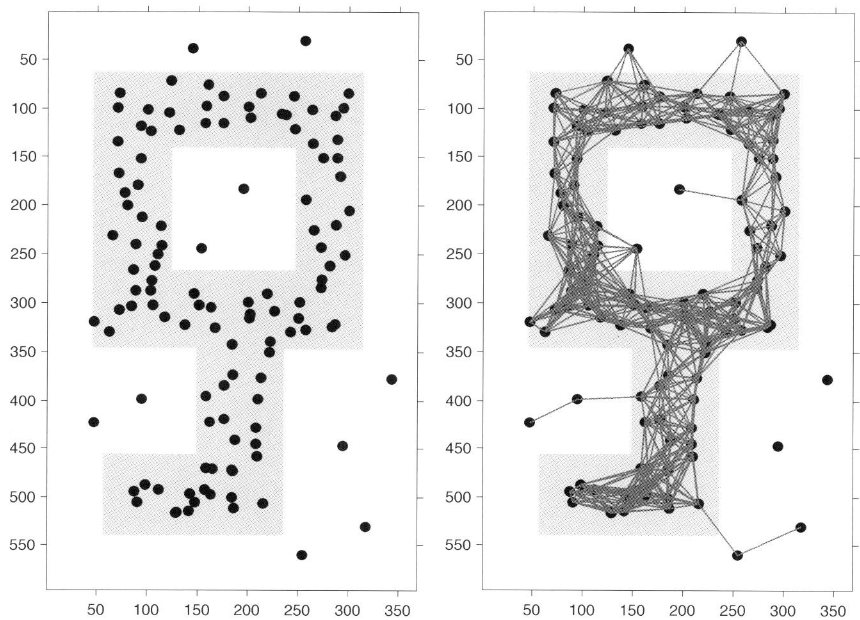

Fig. 10.4 Left: A densely sampled point cloud that approximate the underlying object (gray). Right: The rips complex of the point cloud data. $\epsilon = 70$ is used for construction. There are 119 nodes and 789 links. The increased sampling density increases the complexity of the graph as well the number of outliers.

10.4 Persistence Diagrams

10.4.1 *Morse Functions*

A function is called a Morse function if all critical values are unique and non-degenerate, i.e. the Hessian does not vanish (Milnor, 1973). We note that for integer-valued digital images, critical values of intensity may not be all unique; however, the underlying continuous signal μ in (10.1) is likely and assumed to be a Morse function. We estimate the signal using a kernel function and obtain a smooth estimate. For illustrative purposes, we will show how to construct the persistence diagram for a 1D Morse function.

Assuming μ is a Morse function with a finite number of critical values, define a sublevel set

$$R(y) = \mu^{-1}(-\infty, y].$$

The sublevel set is the subset of $\mathbb{R}$ that satisfies $\mu(x) \leq y$. The sublevel set can have many disjoint components.

Let $\#R(y)$ be the number of connected components in the sublevel set. Let us denote the local minimums as $g_1, \cdots, g_m$ and the local maximums as $h_1, \cdots, h_n$. Since the critical values of the Morse function are all unique, we can strictly order the local minimums from the smallest to the largest as

$$g_{(1)} < g_{(2)} < \cdots < g_{(m)}$$

and similarly for the local maximums as

$$h_{(1)} < h_{(2)} < \cdots < h_{(n)},$$

where $h_{(i)}$ denotes the i-th order statistic, i.e. smallest value. We further collect all the critical values,

$$z_1 = g_1, \ldots, z_m = g_m, z_{m+1} = h_1, \ldots, z_{m+n} = h_n$$

and order them as

$$z_{(1)} < z_{(2)} < \cdots < z_{(m+n)}.$$

At each minimum, we have the birth of a new component, i.e.

$$\#R(g_i) = \#R(g_i - \varepsilon) + 1$$

for sufficiently small ε. The new component is identified with the local minimum g_i. Similarly at each maximum, we have the death of a component, i.e.

$$\#R(h_i) = \#R(h_i - \varepsilon) - 1,$$

and two components will merge as one. The number of connected components will only change if we pass through critical points and we can iteratively compute $\#R$ at each critical value as

$$\#R(z_{(i+1)}) = \#R(z_{(i)}) \pm 1.$$

The sign depends on whether $z_{(i+1)}$ is a maximum (-1) or a minimum $(+1)$. This is the basis of Morse theory, which states the topological characteristics of a topological space is characterized by the local behavior at critical points of a Morse function on that space (Milnor, 1973). Persistent homology then produces pairs (g_i, h_j) of critical values so that a component is born at g_i and dies at h_j. Of course these are the topological parameters of interest which are unknown and to be statistically estimated with data generated according to (10.1).

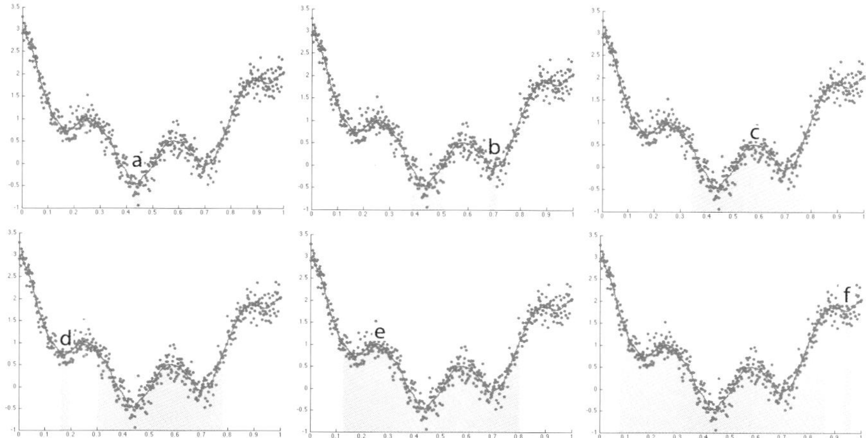

Fig. 10.5   The births and deaths of components in sublevel sets. We have critical values a, b, c, d, e, f, where $a < b < d < f$ are minimums and $c < e$ are maximums. At $y = a$, we have a single component marked by a single gray area. When we increase the level to $y = b$, we have the birth of a new component in addition to the existing component born at a. At the maximum $y = c$, the two components merge together to form a single component. Following the pairing rule given in Edelsbrunner and Harer (2008), we pair (b, c) and (d, e). Other critical values are paired similarly.

Example. The birth and death processes are illustrated in Figures 10.5 and 10.6, where the gray dots are simulated with Gaussian noise with mean 0 and variance 0.2^2 as

$$f(x) = \mu(x) + N(0, 0.2^2) \tag{10.2}$$

with signal $\mu(t) = 10(t - 1/2)^2 + \cos(7\pi t)/2$. The signal μ is estimated using the 1D version of heat kernel smoothing (Chung *et al.*, 2007). Now we increase y from $-\infty$ to ∞. When we hit the first critical value $y = a$, the sublevel set consists of a single point, i.e. $\#R(a) = 1$. When we hit the minimum at $y = b$, we have the birth of a new component at b, i.e. $\#R(b) = 2$. When we hit the maximum at $y = c$, the two components identified by a and b are merged together to form a single component, i.e. $\#R(c) = 1$.

10.4.2   Persistence Diagrams

Since the birth and death of critical values are difficult to visualize, we present a new way of data visualization using the persistent diagram that

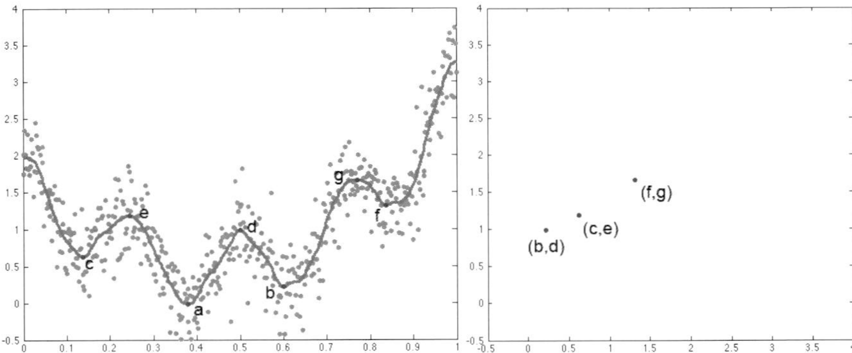

Fig. 10.6   The birth and death process of sublevel sets. In this slightly different example, $a < b < c < f$ are minimums and $d < e < g$ are maximums. At $y = b$, we add a new component to the sublevel set. When we increase the level to $y = d$, we have the death of the component so we pair them. We pair (f, g), (c, e) and (b, d) and plot them to produce the persistence diagram on the right.

represent paired critical values in 2D. It requires the following pairing rule:

When we pass a maximum and merge two components, we pair the maximum with the higher of the minimums of the two components (Edelsbrunner and Harer, 2008).

Doing so we are pairing the birth of a component to its death. Obviously the paired extremes do not have to be adjacent to each other. If there is a boundary, the function value evaluated at the boundary is treated as a critical value. The persistence diagram is then the scatter plot of these pairings. In the simulation (10.2), we need to pair (b, c) and (d, e) (Figure 10.6). Other critical values are paired similarly. For technical reasons, the persistence diagram also include all of the points (a, a), where $a \in \mathbb{R}$.

High Dimensional Pairing.   For higher dimensional Morse functions, saddle points can also create or merge sublevel sets so we also have to be concerned with them. For higher dimensions, persistence diagrams will have more pairs compared to 1D cases. The addition of the saddle points makes the construction of the persistence diagrams much more complex. Currently there is only one publicly available algorithm called **PLEX** for generating persistence diagrams based on the filtration of Morse complexes (Edelsbrunner *et al.*, 2002; Zomorodian and Carlsson, 2005).

For a 2D Morse function defined on a cortical manifold $\mathcal{M} \subset \mathbb{R}^3$, we also need to consider saddle points so the situation is more complicated. At a saddle point, we can have two possible pairings corresponding to either birth or death. A saddle point may join two components. This case is analogous to the local maximum in the 1D case. In this case, persistent homology pairs the value of the saddle point with the larger of the minimums of the two components. This pair is recorded as the persistence diagram of degree 0.

If the saddle point does not join two disconnected components, then a hole is born in the sublevel set. Persistent homology pairs the value at this saddle point with the value of the local maximum where this hole disappears. This pair is recorded as the persistence diagram of degree 1. This complication makes generalizing the iterative pairing and deletion algorithm to higher dimension difficult. Available topologically oriented algorithms is based on constructing filtered simplicial complexes and finding a rule for adding and deleting one simplex at a time (Edelsbrunner *et al.*, 2002; Zomorodian and Carlsson, 2005).

10.4.3 *Persistence Diagram for Cortical Thickness*

Among various cortical measures, we consider cortical thickness, which has been used in characterizing various clinical populations (Chung *et al.*, 2005a; Fischl and Dale, 2000; Luders *et al.*, 2006a; Miller *et al.*, 2000; Yezzi and Prince, 2003). Cortical thickness f is defined as the distance between the outer and inner cortical surfaces and projected onto the outer cortical surface $\mathcal{M}$. Cortical thickness is assumed to follow

$$f(x) = \mu(x) + \epsilon(x),$$

where μ is the unknown cortical thickness and ϵ is the noise. Since cortical thickness is highly noisy, heat kernel smoothing is applied to remove high frequency spatial noise and to estimate μ. Let $\zeta : \mathcal{M} \to S^2$ be a sufficiently smooth surface flattening which can be obtained , for instance, from the deformable surface algorithm. Then the pullback $(\zeta^{-1})^*\mu = \mu \circ \zeta^{-1}$ projects the cortical thickness from the cortical surface $\mathcal{M}$ to the unit sphere. Figure 10.7 shows the pull back and the corresponding heat kernel smoothing on S^2. Note that in the process of flattening, the critical values do not change so the persistence diagram should be identical for f and its pullback $(\zeta^{-1})^*\mu$. Therefore, we can construct the persistence diagram on the unit 2–sphere by projecting the cortical data to the sphere (Figures 10.7 and 10.8). See Chung *et al.* (2009b) for the detailed construction.

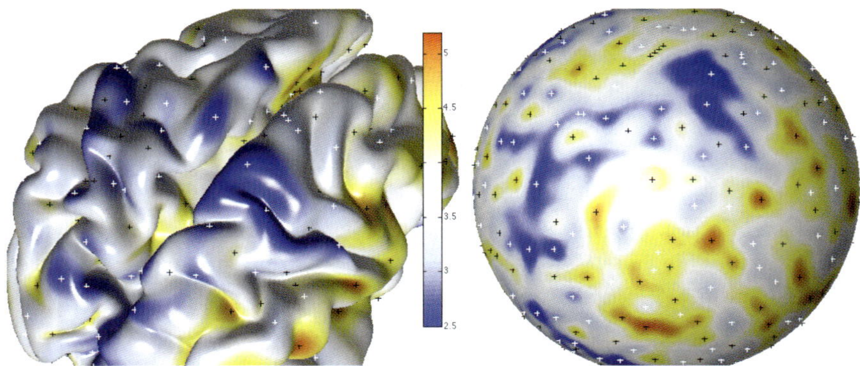

Fig. 10.7 Heat kernel smoothing of cortical thickness and surface coordinates with bandwidth $\sigma = 0.001$ and degree $k = 42$. It has been been flattened onto the sphere for better visualization. The white (black) crosses are local minimums (maximums). They are paired in a special manner to obtain the persistence and min-max diagrams, which are invariant to whether it is constructed from the cortical surface or from the unit sphere.

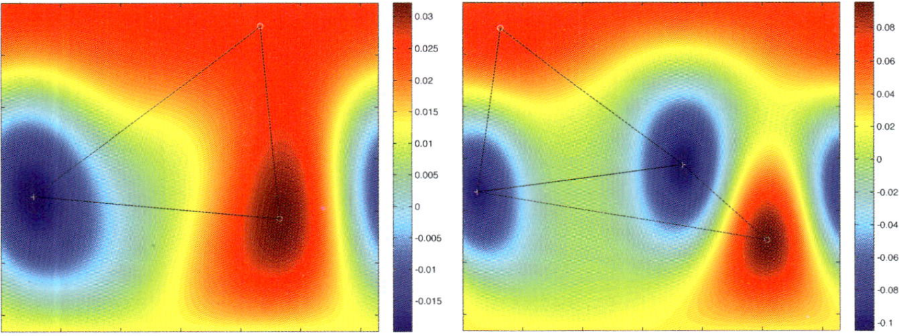

Fig. 10.8 Given smoothed 2D image, we construct the Delaunay triangulation consisting of critical points. This gives an information about neighborhood and the subsequent pairing rules.

Persistence Diagrams for Cortical Mesh. For a sample of size n, define the estimator $\widehat{\mu}_n$ of unknown cortical thickness μ in the following way. For each face in a triangulation, we define $\widehat{\mu}_n$ on the face by affine interpolation from the values on the vertices. This construction is well defined on the edges, and defines a function on the triangulation T. It remains to calculate the persistence diagrams of the sublevel sets of $\widehat{\mu}_n$ on the triangulated surface. Because of the way $\widehat{\mu}_n$ is constructed, we can calculate its persistence diagrams using our triangulation.

We filter T using $\widehat{\mu}_n$ as follows. Let $\epsilon_1 \leq \epsilon_2 \leq \cdots \leq \epsilon_m$ be the ordered list of values of $\widehat{\mu}_n$ on the vertices of the triangulation. Let T_i be the subcomplex of T containing all vertices v with $\widehat{\mu}_n(v) \leq \epsilon_i$ and all edges whose boundaries are in T_i and all faces whose boundaries are in T_i. Then we obtain the following filtration of T,

$$\phi = T_0 \subset T_1 \subset T_2 \subset \cdots \subset T_m = T.$$

The end result is that the topological properties of the sublevel sets of $\widehat{\mu}_n$ will equal the topological properties of the above filtration of T.

We calculated the persistent homology, in degrees 0, 1 and 2 of the triangulation T filtered according to the estimator for each of the 27 subjects (Figure 10.9). Since the data is two–dimensional, we do not expect any interesting homology in higher degrees. In degree two, the persistent homology consists of a single persistence pair (a, ∞), where a is the maximum of $\widehat{\mu}_n$.

The stability of the persistent diagram under small perturbation is established in Cohen-Steiner *et al.* (2007) and Edelsbrunner and Harer (2008). Let $D(\mu)$ and $D(\nu)$ be the persistence diagrams of μ and ν respectively. A metric on the space of persistence diagrams is the bottleneck distance d which bounds the Hausdorff distance. It is given by

$$d(D(\mu), D(\nu)) = \inf_{\gamma} \sup_{p \in D(\mu)} \|p - \gamma(p)\|_\infty, \tag{10.3}$$

where the infimum is taken over all bijections $\gamma : D(\mu) \to D(\nu)$ and $\| \cdot \|_\infty$ is the sup-norm metric. In Cohen-Steiner *et al.* (2007), the following result is proven:

$$d(D(\mu), D(\nu)) \leq \|\mu - \nu\|_\infty. \tag{10.4}$$

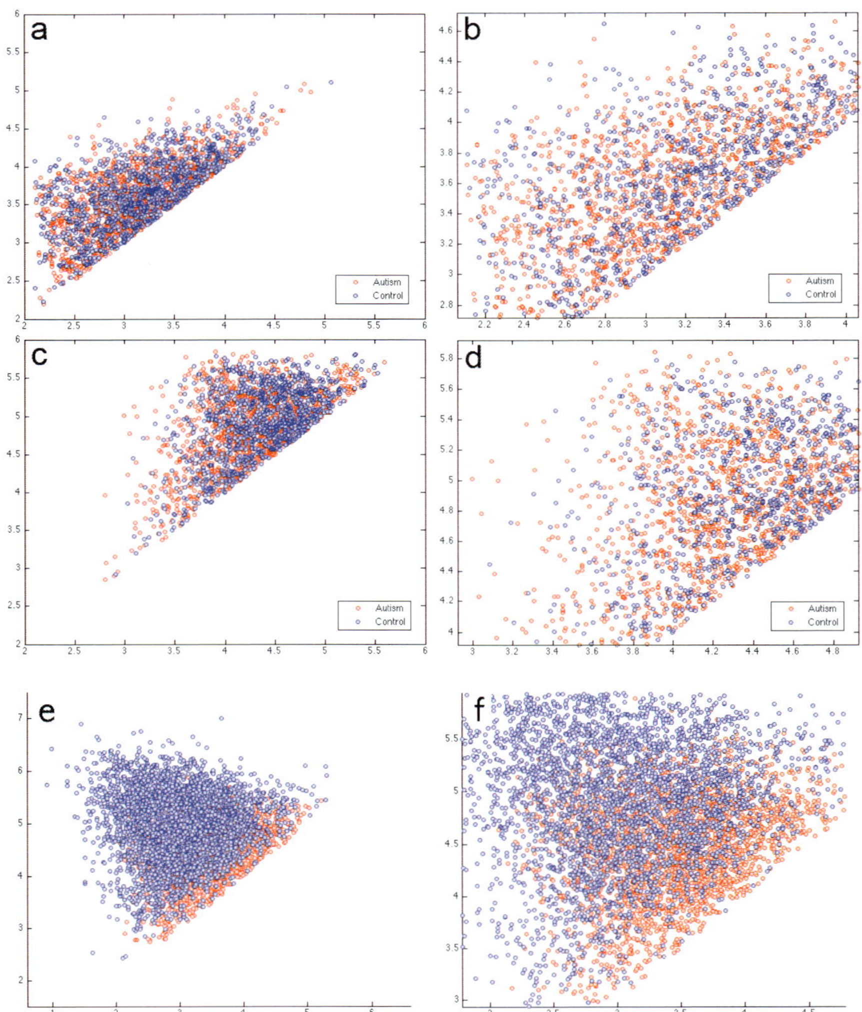

Fig. 10.9   The persistence diagrams for 11 control (blue) and 16 autistic (red) subjects in degree 0 (a) and degree 1 (c). The min-max diagram without saddle points (e). The second columns are the enlargement of the first columns.

10.4.4 *Inference on Persistent Diagrams*

At this point, it is unclear how one determines the possible statistical significance of persistent diagram difference. Here we present a case study of discriminating autistic subjects from normal controls (Chung *et al.*, 2009a). One may be tempted to use hypothesis-free classification frameworks for inference, however, Figure 10.9 shows that classification based on possibly discriminating spatial pattern is likely to be challenging. Note that the autistic scatter plots basically encompass the control scatter plots for the degree 0 and degree 1 persistence diagrams. Since there is considerable overlap, machine learning techniques would need to be adapted for this challenge. On the other hand, there seems to be spatial concentration difference in the pairings. Therefore, we have computed the pairing concentration by computing the number of parings within a circle of radius 0.2 at the point $x \in [1, 7]^2$. The average pairing concentration maps are shown in Figure 10.10, where we can see concentration difference for both the degree 0 and 1 persistence diagrams. The significance of the concentration map difference is determined using a permutation test. We first constructed the two sample t statistic map $T(p)$. The type-I error for correcting for multiple

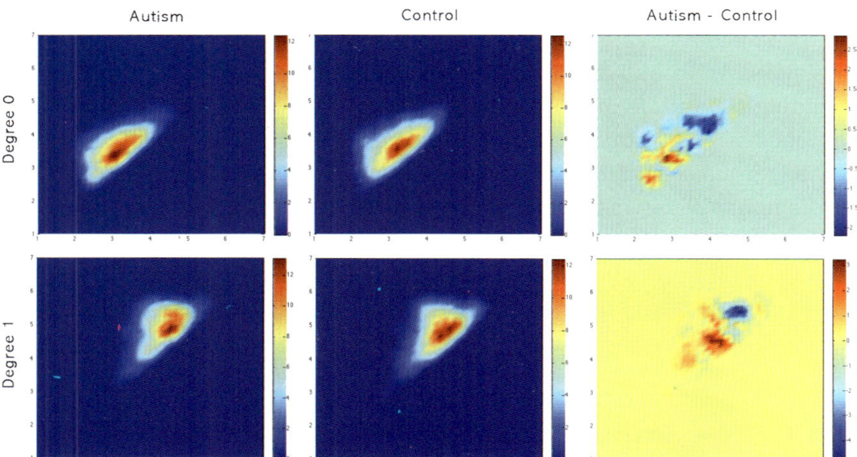

Fig. 10.10 The pairing concentration is computed by counting the number of pairings within a circle of fixed radius 0.2 at the point $x \in [1, 7]^2$. The first (second) row is the mean concentration map for degree 0 (1) persistence. The first (second) column is the concentration map of autistic (control). The concentration difference (autism - control) is given in the last column which shows concentration difference between the groups.

comparisons of a one-sided test is given by $\sup_{p \in [1,7]^2} T(p)$ (Worsley *et al.*, 1996b). The empirical distribution of $\sup_{p \in [1,7]^2} T(p)$ is then estimated from 5000 random permutations. For the degree-0 persistence, we obtain the maximum T-stat value of 3.51 corresponding to the corrected p-value of 0.078 at the position (2.3, 4.2). For the degree-1 persistence, the maximum T-stat value is 3.95 corresponding to the corrected p-value of 0.021 at the position (5.5, 5.8).

Our finding is consistent with previous neuroanatomical studies that show the abnormal neuroanatomical structures for autistic subjects (Chung *et al.*, 2005a). Here we only presented a simple nonparametric approach for determining statistical significance based on the pairing concentration. Possibly a better statistical inference procedure is needed. It is hoped that this paper presents itself as a spring board for further investigation of persistence diagram based characterization of medical images. There are many methodological issues we have not discussed such as rigorous inferential procedures or the estimation of confidence regions around paired points possibly via the bootstrap. These are the next challenges in future works.

10.5   Min-Max Diagrams

It is possible to obtain a simplified version of persistent diagram by not including the saddle points in the pairing rule since the saddle points does not yield a clear statistical interpretation compared to local minimums and maximums. In fact, there is no statistical methodology developed for saddle points so far. This makes the construction of the persistent diagrams substantially simpler. The resulting reduced persistence diagram should be viewed as an approximation to the true persistence diagram. Figure 10.9 is an example of the min-max diagram. For the detailed exposition of the min-max diagram, see Chung *et al.* (2009b).

10.5.1   *Why Critical Values?*

The use of critical values of measurements within classical image analysis and computer vision has been relatively limited so far, and typically appear as part of simple preprocessing tasks such as feature extraction and identification of edge pixels in an image. For example, first or second order image derivatives may be used to identify the edges of objects to serve as the contour of an anatomical shape, possibly using priors to provide additional shape context. Specific properties of critical values as a topic on its own, however, has received less attention. Whether critical points may serve a more central role in the design of image processing algorithms is a question that has not been investigated in sufficient detail.

Critical points of measurements are not used in classical image analysis and computer vision very frequently. One reason is that it is difficult to construct a streamlined linear analysis framework using critical points, or values of images. Also, the computation of critical values is a nonlinear process and almost always requires the numerical estimation of derivatives. In some applications where this is necessary, the discretization scheme must be chosen carefully, and remains an active area of research (Osher and Fedkiw, 2003). It is noticed that in most of these applications, the interest is only in the stable estimation of these points rather than their properties, and how these properties vary as a function of images.

In brain imaging, on the other hand, the use of extreme values has been quite popular in other types of problems. For example, these ideas are employed in the context of multiple comparison correction using random field theory (Worsley *et al.*, 1996b; Taylor and Worsley, 2008; Kiebel *et al.*, 1999). Recall that in the random field theory, the extreme value of a statistic is obtained from an ensemble of images, and is used to compute the p-value for correcting for correlated noise across neighboring voxels.

Critical points have been also been used in image processing, and serve as tools for feature extraction (Cootes *et al.*, 1993; Sato *et al.*, 1998; Antoine *et al.*, 1996). In this context, image derivatives are computed after image smoothing and thresholded to obtain edges and ridges of images, that are used to identify pixels likely to lie on boundaries of anatomical objects. Then, the collection of critical points are used as a geometric feature that characterize anatomical shape.

10.5.2 *Iterative Pairing and Deletion Algorithm*

Our interest in this section is to take a topologically oriented view of the image data. We seek to interpret the critical values in this context and assess their response as a function of anatomy. In particular, we explore specific representation schemes and evaluate the benefits they afford with respect to different applications. The image processing and analysis steps are as follows.

(1) Given a function of images, e.g. image intensities, cortical thickness, curvature maps etc., we smooth the functional data using heat kernel smoothing (Chung *et al.*, 2007).

(2) Determine critical values numerically on the smoothed functional data. Heat kernel smoothing will increase the stability of estimation.

(3) The obtained critical values are paired in a nonlinear fashion following a specific pairing rule to produce min-max diagrams.

(4) Perform inference on the min-max diagrams.

Min-max diagrams are similar to the theoretical construct of persistence diagrams in algebraic topology and computational geometry, but have notable differences (Edelsbrunner and Harer, 2008; Zomorodian, 2001; Cohen-Steiner *et al.*, 2007; Morozov, 2008). The persistence diagram is a scatter plot of particular pairing that has been used to show the topological characteristics of signal. However, we wish to make it clear that this pairing rule is not that of persistence although there are similarities.

Min-max diagrams resemble scatter plots, and lead to a powerful representation of the key characteristics of their corresponding images. We discuss these issues in detail, and provide a number of examples and experiments to highlight their key advantages, limitations, and possible applications to a wide variety of medical imaging problems.

Iterative Pairing and Deletion Algorithm. We have developed a new simpler pairing rule called *iterative pairing and deletion* for pairing critical values in the reduced diagram (Chung *et al.*, 2009b). This is a new $\mathcal{O}(n \log n)$ algorithm for generating such diagrams without having to modify or adapt the complicated machinery used for constructing persistence diagrams (Chung *et al.*, 2009a; Edelsbrunner and Harer, 2008; Zomorodian and Carlsson, 2005). At first glance, the nonlinear nature of pairing does not seem to yield a straightforward algorithm. The trick is to start with the maximum of minimums and go down to the next largest minimum in an iterative fashion.

Algorithm 10.1. Iterative Pairing and Deletion

(1) $H \leftarrow \{h_1, \cdots, h_n\}$.
(2) $i \leftarrow m$.

(3) $h_i^* = \arg\min_{h_j \in H}\{h_j | h_j > g_{(i)}, h_j \sim g_{(i)}\}$.

(4) If $h_i^* \neq \emptyset$, pair $(g_{(i)}, h_i^*)$

(5) $H \leftarrow H - h_i^*$.

(6) If $i > 1$, $i \leftarrow i - 1$ and go to Step 3.

The algorithm starts with $g_{(m)}$ (step 3). We only need to consider maximums above $g_{(m)}$ for pairing. We check if maximums h_j are in a neighborhood of $g_{(m)}$. If they are neighbors, the relationship will be denoted as $h_j \sim g_{(m)}$. The only possible scenario of not having any larger maximum is when the function is unimodal and obtains the global minimum $g_{(m)}$. In this situation we have to pair $(g_{(m)}, \infty)$. Since ∞ falls outside our 'plot', we leave out $g_{(m)}$ without pairing. Other than this special case, there exists at least one smallest maximum h_m^* in a neighborhood of $g_{(m)}$ (intuitively, if there is a valley, there must be mountains nearby). Once we paired them (step 4), we delete the pair from the set of extreme values (step 5) and go to the next maximum of minimums $g_{(m-1)}$ and proceed until we exhaust the set of all critical values (step 6). Due to the sorting of minimums and maximums, the running time is $\mathcal{O}(n \log n)$.

This may also be implemented using a plane-sweep approach, which also gives a running time of $\mathcal{O}(n \log n)$. In this case, pairing will be based on how points enter or leave the queue of events' as the plane (or line) sweeps in the vertical direction. Higher dimensional implementation is identical to the 1D version except how we define neighbors of a critical point. The neighborhood relationship $\sim$ can be established by constructing the Delaunay triangulation on all critical points.

10.5.3 *Statistical Inference on Mix-Max Diagrams*

We used an MRI dataset of 16 highly functional autistic subjects and 11 normal control subjects (aged-matched right-handed males). High resolution magnetic resonance images were obtained using a 3-Tesla GE SIGNA scanner. The images went through intensity nonuniformity correction (Sled *et al.*, 1988) and spatially normalized into the MNI stereotaxic space *via* a global affine transformation, and tissue segmentation (Collins *et al.*, 1994). Subseqeuntly a supervised neural network classifier was used for tissue segmentation. Brain substructures such as the brain stem were removed to make the both outer and the inner surfaces to be topologically equivalent to a sphere. A deformable surface algorithm was used to obtain the inner cortical surface by deforming from a spherical mesh (MacDonald *et al.*, 2000).

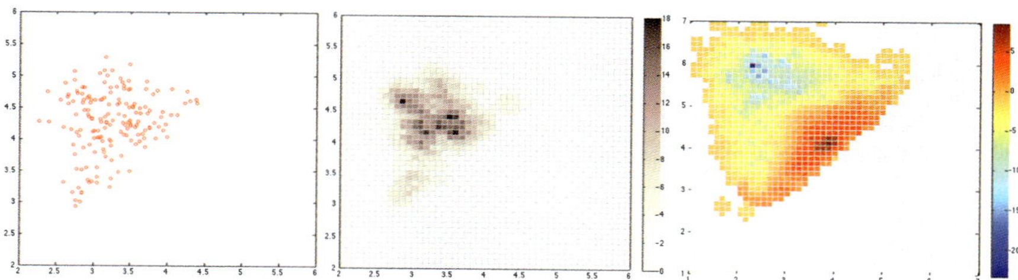

Fig. 10.11   Left: Min-max diagram of an autistic subject from Figure 10.9 e. Middle: The concentration map of the min-max diagram is constructed by discretizing the square $[1, 7]^2$ into 50^2 uniform pixels and evaluating the number of pairs within a circle ($r = 0.2$) centered on the pixel. Right: The t-test statistic (autism - control) shows significant group differences in red ($t \geq 3.61$) and blue ($t \leq -4.05$) regions at level 0.05 (corrected).

The outer surface $\mathcal{M}$ was obtained by deforming the inner surface further. The cortical thickness f is then defined as the distance between the two surfaces, this measure is known to be relevant for autism (Figure 10.7).

Since the critical values do not change even if we geometrically change the underlying manifold from $\mathcal{M}$ to S^2, the min-max diagram must be topologically invariant as well. Therefore, the min-max diagram is constructed on the unit sphere by projecting the cortical data on to the sphere. Figure 10.9 shows the superimposed min-max diagram for 11 control (blue) and 16 autistic (red) subjects. A single subject example is shown in Figure 10.11. Pairings for autistic subjects are more clustered near $y = x$ indicating higher frequency noise in autism. More pairing occurs at high and low thickness values in the controls showing additional topological structures not present in autism.

Permutation Test. We have formally tested our hypothesis of different topological structures between the groups. Given a min-max diagram in the square $[1, 7]^2$, we have discretized the square with the uniform grid such that there are a total of 50^2 pixels (see Figure 10.11 b). A concentration map of the pairings was obtained by counting the number of pairs in a circle of radius 0.2 centered at each pixel.

Notice that this approach is somewhat similar to the voxel-based morphometry (Ashburner and Friston, 2000), where brain tissue density maps are used as a shapeless metric for characterizing concentration of the amount of tissue.

The concentration maps are constructed for all min-max diagrams and the two sample t-statistic map $T(t)$ (with equal variance) is constructed (Figure 10.11). Unfortunately, the concentration maps do not follow Gaussian distributional assumptions. So we have performed a permutation test with 5000 random permutations on the maximum of t-statistic of concentration maps to empirically estimate the distribution of $\sup_{t \in [1,7]^2} T(t)$ and $\inf_{t \in [1,7]^2} T(t)$ and determine the statistical significance (Figure 10.11). Note that this is the usual multiple comparison problem due to correlated t statistic values across neighboring pixels (Worsley *et al.*, 1996b).

By thresholding the tails of the empirical distribution at 0.05, we obtain the quantile points 3.61 and -4.05. We have detected two main clusters of pairing concentration difference. The blue cluster below -4.05 is the region of high pairing concentration for controls while the red cluster above 3.61 is the region of high pairing concentration for autism. The implication is that more pairing occurs at high and low thickness values in the control subjects. If data is white noise, pairings occur close to $y = x$ line. The deviation from $y = x$ indicates signal. In the t-test result, we detected two main clusters of pairing difference. High number of pairings occurs around (2,6) for controls and (4,4) for autism. This is only possible if surfaces have more geometric features/signal in the controls. On the other hand, the autism shows noisier characteristic.

10.6 Graph Filtrations

In the previous chapter, we have explored many different weighted network models obtained from DTI and MRI using various methods. In this section, we will present a more general framework for modeling weighted brain networks motivated by Rips filtration Chung *et al.* (2011a) and Lee *et al.* (2011b). This section summarizes the framework first given in Lee *et al.* (2011b).

The brain connectivity studies based on graph theory have provided new understanding of human brain (Bassett, 2006; Sporns *et al.*, 2005). The characteristic of the brain network is quantified by the global topological measures such as clustering coefficient, characteristic path length and modularity (Rubinov and Sporns, 2010; Bullmore and Sporns, 2009). The network comparison is then performed by determining the differences in these topological measures at a fixed scale. However, it is unclear at what scale the comparison should be performed. To remedy the problem, we propose a radically different computational framework for determining network difference. Instead of trying to find one particular characteristic of network at a given scale, one can also look at the overall change of topological features through persistent homology (Adler *et al.*, 2010; Edelsbrunner and Harer, 2008).

In the persistent homology, topological features such as the connected components and cycles of the network are tabulated in terms of the Betti numbers. The network difference is then quantified over every possible scales using *graph filtration*. The graph filtration is a new graph simplification technique that iteratively build a nested subgraphs of the original graph. The algorithm simplifies a complex graph by piecing together the patches of locally connected nearest nodes. The process of graph filtration can be shown to be mathematically equivalent to the single linkage hierarchical clustering and dendrogram construction.

Once the graph filtration is obtained, we transform it into an algebraic form called the single linkage matrix. The single linkage matrix is subsequently used in computing the network difference using the Gromov-Hausdorff (GH) metric. The GH metric is a deformation-invariant dissimilarity measure often used in matching deformable shapes (Mémoli, 2008; Bronstein *et al.*, 2006). The GH metric was never used in measuring the distance between brain networks before. The analysis steps are as follows:

(1) From the weighted graph, construct the graph filtration.

(2) Construct the single linkage distance matrix that is equivalent to the graph filtration.

(3) Determine the distance between brain networks using the GH-metric on the single linkage distance.

(4) Inference on the GH-metric is done by the Jackknife resampling technique.

10.6.1 *Weighted Graphs*

Many previous network studies try to find hidden patterns in already constructed weighted networks (Lee *et al.*, 2011b; Li *et al.*, 2009; McIntosh and Gonzalez-Lima, 1994; Newman and Watts, 1999; Song *et al.*, 2005). The edge weights are usually given by some similarity measure between nodes.

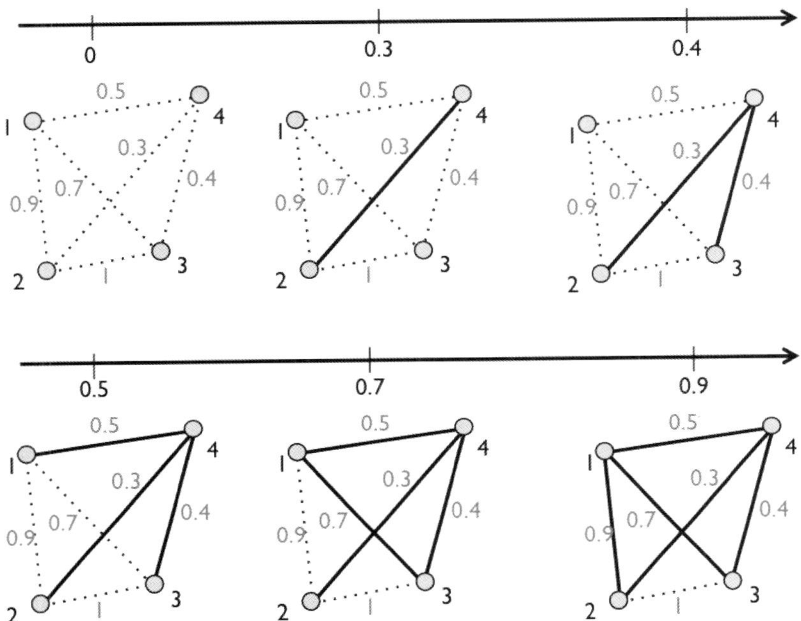

Fig. 10.12 Decomposition of a weighted graph. We may assume the edge weights are all unique, which is likely the case in weighted brain networks. We sort the edge weights in an increasing order. Then we add an edge one at a time in the increasing order. At 0.5, we are connecting all the nodes without introducing a cycle. When we combine all the added edges up to 0.5, we obtain the minimum spanning tree.

By motivated by the Rips filtration in the persistent homology, we present a different network modeling and visualization framework for weighted networks by introducing the concept of *graph filtration*, which is a sequence of finite number of nested subnetworks obtained from the original weighted network. The network filtration simplifies a complex weighted network by decomposing it into the finite number of unweighted networks with special properties. We first define the weighted networks as a metric space. Then the concept of network filtration is defined in the metric space using the persistent homology.

Consider a weighted network with the node set $V = \{1, \ldots, p\}$ and the edge weights $\rho = (\rho_{ij})$, where ρ_{ij} is the weight between nodes i and j. Figure 10.12 shows an example. The edge weight ρ_{ij} is usually given by a similarity measure between the observed data x_i and x_j on the nodes i and j. Various similarity measures have been proposed. The correlation or mutual information between measurements for the biological or metabolic network have been used as edge weights (Lee *et al.*, 2011b).

We will assume that the edge weights satisfy the metric properties: nonnegativity, identity, symmetry and the triangle inequality so that

$$\rho_{i,j} \geq 0, \ \rho_{ii} = 0 \ \rho_{ij} = \rho_{ji}, \ \rho_{ij} \leq \rho_{ik} + \rho_{kj}.$$

With this condition $X = (V, \rho)$ forms a metric space. Many real-world networks satisfy the metric properties. Suppose we have measurement vector x_i on the node i. If we center and rescale the measurement x_i such that

$$\| x_i \|^2 = x_i^\top x_i = 1,$$

the correlation between the nodes i and j is given by $x_i^\top x_i$. Then $\rho_{ij} = 1 - x_i^\top x_j$ satisfies the metric properties. The triangle inequality can be easily derived from

$$\| x_i - x_j \|^2 \leq \| x_i - x_k \|^2 + \| x_k - x_j \|^2 .$$

Rips and Graph Filtrations. By thresholding the edge weights ρ at certain level ϵ, we can construct an unweighted graph. Given the weighted network $X = (V, \rho)$, the unweighted network B_ϵ is a graph consisting of the node set V and the edge set, which is given by connecting nodes i and j if $\rho_{ij} \leq \epsilon$ for some threshold ϵ. The unweighted network B_ϵ is a simplicial complex consisting of 0-simplices (nodes) and 1-simplices (edges). The unweighted network is a special case of the Rips complex.

In the metric space $X = (V, \rho)$, the Rips complex R_ϵ is a simplicial complex whose $(p-1)$-simplices correspond to unordered p-tuples of points that satisfy $\rho_{ij} \leq \epsilon$ in a pairwise fashion (Ghrist, 2008). While the unweighted network B_ϵ has at most 1-simplices, the Rips complex can have at most $(p - 1)$-simplices. Therefore, we have $B_\epsilon \subset R_\epsilon$. The Rips complex has the property that

$$R_{\epsilon_0} \subset R_{\epsilon_1} \subset R_{\epsilon_2} \subset \cdots$$

for $0 = \epsilon_0 \leq \epsilon_1 \leq \epsilon_2 \leq \cdots$. When $\epsilon = 0$, the Rips complex is simply the node set V. By increasing the ϵ value, we are connecting more nodes so the size of the edge set increases. Such the nested sequence of the Rips complexes is called a Rips filtration, the main object of interest in the persistent homology (Edelsbrunner and Harer, 2008). The increasing ϵ values are called the filtration values.

Since a unweighted network is a special case of the Rips complex, it inherits all the topological properties of the Rips complex and filtration. Therefore, we have the nested sequence of networks

$$B_{\epsilon_0} \subset B_{\epsilon_1} \subset B_{\epsilon_2} \subset \cdots$$

for $0 = \epsilon_0 \leq \epsilon_1 \leq \epsilon_2 \cdots$. The sequence of such nested network will be defined as the *graph filtration*. If we order the edge weights in the increasing order, we have the sorted edge weights:

$$\min_{i,j} \rho_{ij} = \rho_{(1)} < \rho_{(2)} < \cdots < \rho_{(q)} = \max_{i,j} \rho_{ij},$$

where $q \leq (p^2 - p)/2$. We assume there are q unique edge weights among the maximum possible $(p^2 - p)/2$ weights. The subscript $_{()}$ denotes the order statistic. Then the weighted graph $X = (V, \rho)$ can be uniquely decomposed as the network filtration:

$$B_0 \subset B_{\rho_{(1)}} \subset \cdots \subset B_{\rho_{(q)}}.$$

10.6.2 *Single Linkage Matrix*

The graph filtration corresponds to the single linkage hierarchical clustering. The equivalence to the graph filtration and the dendrogram is self-evident (Lee *et al.*, 2011b). The linking of nodes i and j corresponds to the linking of leaves in the dendrogram (Figure 10.13). Increasing the ϵ value in the graph filtration corresponds to increasing the height of the dendrogram.

In the hierarchical clustering, the distance between patches of nodes C_1 and C_2 is given by the distance between the closest members in C_1 and C_2:

$$d_{SL}(C_1, C_2) = \min_{i \in C_1, j \in C_2} \rho_{ij}.$$

The limitation of the single linkage matrix is the inability to discriminate a cycle in a graph. Consider two graphs with three nodes (Figure 10.14). By performing the graph filtration, we obtain the corresponding dendrograms which are identical regardless of if there is a cycle in the graph. The single linkage matrices are then given by

$$\begin{pmatrix} 0 & 0.2 & 0.5 \\ 0.2 & 0 & 0.5 \\ 0.5 & 0.5 & 0 \end{pmatrix} \quad \text{and} \quad \begin{pmatrix} 0 & 0.2 & 0.5 \\ 0.2 & 0 & 0.5 \\ 0.5 & 0.5 & 0 \end{pmatrix}.$$

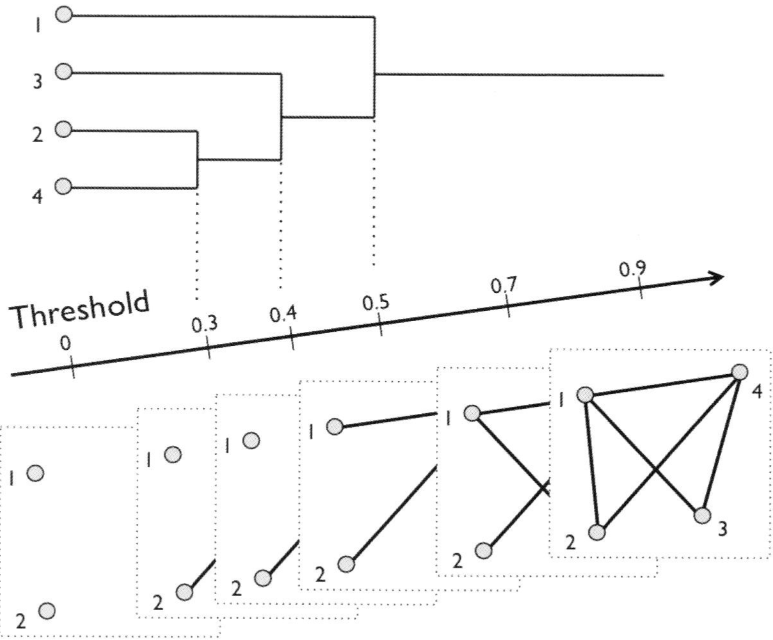

Fig. 10.13   The weighted graph in Figure 10.12 is decomposed into a sequence of nested unweighted graphs. By recording the sequence of deleted edges, we can construct the corresponding single linkage dendrogram.

They again produce the identical single linkage matrix. The limitations of the dendrogram representation of brain networks are obvious from this example. The dendrogram representation is based on the minimum spanning tree (MST) of a graph, which is basically a tree presentation. Hence dendrogram cannot properly represent cycles and loops in the network.

Instead of using the single linkage distance, we can also use the geodesic distance matrix. The geodesic distance is defined as the sum of edge weights along the shortest path in the graph (Lee *et al.*, 2011b). After obtaining the single linkage distance, we need to compute the distance between the networks for quantification.

Given two networks (X, ρ^X) and (Y, ρ^Y), the Gromov-Hausdorff Distance (GH) distance between X and Y is defined as (Lee *et al.*, 2011b; Mémoli, 2008):

$$d_{GH}(X, Y) = \frac{1}{2} \max_{\forall i,j} |\rho_{ij}^X - \rho_{ij}^Y|.$$

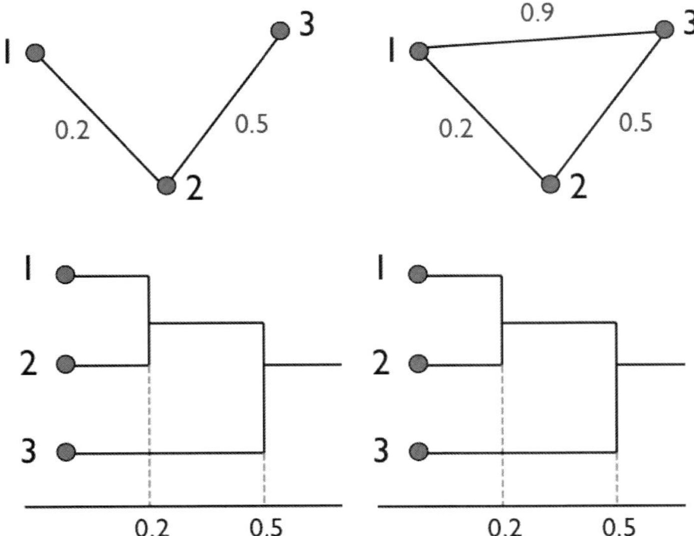

Fig. 10.14 Using $1 - \mathrm{corr}(x_i, x_j)$, we change the edge weights. The corresponding dendrograms are identical showing the weakness of the dendrogram representation. The dendrogram representation is based on the minimum spanning tree (MST) of a network, which is basically a tree presentation. Hence dendrogram cannot properly represent cycles and loops in the network.

10.6.3 *Persistent Brain Networks*

In Lee *et al.* (2011b), the method was applied in differentiating PET images of 24 attention-deficit hyperactivity disorder (ADHD) (19 boys, mean age 8.2 ± 1.6 years), 26 autistic (24 boys, mean age: 6.0 ± 1.8 years) and 11 controls (7 boys, mean age: 9.7 ± 2.5 years). After a sequence of image processing, mean FDG uptake within 96 ROIs were extracted.

The edge weights from correlation and single linkage distance d_{SL} are shown in Figure 10.15. The corresponding barcode and dendrogram representations are shown in Figure 10.16. The group difference is more evident in the single linkage distance. The maximum single linkage distances of the ADHD, autism and control subjects are 0.62, 0.51, 0.48. This implies that the control network become much faster to a single connected component than other groups over filtration. The most regions in ADHD are weakly connected except a few strongly connected regions within the occipital (O) and left frontal (F) regions and between the right and the left frontal regions

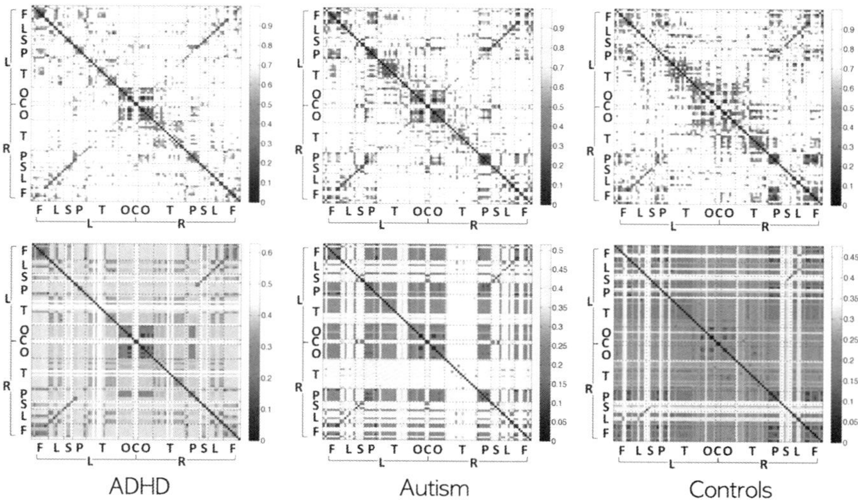

Fig. 10.15　Top: Edge weights ρ for the three groups: attention-deficit hyperactivity disorder (ADHD), autism and pediatric controls. Bottom: Single linkage distance d_{SL} for three groups showing a better group separation compared to the edge weights ρ. See Lee *et al.* (2011b) for details. The figure was generated by Hyekyoung Lee of Seoul National University.

(Kraina and Castellanos, 2006). On the other hand, the normal network is well-connected in the whole brain regions. In the autistic network, the connection is segmented according to lobes and temporal (T) asymmetry is obviously visible (Minshew and Williams, 2007).

We have compared the performance of graph filtration against other widely used graph distances: bottleneck distance, assortativity, centrality, clustering coefficient, characteristic path length, small-worldness and modularity (Edelsbrunner and Harer, 2008; Rubinov and Sporns, 2010; Bullmore and Sporns, 2009).

Since each group generates a single network, it is difficult to compare the performance of different techniques on a single network. Comparison is done the Jackknife resampled networks. For a group with n subjects, one subject is removed and the remaining $n - 1$ subjects are used to construct a network. This process is repeated for each subject to produce n networks for the group. Therefore, 24, 26 and 11 networks for the ADHD, autistic and control subjects.

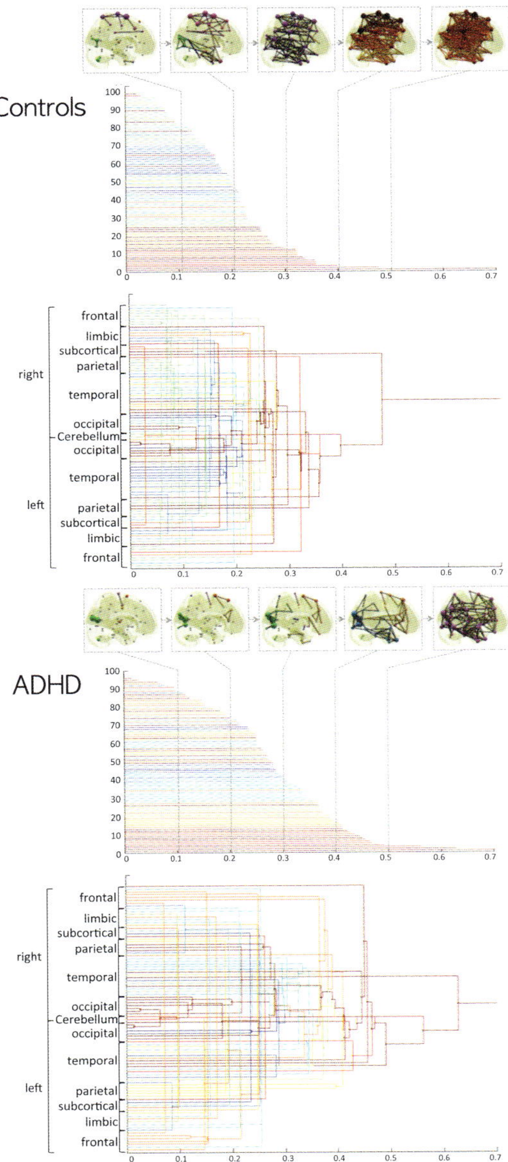

Fig. 10.16   The barcode and dendrogram representation of the brain networks of ADHD and normal control subjects. Nodes belong to form a connected component are colored identically. See Lee *et al.* (2011c) for details. The figure was generated by Hyekyoung Lee of Seoul National University.

After constructing the distance matrices, the networks are divided into three clusters using the hierarchical clustering and evaluated the clustering accuracy by comparing the assigned labels with the true labels. The clustering accuracies of GH distance, characteristic path length and small-worldness are all 100 %. Other than these three metrics, all other graph distances show low clustering accuracy. See Lee *et al.* (2011b) for details. The average between-group distance is much larger than the within group-distance in the GH-metric at 0.49 while all other distances are 0.02 to 0.34 range indicating the superior performance of the GH-metric.

Bibliography

Abdi, H. (2007). *The RV coefficient and the congruence coefficient* (Sage, Thousand Oaks, CA).

Abell, F., Krams, M., Ashburner, J., Passingham, R., Friston, K., Frackowiak, R., Happé, F., Frith, C. and Frith, U. (1999). The neuroanatomy of autism: a voxel-based whole brain analysis of structural scans, *NeuroReport* **10**, pp. 1647–1651.

Achard, S. and Bullmore, E. (2007). Efficiency and cost of economical brain functional networks, *PLoS computational biology* **3**, 2, p. e17.

Adler, R. (1981). *The Geometry of Random Fields* (John Wiley & Sons).

Adler, R. (1990). *An Introduction to Continuity, Extrema, and Related Topics for General Gaussian Processes* (IMS, Hayward, CA).

Adler, R. (2000). On excursion sets, tube formulas and maxima of random fields, *Annals of Applied Probability* **10**, pp. 1–74.

Adler, R., Bobrowski, O., Borman, M., Subag, E. and Weinberger, S. (2010). Persistent homology for random fields and complexes, *ArXiv e-prints* .

Adler, R. and Hasofer, A. (1976). Level crossings for random fields, *The annals of Probability* **4**, pp. 1–12.

Adler, R., Samorodnitsky, G. and Gadrich, T. (1993). The expected number of level crossings for stationary, harmonisable, symmetric, stable processes, *The Annals of Applied Probability* **3**, pp. 553–575.

Adler, R. and Taylor, J. (2007). *Random fields and geometry* (Springer Verlag).

Aldous, D. (1989). *Probability Approximations via the Poisson Clumping Heuristic* (Springer-Verlag, New York).

Allison, P. (2000). Multiple imputation for missing data: A cautionary tale, *Sociological Methods and Research* **28**, pp. 301–309.

Anderson, E., Bai, Z., Bischof, C., Blackford, L., Demmel, J., Dongarra, J., Du Croz, J., Hammarling, S., Greenbaum, A., McKenney, A. *et al.* (1999). *LAPACK Users' guide* (Society for Industrial and Applied Mathematics Philadelphia, PA, USA).

Anderson, T. (1984). *An Introduction to Multivariate Statistical Analysis*, 2nd edn. (Wiley.).

Andrade, A., Kherif, F., Mangin, J., Worsley, K., Paradis, A., Simon, O., Dehaene, S., Le Bihan, D. and Poline, J.-B. (2001). Detection of fmri activation using cortical surface mapping, *Human Brain Mapping* **12**, pp. 79–93.

Andresen, P. R., Bookstein, F. L., Conradsen, K., Ersbøll, B. K., Marsh, J. L. and Kreiborg, S. (2000). Surface-bounded growth modeling applied to human mandibles, **19**, pp. 1053–1063.

Angelopoulou, E. (1999). Gaussian curvatures from photometric scatter plots, *Workshop on Photometric Modeling for Computer Vision and Graphics*, pp. 12–19.

Angenent, S., Hacker, S., Tannenbaum, A. and Kikinis, R. (1999). On the laplace-beltrami operator and brain surface flattening, *IEEE Transactions on Medical Imaging* **18**, pp. 700–711.

Antoine, J., Petra, A. and Max, A. (1996). Evaluation of ridge seeking operators for multimodality medical image matching, *IEEE Transactions on Pattern Analysis and Machine Intelligence* .

Arfken, G. (2000). *Mathematical Methods for Physicists*, 5th edn. (Academic Press).

Arsigny, V., Fillard, P., Pennec, X. and Ayache, N. (2005). Fast and simple calculus on tensors in the Log-Euclidean framework, *Lecture Notes in Computer Science* **3749**, pp. 115–122.

Ashburner, J., Andersson, J. and Friston, K. (1999). High-dimensional image registration using symmetric priors, *NeuroImage* **9**, 6, pp. 619–628.

Ashburner, J. and Friston, K. (2000). Voxel-based morphometry - the methods, *NeuroImage* **11**, pp. 805–821.

Ashburner, J. and Friston, K. (2001). Why voxel-based morphometry should be used, *NeuroImage* **14**, pp. 1238–1243.

Ashburner, J., Good, C. and Friston, K. (2000). Tensor based morphometry, *NeuroImage* **11S**, p. 465.

Ashburner, J., Hutton, C., Frackowiak, R. S. J., Johnsrude, I., Price, C. and Friston, K. J. (1998). Identifying global anatomical differences: deformation-based morphometry, *Human Brain Mapping* **6**, pp. 348–357.

Ashburner, J., Neelin, P., Collins, D., Evans, A. and Friston, K. (1997). Incorporating prior knowledge into image registration, *NeuroImage* **6**, pp. 344–352.

Athreya, S. (2000). Monotonicity property for a class of semilinear partial differential equations, *Séminaire de Probabilités XXXIV* , pp. 388–392.

Avants, B., Epstein, C., Grossman, M. and Gee, J. (2008). Symmetric diffeomorphic image registration with cross-correlation: Evaluating automated labeling of elderly and neurodegenerative brain, *Medical image analysis* **12**, pp. 26–41.

Aylward, E., Minshew, N., Goldstein, G., Honeycutt, N., Augustine, A., Yates, K., Bartra, P. and Pearlson, G. (1999). Mri volumes of amygdala and hippocampus in nonmentally retarded autistic adolescents and adults, *Neurology* **53**, pp. 2145–2150.

Babuška, I., Tempone, R. and Zouraris, G. (2004). Galerkin finite element approximations of stochastic elliptic partial differential equations, *Siam J. Numer. Anal* **42**, pp. 800–825.

Banerjee, O., El Ghaoui, L. and d'Aspremont, A. (2008). Model selection through sparse maximum likelihood estimation for multivariate Gaussian or binary data, *The Journal of Machine Learning Research* **9**, pp. 485–516.

Banerjee, O., Ghaoui, L., d'Aspremont, A. and Natsoulis, G. (2006). Convex optimization techniques for fitting sparse Gaussian graphical models, in *Proceedings of the 23rd international conference on Machine learning*, p. 96.

Banuelos, R. and Burdzy, K. (1999). On the Hot Spots Conjecture of J Rauch, *Journal of Functional Analysis* **164**, pp. 1–33.

Barrick, T., Mackay, C., Prima, S., maes, F., Vandermeulen, D., Crow, T. and Roberts, N. (2005). Automatic analysis of cerebral asymmetry: an exploratory study of the relationship between brain torgue and planum temporale asymmetry, *NeuroImage* **24**, pp. 678–691.

Barta, P., Miller, M. and Qiu, A. (2005). A stochastic model for studying the laminar structure of cortex from mri, *IEEE Transactions on Medical Imaging* **24**, pp. 728–742.

Barton, C. and Cramer, E. (1989). Hypothesis testing in multivariate linear models with randomly missing data, *Communications in Statistics-Simulation and Computation* **18**, pp. 875–895.

Basawa, I. and Rao, B. (1980). *Statistical Inference for Stochastic Processes* (Academic Press, London).

Basser, P., Mattiello, J. and LeBihan, D. (1994). MR diffusion tensor spectroscopy and imaging, *Biophys J.* **66**, pp. 259–267.

Basser, P., Pajevic, S., Pierpaoli, C., Duda, J. and Aldroubi, A. (2000). In vivo tractography using dt-mri data, *Magnetic Resonance in Medicine* **44** pp. 625–632.

Basser, P. and Pierpaoli, C. (1996). Microstructural and physiological features of tissues elucidated by quantitative-diffusion-tensor MRI, *Journal of Magnetic Resonance, Series B* **111**, pp. 209–219.

Bassett, D. (2006). Small-world brain networks, *The Neuroscientist* **12**, pp. 512–523.

Batchelor, P., Calamante, F., Tournier, J., Atkinson, D., Hill, D. and Connelly, A. (2006). Quantification of the shape of fiber tracts, *Magnetic Resonance in Medicine* **55**, pp. 894–903.

Batchelor, P., Hill, D., Calamante, F. and Atkinson, D. (2001). Study of connectivity in the brain using the full diffusion tensor from MRI, *Lecture Notes in Computer Science* , pp. 121–133.

Behrens, T., Berg, H., Jbabdi, S., Rushworth, M. and Woolrich, M. (2007). Probabilistic diffusion tractography with multiple fibre orientations: what can we gain? *NeuroImage* **34**, pp. 144–155.

Belkin, M. and Niyogi, P. (2002). Laplacian eigenmaps and spectral techniques for embedding and clustering, *Advances in Neural Information Processing Systems* **1**, pp. 585–592.

Belsley, D., Kuh, E. and Welsch, R. (2004). *Regression diagnostics: Identifying influential data and sources of collinearity* (Wiley-IEEE).

Benjamini, Y. and Hochberg, Y. (1995). Controlling the false discovery rate: a practical and powerful approach to multiple testing, *J. R. Stat. Soc, Ser. B* **57**, pp. 289–300.

Benjamini, Y. and Yekutieli, D. (2001). The control of the false discovery rate in multiple testing under dependency, *Annals of statistics* , pp. 1165–1188.

Berge, A., Jensen, A. and Solberg, A. (2007). Sparse inverse covariance estimates for hyperspectral image classification, *IEEE Transactions on Geoscience and Remote Sensing* **45**, p. 1399.

Berline, N., Getzler, E. and M., V. (1991). *Heat kernels and dirac operators* (Springer-Verlag).

Bernal-Rusiel, J., Atienza, M. and Cantero, J. (2008). Detection of focal changes in human cortical thickness: spherical wavelets versus gaussian smoothing, *NeuroImage* **41**, pp. 1278–1292.

Betounes, D. (1998). *Partial differential equations for computational science: with Maple and vector analysis* (Springer).

Bocher, M. (1906). Introduction to the theory of Fourier's series, *Ann. Math* **7**, pp. 81–152.

Bookstein, F. (1989). Principal warps: thin-plate splines and the decomposition of defomrations, *IEEE Transactions on Pattern Analysis and Machine Intelligence* **11**, pp. 567–585.

Bookstein, F. (1991). *Morphometric Tools for Landmark Data:Geometry and Biology* (Cambridge University Press, Cambridge).

Bookstein, F. (2001). Voxel-based morphometry should not be used with imperfectly registered images, *NeuroImage* **14**, pp. 1454–1462.

Boothby, W. (1986). *An Introduction to Differential Manifolds and Riemannian Geometry*, second edition edn. (Academic Press, London).

Boykov, Y. and Kolmogorov, V. (2003). Computing geodesics and minimal surfaces via graph cuts, in *International Conference on Computer Vision*, Vol. 1, pp. 26–33.

Boyles, R. (1983). On the convergence of the EM algorithm, *Journal of the Royal Statistical Society. Series B (Methodological)* **45**, pp. 47–50.

Brambilla, P., Nicoletti, M., Sassi, R., Mallinger, A., Frank, E., Kupfer, D., Keshavan, M. and Soares, J. (2003). Magnetic resonance imaging study of corpus callosum abnormalities in patients with bipolar disorder, *Biological psychiatry* **54**, pp. 1294–1297.

Brechbuhler, C., Gerig, G. and Kubler, O. (1995). Parametrization of closed surfaces for 3d shape description, *Computer Vision and Image Understanding* **61**, pp. 154–170.

Brezinski, C. (2004). Extrapolation algorithms for filtering series of functions, and treating the Gibbs phenomenon, *Numerical Algorithms* **36**, pp. 309–329.

Brickman, A., Habeck, C., Zarahn, E., Flynn, J. and Stern, Y. (2007). Structural MRI covariance patterns associated with normal aging and neuropsychological functioning, *Neurobiology of aging* **28**, pp. 284–295.

Bronstein, A. M., Bronstein, M. M. and Kimmel, R. (2006). Efficient computation of isometry-invariant distances between surfaces, *SIAM Journal on Scientific Computing* **28**, pp. 1812–1836.

Bubenik, P. and Kim, P. (2007). A statistical approach to persistent homology, *Homology Homotopy and Applications* **9**, pp. 337–362.

Bullmore, E. and Sporns, O. (2009). Complex brain networks: graph theoretical analysis of structural and functional systems, *Nature Review Neuroscience* **10**, pp. 186–98.

Bulow, T. (2004). Spherical diffusion for 3D surface smoothing, *IEEE Transactions on Pattern Analysis and Machine Intelligence* **26**, pp. 1650–1654.

Cachia, A., Mangin, J.-F., Riviere, D., Kherif, F., Boddaert, N., Andrade, A., Papadopoulos-Orfanos, D., Poline, J.-B., Bloch, I., Zilbovicius, M., Sonigo, P., Brunelle, F. and Regis, J. . (2003a). A primal sketch of the cortex mean curvature: a morphogenesis based approach to study the variability of the folding patterns, *IEEE Transactions on Medical Imaging* **22**, pp. 754–765.

Cachia, A., Mangin, J.-F., Riviére, D., Papadopoulos-Orfanos, D., Kherif, F., Bloch, I. and Régis, J. (2003b). A generic framework for parcellation of the cortical surface into gyri using geodesic voronoï diagrams, *Image Analysis* **7**, pp. 403–416.

Candes, E. and Wakin, M. (2008). People hearing without listening: An introduction to compressive sampling, *IEEE Signal Processing Magazine* **25**, pp. 21–30.

Cao, J. (1999). The size of the connected components of excursion sets of χ^2, t and F fields, *Advances in Applied Probability* **31**, pp. 579–595.

Cao, J. and Worsley, K. (1999a). The geometry of correlation fields with an application to functional connectivity of the brain, *Annals of Applied Probability* **9**, pp. 1021–1057.

Cao, J. and Worsley, K. (2001). Applications of random fields in human brain mapping, *Spatial Statistics: Methodological Aspects and Applications* **159**, pp. 170–182.

Cao, J. and Worsley, K. J. (1999b). The detection of local shape changes via the geometry of Hotelling's t2 fields, *Annals of Statistics* **27**, pp. 925–942.

Carper, R., Moses, P., Tigue, Z. and Courchesne, E. (2002). Cerebral lobes in autism: Early hyperplasia and abnormal age effects, *NeuroImage* **16**, pp. 1038–1051.

Carr, J., Fright, W. and Beatson, R. (1997). Surface interpolation with radial basis functions for medical imaging, *IEEE Transactions on Medical Imaging* **16**, pp. 96–107.

Carrion, V., Weems, C. and Reiss, A. (2007). Stress predicts brain changes in children: A pilot longitudinal study on youth stress, posttraumatic stress disorder, and the hippocampus, *Pediatrics* **119**, p. 509.

Catani, M., Howard, R., Pajevic, S. and Jones, D. (2002). Virtual in vivo interactive dissection of white matter fasciculi in the human brain, *NeuroImage* **17**, pp. 77–94.

Cates, J., Fletcher, P., Styner, M., Hazlett, H. and Whitaker, R. (2008). Particle-Based Shape Analysis of Multi-Object Complexes, in *Medical image computing and computer-assisted intervention: MICCAI... International Conference on Medical Image Computing and Computer-Assisted Intervention*, Vol. 11, pp. 477–485.

Chandrasekharaiah, D. and Debnath, L. (1994). *Continuum Mechanics* (Academic Press, San Diego).

Chaudhuri, P. and Marron, J. S. (2000). Scale space view of curve estimation, *The Annals of Statistics* **28**, pp. 408–428.

Chavel, I. (1984). *Eigenvalues in Riemannian Geometry* (Academic Press, New York).

Christensen, G., Joshi, S. and Miller, M. (1997). volumetric transformation of brain anatomy, *IEEE Transactions on Medical Imaging* **16**, pp. 864–877.

Christensen, G., Rabbitt, R. and Miller, M. (1993). A deformable neuroanatomy text-book based on viscous fluid mechanics, *Proc. of the 27th Annual Conference on Information Science and Systems* , pp. 211–216.

Chung, M. (2001). *Statistical Morphometry in Neuroanatomy* (Ph.D. Thesis, McGill University).

Chung, M. (2006). Heat kernel smoothing on unit sphere, in *Proceedings of IEEE International Symposium on Biomedical Imaging (ISBI)*, Vol. I, pp. 467–473.

Chung, M., Adluru, N., Dalton, K., Alexander, A. and Davidson, R. (2011a). Scalable brain network construction on white matter fibers, in *Proc. of SPIE*, Vol. 7962, p. 79624G.

Chung, M., Adluru, N., Dalton, K. M., Alexander, A. and Davidson, R. (2010a). Characterization of structural connectivity in autism using graph networks with DTI, *16th Annual Meeting of the Organization for Human Brain Mapping* , 938.

Chung, M., Adluru, N., Lee, J., Lazar, M., Lainhart, J. and Alexander, A. (2010b). Cosine series representation of 3d curves and its application to white matter fiber bundles in diffusion tensor imaging, *Statistics and Its Interface* **3**, pp. 69–80.

Chung, M., Bubenik, P. and Kim, P. (2009a). Persistence diagrams of cortical surface data, *Proceedings of the 21st International Conference on Information Processing in Medical Imaging (IPMI), Lecture Notes in Computer Science (LNCS)* **5636**, pp. 386–397.

Chung, M., Dalton, K., Alexander, A. and Davidson, R. (2004). Less white matter concentration in autism: 2D voxel-based morphometry, *NeuroImage* **23**, pp. 242–251.

Chung, M., Dalton, K. and Davidson, R. (2008a). Tensor-based cortical surface morphometry via weighted spherical harmonic representation, *IEEE Transactions on Medical Imaging* **27**, pp. 1143–1151.

Chung, M., Dalton, K., Shen, L., Evans, A. and Davidson, R. (2007). Weighted Fourier representation and its application to quantifying the amount of gray matter, *IEEE Transactions on Medical Imaging* **26**, pp. 566–581.

Chung, M., Hanson, J., Avants, B., Gee, J., Davidson, R. and Pollak, S. (2010c). Structural connectivity mapping via the tensor-based morphometry, *16th Annual Meeting of the Organization for Human Brain Mapping* , 481.

Chung, M., Hanson, J., Davidson, R. and Pollak, S. (2011b). Effect of family income on hippocampus growth: longitudinal study, *17th Annual Meeting of the Organization for Human Brain Mapping* , 2697.

Chung, M., Hartley, R., Dalton, K. and Davidson, R. (2008b). Encoding cortical surface by spherical harmonics, *Satistica Sinica* **18**, pp. 1269–1291.

Chung, M., Lazar, M., Alexander, A., Lu, Y. and Davidson, R. (2003a). Probabilistic connectivity measure in diffusion tensor imaging via anisotropic kernel smoothing, *University of Wisconsin, Department of Statistics, Technical Report* **1081**.

Chung, M., Lee, H., Kim, P. and Ye, J. (2011c). Sparse topological data recovery in medical images, in *Biomedical Imaging: From Nano to Macro, 2011 IEEE International Symposium on*, pp. 1125–1129.

Chung, M., Nacewicz, B., Wang, S., Dalton, K., Pollak, S. and Davidson, R. (2008c). Amygdala Surface Modeling with Weighted Spherical Harmonics, *Lecture Notes in Computer Science* **5128**, pp. 177–184.

Chung, M., Robbins, S., Dalton, D. R. A. A., K.M. and Evans, A. (2005a). Cortical thickness analysis in autism with heat kernel smoothing, *NeuroImage* **25**, pp. 1256–1265.

Chung, M., Robbins, S. and Evans, A. (2005b). Unified statistical approach to cortical thickness analysis, *Information Processing in Medical Imaging (IPMI)*, *Lecture Notes in Computer Science* **3565**, pp. 627–638.

Chung, M., Shen, L., Dalton, K. and Davidson, R. (2006). Multi-scale voxel-based morphometry via weighted spherical harmonic representation, *Medical Imaging and Augmented Reality, Lecture Notes in Computer Science* **4091**, pp. 36–43.

Chung, M., Singh, V., Kim, P., Dalton, K. and Davidson, R. (2009b). Topological Characterization of Signal in Brain Images Using Min-Max Diagrams, *MICCAI, Lecture Notes in Computer Science (LNCS)* **5762**, pp. 158–166.

Chung, M. and Taylor, J. (2004). Diffusion smoothing on brain surface via finite element method, in *Proceedings of IEEE International Symposium on Biomedical Imaging (ISBI)*, Vol. 1, pp. 432–435.

Chung, M., Worsley, K., Brendon, M., Dalton, K. and Davidson, R. (2010d). General Multivariate Linear Modeling of Surface Shapes Using SurfStat, *NeuroImage* **53**, pp. 491–505.

Chung, M., Worsley, K., Paus, T., Cherif, D., Collins, C., Giedd, J., Rapoport, J., and Evans, A. (2001a). A unified statistical approach to deformation-based morphometry, *NeuroImage* **14**, pp. 595–606.

Chung, M., Worsley, K., Robbins, S. and Evans, A. (2003b). Tensor-based brain surface modeling and analysis, in *IEEE Conference on Computer Vision and Pattern Recognition (CVPR)*, Vol. I, pp. 467–473.

Chung, M., Worsley, K., Robbins, S., Paus, T., Taylor, J., Giedd, J., Rapoport, J. and Evans, A. (2003c). Deformation-based surface morphometry applied to gray matter deformation, *NeuroImage* **18**, pp. 198–213.

Chung, M., Worsley, K., Taylor, J., Ramsay, J., Robbins, S. and Evans, A. (2001b). Diffusion smoothing on the cortical surface, *NeuroImage* **13**, 6S1, p. 95.

Chung, M., Wu, Y. and Alexander, A. (2009c). 3d eigenfunction expansion of sparsely sampled 2D cortical data, in *IEEE International Symposium on Biomedical Imaging (ISBI): From Nano to Macro*, pp. 113–116.

Clayden, J., Storkey, A. and Bastin, M. (2007). A probabilistic model-based approach to consistent white matter tract segmentation, *IEEE Transactions on Medical Imaging* **11**, pp. 1555–1561.

Cohen-Steiner, D., Edelsbrunner, H. and Harer, J. (2007). Stability of persistence diagrams, *Discrete and Computational Geometry* **37**, pp. 103–120.

Collins, D. and Evans, A. (1999). ANIMAL:automatic nonlinear image matching and anatomical labeling, *Brain Warping* , pp. 133–142.

Collins, D., Holmes, C., Peters, T. and Evans, A. (1995). Automatic 3d model-based neuroanatomical segmentation, *Human Brain Mapping* **3**, pp. 190–208.

Collins, D., Neelin, P., Peters, T. and Evans, A. (1994). Automatic 3d intersubject registration of mr volumetric data in standardized talairach space, *J. Comput. Assisted Tomogr.* **18**, pp. 192–205.

Collins, D. L., Paus, T., Zijdenbos, A., Worsley, K. J., Blumenthal, J., Giedd, J. N., Rapoport, J. L. and Evans, A. C. (1998). Age related changes in the shape of temporal and frontal lobes: An mri study of children and adolescents, *Soc. Neurosci. Abstr.* **24**, p. 304.

Conover, W. (1980). *Practical nonparametric statistics* (Wiley New York).

Conturo, T., Lori, N., Cull, T., Akbudak, E., Snyder, A., Shimony, J., McKinstry, R., Burton, H. and Raichle, M. (1999). Tracking neuronal fiber pathways in the living human brain, in *Natl Acad Sci USA*, Vol. 96.

Conway, J. (1990). *A course in functional analysis* (Springer).

Cook, P., Bai, Y., Nedjati-Gilani, S., Seunarine, K., Hall, M., Parker, G. and Alexander, D. (2006). Camino: Open-source diffusion-MRI reconstruction and processing, in *14th Scientific Meeting of the International Society for Magnetic Resonance in Medicine*.

Cootes, T., Hill, A., Taylor, C. and Haslam, J. (1993). The Use of Active Shape Models for Locating Structures in Medical Images, *Lecture Notes in Computer Science* , pp. 33–33.

Cootes, T., Taylor, C., Cooper, D., Graham, J. *et al.* (1995). Active shape models-their training and application, *Computer vision and image understanding* **61**, pp. 38–59.

Corouge, I., Gouttard, S. and Gerig, G. (2004). Towards a shape model of white matter fiber bundles using diffusion tensor MRI, in *IEEE International Symposium on Biomedical Imaging: Nano to Macro*, pp. 344–347.

Courant, R. and Hilbert, D. (1953). *Methods of Mathematical Physics*, english edn. (Interscience, New York).

Csernansky, J., Wang, L., Joshi, S., Tilak Ratnanather, J. and Miller, M. (2004). Computational anatomy and neuropsychiatric disease: probabilistic assessment of variation and statistical inference of group difference, hemispheric asymmetry, and time-dependent change, *NeuroImage* **23**, pp. 56–68.

Dale, A. and Fischl, B. (1999). Cortical surface-based analysis i. segmentation and surface reconstruction, *NeuroImage* **9**, pp. 179–194.

Dalton, K., Anderle, M., Fisher, R., Schaeffer, H., Alexander, A. and Davidson, R. (2003). Brain function in individuals diagnosed with autism during discrimination of emotion, in *The proceeding of the 9th Annual Meeting of the Organization for Human Brain Mapping*.

Dalton, K., Nacewicz, B., Johnstone, T., Schaefer, H., Gernsbacher, M., Goldsmith, H., Alexander, A. and Davidson, R. (2005). Gaze fixation and the neural circuitry of face processing in autism, *Nature Neuroscience* **8**, pp. 519–526.

Darbon, J. (2007). A note on the discrete binary mumford-shah model, *Lecture Notes in Computer Science* **4418**, p. 283.

Davatzikos, C. (1997). Spatial transformation and registration of brain images using elastically deformable models, *Comput. Vis. Image Understanding* **66**, pp. 207–222.

Davatzikos, C. (1999). Brain morphometrics using geometry-based shape transformations, *Proc. of Workshop on Biomed. Image Registration, Slovenia* .

Davatzikos, C. and Bryan, R. (1995). Using a deformable surface model to obtain a shape representation of the cortex, *Proceedings of the IEEE International Conference on Computer Vision* **9**, pp. 2122–2127.

Davatzikos, C., Genc, A., Xu, D. and Resnick, S. (2001). Voxel-based morphometry using the ravens maps: Methods and validation using simulated longitudinal atrophy, *NeuroImage* **14**, pp. 1361–1369.

Davatzikos, C., Vaillant, M., Resnick, S., Prince, J., Letovsky, S. and Bryan, N. (1996). A computerized approach for morphological analysis of the corpus callosum, *Journal of Computer Assisted Tomography* **20**, pp. 88–97.

David, O., Kiebel, S., Harrison, L., Mattout, J., Kilner, J. and Friston, K. (2006). Dynamic causal modeling of evoked responses in eeg and meg, *NeuroImage* **30**, pp. 1255–1272.

de Silva, V. and Ghrist, R. (2007). Homological sensor networks, *Notic Amer Math Soc* **54**, pp. 10–17.

Dekaban, A. (1977). Tables of cranial and orbital measurements cranial volume and derived indexes in males and females from 7 days to 20 years of age, *Ann. Neurology* **2**, pp. 485–491.

Dekaban, A. and Shadowsky, D. (1978). Changes in brain weights during the span of human life: relation of brain weights to body heights and body weights, *Ann. Neurology* **4**, pp. 345–356.

Dempster, A., Laird, N., Rubin, D. *et al.* (1977). Maximum likelihood from incomplete data via the EM algorithm, *Journal of the Royal Statistical Society. Series B (Methodological)* **39**, pp. 1–38.

Desrun, M., Meyer, M., Sschroder, P. and Barr, A. (1999). Implicit fairing of irregular meshes using diffusion and curvature flow, in *ACM SIGGRAPH*, pp. 317–324.

Dirac, P. (1981). *The principles of quantum mechanics* (Oxford University Press, USA).

do Carmo, M. (1992). *Riemannian Geometry* (Prentice-Hall, Inc.).

Dobra, A., Hans, C., Jones, B., Nevins, J., Yao, G. and West, M. (2004). Sparse graphical models for exploring gene expression data, *Journal of Multivariate Analysis* **90**, pp. 196–212.

Dong, S., Bremer, P., Garland, M., Pascucci, V. and Hart, J. (2006). Spectral surface quadrangulation, in *ACM SIGGRAPH 2006 Papers* (ACM), pp. 1057–1066.

Donoho, D. and Tsaig, Y. (2006). *Fast solution of l_1-norm minimization problems when the solution may be sparse* (Citeseer).

Dougherty, E. (1999). *Random Processes for Image and Signal Processing* (IEEE Press).

Drew, D. (1991). *Theory of multicomponent fluids* (Springer-Verlag, New York).

Dryden, I. and Mardia, K. (1998). *Statistical Shape Analysis* (John Wiley & Sons).

Edelsbrunner, H., Dequent, M.-L., Mileyko, Y. and Pourquie, O. (2008). Assessing periodicity in gene expression as measured by microarray data, *Preprint* .

Edelsbrunner, H. and Harer, J. (2008). Persistent homology - a survey, *Contemporary Mathematics* **453**, pp. 257–282.

Edelsbrunner, H. and Harer, J. (2009). *Computational Topology: An Introduction* (American Mathematical Society Press).

Edelsbrunner, H., Letscher, D. and Zomorodian, A. (2002). Topological persistence and simplification, *Discrete and Computational Geometry* **28**, pp. 511–533.

Egaas, B., Courchesne, E. and Saitoh, O. (1995). Reduced size of corpus callosum in autism, *Archives of Neurology* **52**, p. 794.

Embrechts, P., Resnick, S. and Samorodnitsky, G. (1999). Extreme value theory as a risk management tool, *North American Actuarial Journal* **3**, pp. 30–41.

Erdös, P. and Rényi, A. (1961). On the evolution of random graphs, *Bull. Inst. Internat. Statist* **38**, 4, pp. 343–347.

Evans, L. (1998). *Partial differential equations* (American Mathematical Society).

Fan, J. and Gijbels, I. (1996). *Local Polynomial Modelling and Its Applications* (Chapman & Hall/CRC).

Feller, W. (1968). *Introduction to probability theory and its applications, Vol. 1* (Wiley, New York).

Fiedler, M. (1973). Algebraic connectivity of graphs, *Czechoslovak Mathematical Journal* **23**, pp. 298–305.

Figueiredo, M., Nowak, R. and Wright, S. (2008). Gradient projection for sparse reconstruction: Application to compressed sensing and other inverse problems, *Selected Topics in Signal Processing, IEEE Journal of* **1**, pp. 586–597.

Fischl, B. and Dale, A. (2000). Measuring the thickness of the human cerebral cortex from magnetic resonance images, *Proceedings of the National Academy of Sciences (PNAS)* **97**, pp. 11050–11055.

Fisher, R. (1915). Frequency distribution of the values of the correlation coefficient in samples of an indefitely large population, *Biometrika* **10**, pp. 507–521.

Flury, B. (1997). *A First Course in Multivariate Statistics* (Springer).

Fornefett, M., Rohr, K. and Stiehl, H. (1999). Elastic registration of medical images using radial basis functions with compact support, in *IEEE Computer Society Conference on Computer Vision and Pattern Recognition*, pp. 402–407.

Fornito, A., Zalesky, A. and Bullmore, E. (2010). Network scaling effects in graph analytic studies of human resting-state fMRI data, *Frontiers in Systems Neuroscience* **4**, pp. 1–16.

Foster, J. and Richards, F. (1991). The Gibbs phenomenon for piecewise-linear approximation, *American Mathematical Monthly* **98**.

Fox, J. (2002). *An R and S-Plus companion to applied regression* (Sage Publications, Inc).

Fox, J., Friendly, M. and Monette, G. (2009). Visualizing hypothesis tests in multivariate linear models: the heplots package for R, *Computational Statistics* **24**, pp. 233–246.

Freeman, L. (1977). A set of measures of centrality based on betweenness, *Sociometry* **40**, pp. 35–41.

Friedman, J., Bentley, J. and Finkel, R. (1997). An algorithm for finding best matches in logarithmic expected time, *ACM transactions on mathematics software* **3**, pp. 209–226.

Friedman, J., Hastie, T. and Tibshirani, R. (2008). Sparse inverse covariance estimation with the graphical lasso. *Biostatistics* **9**, p. 432.

Frigge, M., Hoaglin, D. and Iglewicz, B. (1989). Some implementations of the boxplot, *American Statistician* , pp. 50–54.

Friston, K. (1994). Functional and effective connectivity in neuroimaging: a synthesis, *Human Brain Mapping* **2**, pp. 56–78.

Friston., K. (2002). A short history of statistical parametric mapping in functional neuroimaging, Tech. Rep. Technical report, Wellcome Department of Imaging Neuroscience, ION, UCL., London, UK.

Friston, K., Frith, C., Fletcher, P., Liddle, P. and Frackowiak, R. (1996). Functional topography: multidimensional scaling and functional connectivity in the brain, *Cerebral Cortex* **6**, pp. 156–164.

Friston, K., Frith, C. and Frackowiak, R. (1993a). Time-dependent changes in effective connectivity measured with PET, *Human Brain Mapping* **1**, pp. 69–79.

Friston, K., Frith, C., Liddle, P. and Frackowiak, R. (1993b). Functional connectivity: the principal-component analysis of large(PET) data sets, *Journal of Cerebral Blood Flow and Metabolism* **13**, pp. 5–14.

Friston, K., Harrison, L. and Penny, W. (2003). Dynamic causal modelling, *NeuroImage* **19**, pp. 1273–1302.

Gaser, C., Luders, E., Thompson, P., Lee, A., Dutton, R., Geaga, J., Hayashi, K., Bellugi, U., Galaburda, A., Korenberg, J., Mills, D., Toga, A. and Reiss, A. (2006). Increased local gyrification mapped in williams syndrome, *NeuroImage* **33**, pp. 46–54.

Gaser, C., Volz, H.-P., Kiebel, S., Riehemann, S. and Sauer, H. (1999). Detecting structural changes in whole brain based on nonlinear deformations-application to schizophrenia research, *NeuroImage* **10**, pp. 107–113.

Gebal, K., Bærentzen, J., Aanæs, H. and Larsen, R. (2009). Shape analysis using the auto diffusion function, in *Computer Graphics Forum*, Vol. 28 (Wiley Online Library), pp. 1405–1413.

Gee, J. and Bajcsy, R. (1999). Elastic matching: Continuum mechanical and probabilistic analysis, *Brain Warping* , pp. 183–198.

Gee, J., Reivich, M. and Bajcsy, R. (1993). Elastically deforming an atlas to match anatomical brain images, *Journal of Computer Assisted Tomography* **17**, pp. 225–236.

Gelb, A. (1997). The resolution of the gibbs phenomenon for spherical harmonics, *Mathematics of Computation* **66**, pp. 699–717.

Gel'fand, I., Shilov, G. and Saletan, E. (1964). *Generalized functions* (Academic Press New York).

Genovese, C., Lazar, N. and Nichols, T. (2002). Thresholding of statistical maps in functional neuroimaging using the false discovery rate, *NeuroImage* **15**, pp. 870–878.

Gerig, G., Styner, M., Jones, D., Weinberger, D. and Lieberman, J. (2001). Shape analysis of brain ventricles using spharm, in *MMBIA*, pp. 171–178.

Ghrist, R. (2008). Barcodes: The persistent topology of data, *Bulletin of the American Mathematical Society* **45**, pp. 61–75.

Gibbs, J. (1898). Fourier's series, *Nature* **59**, p. 200.

Gibbs, J. (1899). Fourier's series, *Nature* **59**, p. 606.

Giedd, J., Blumenthal, J., Jeffries, N., Rajapakse, J., Vaituzis, A., Liu, H., Y.C., B., Tobin, M., Nelson, J. and Castellanos, F. (1999). Development of the human corpus callosum during childhood and adolescence: a longitudinal mri study. *Progress in Neuro-Psychopharmacology & Biological Psychiatry* **23**, pp. 571–588.

Giedd, J., Snell, J., Lange, N., Rajapakse, J., Kaysen, D., Vaituzis, A., Vauss, Y., Hamburger, S., Kozuch, P. and Rapoport, J. (1996). Quantitative magnetic resonance imaging of human brain development: Ages 4-18, *Cerebral Cortex* **6**, pp. 551–160.

Girvan, M. and Newman, M. (2002). Community structure in social and biological networks, *Proceedings of the National Academy of Sciences* **99**, p. 7821.

Gladwell, G. and Zhu, H. (2002). Courant's nodal line theorem and its discrete counterparts, *The Quarterly Journal of Mechanics and Applied Mathematics* **55**, pp. 1–15.

Goldsmith, J., Crainiceanu, C., Caffo, B. and Reich, D. (2011). Penalized functional regression analysis of white-matter tract profiles in multiple sclerosis, *NeuroImage* **57**, pp. 431–439.

Goldsmith, J., Crainiceanu, C., Caffo, B. and Reich, D. (2012). Longitudinal penalized functional regression for cognitive outcomes on neuronal tract measurements, *Journal of the Royal Statistical Society: Series C (Applied Statistics)* **61**, p. in press.

Golland, P., Grimson, W., Shenton, M. and Kikinis, R. (2001). Deformation analysis for shape based classification, *Information Processing in Medical Imaging (IPMI), Lecture Notes in Computer Science* **2082**, pp. 517–530.

Gong, G., He, Y., Concha, L., Lebel, C., Gross, D., Evans, A. and Beaulieu, C. (2009). Mapping anatomical connectivity patterns of human cerebral cortex using in vivo diffusion tensor imaging tractography, *Cerebral Cortex* **19**, pp. 524–536.

Good, C., Johnsrude, I., Ashburner, J., Henson, R., Friston, K. and Frackowiak, R. (2001). A voxel-based morphometric study of ageing in 465 normal adult human brains, *NeuroImage* **14**, pp. 21–36.

Gorski, K. (1994). On determining the spectrum of primordial inhomogeneity from the cobe dmr sky maps: I. method, *Astrophysical Journal* **430**, p. L85.

Gottlieb, D. and Shu, C.-W. (1997). On the gibbs phenomenon and its resolution, *SIAM Review* **39**, pp. 644–668.

Green, P. and Silverman, B. (1994). *Non-parametric Regression and Generalized Linear Models: A Roughness Penalty Approach* (Chapman and Hall, London).

Griffin, L. (1994). The intrinsic geometry of the cerebral cortex, *Journal of Theoretical Biology* **166**, pp. 261–273.

Grigoryan, A. (1999). Analytic and geometric background of recurrence and non-explosion of the brownian motion on riemannian manifolds, *Bulletin of the American Mathematical Society* **36**, pp. 135–249.

Groemer, H. (1996). *Geometric Applications of Fourier Series and Spherical Harmonics*, (Cambridge University Press).

Gruen, A. and Akca, D. (2005). Least squares 3D surface and curve matching, *ISPRS Journal of Photogrammetry and Remote Sensing* **59**, pp. 151–174.

Gu, X., Wang, Y., Chan, T., Thompson, T. and Yau, S. (2004). Genus zero surface conformal mapping and its application to brain surface mapping, *IEEE Transactions on Medical Imaging* **23**, pp. 1–10.

Gueziec, A., Pennec, X. and Ayache, N. (1997). Medical image registration using geometeric hashing, *IEEE Computational Science and Engineering* **4**, pp. 29–41.

Guéziec, D. (1996). *Spline Curves and Surfaces for Data Modeling, Advances in Morphometrics* (Plenum Press, New Work).

Gurtin, M. and McFadden, G. (1991). *On the Evolutation of Phase Boundaries* (Springer-Verlag, New York).

Guskov, I. and Wood, Z. J. (2001). Topological noise removal, in *Graphics Interface*, pp. 19–26.

Hagler Jr., S. A. S. M., D.J. (2006). Smoothing and cluster thresholding for cortical surface-based group analysis of fmri data, *NeuroImage* **33**, pp. 1093–1103.

Hagmann, P., Kurant, M., Gigandet, X., Thiran, P., Wedeen, V., Meuli, R. and Thiran, J. (2007). Mapping human whole-brain structural networks with diffusion MRI, *PLoS One* **2**, 7, p. e597.

Hagmann, P., Thiran, J., Vandergheynst, P., Clarke, S., Meuli, R. and Lausanne, S. (2000). Statistical fiber tracking on DT-MRI data as a potential tool for morphological brain studies, in *ISMRM Workshop on Diffusion MRI: Biophysical Issues*.

Hair, J., Tatham, R., Anderson, R. and Black, W. (1998). *Multivariate Data Analysis* (Prentice Hall, Inc.).

Hall, K. (1970). An r-dimensional quadratic placement algorithm, *Management Science* **17**, pp. 219–229.

Ham, J., Lee, D., Mika, S. and Schölkopf, B. (2004). A kernel view of the dimensionality reduction of manifolds, in *Proceedings of the Twenty-first International Conference on Machine Learning*, p. 47.

Ham, J., Lee, D. and Saul, L. (2005). Semisupervised alignment of manifolds in *Proceedings of the Annual Conference on Uncertainty in Artificial Intelligence*, Vol. 10, pp. 120–127.

Hamarneh, G. and Gustavsson, T. (2002). Combining snakes and active shape models for segmenting the human left ventricle in echocardiographic images, in *Computers in Cardiology 2000* (IEEE), pp. 115–118.

Han, J., Kim, J., Chung, C. and Park, K. (2007). Evaluation of smoothing in an iterative lp-norm minimization algorithm for surface-based source localization of meg, *Physics in Medicine and Biology* **52**, pp. 4791–4803.

Han, X., Jovicich, J., Salat, D., van der Kouwe, A., Quinn, B., Czanner, S., Busa, E., Pacheco, J., Albert, M., Killiany, R. *et al.* (2006). Reliability of MRI-derived measurements of human cerebral cortical thickness: The effects of field strength, scanner upgrade and manufacturer, *NeuroImage* **32**, pp. 180–194.

Hanson, J., Chung, M., Avants, B., Shirtcliff, E., Gee, J., Davidson, R. and Pollak, S. (2010). Early Stress Is Associated with Alterations in the Orbitofrontal Cortex: A Tensor-Based Morphometry Investigation of Brain Structure and Behavioral Risk, *Journal of Neuroscience* **30**, pp. 7466–7477.

Hardan, A., Minshew, N. and Keshavan, M. (2000). Corpus callosum size in autism, *Neurology* **55**, p. 1033.

Hart, J. C. (1999). Computational topology for shape modeling, in *Proceedings of the International Conference on Shape Modeling and Applications*, pp. 36–43.

Harville, D. (1997). *Matrix Algebra from a Statistician's Perspective* (Springer-Verlag, New York).

Hastie, T., Tibshirani, R. and Friedman, J. (2003). *The elements of statistical learning* (Springer).

Haupt, J., Bajwa, W., Rabbat, M. and Nowak, R. (2008). Compressed sensing for networked data, *IEEE Signal Processing Magazine* **25**, pp. 92–101.

Hayasaka, S., Peiffer, A., Hugenschmidt, C. and Laurienti, P. (2007). Power and sample size calculation for neuroimaging studies by non-central random field theory, *NeuroImage* **37**, pp. 721–730.

He, Y., Chen, Z. and Evans, A. (2007). Small-world anatomical networks in the human brain revealed by cortical thickness from MRI, *Cerebral Cortex* **17**, pp. 2407–2419.

He, Y., Chen, Z. and Evans, A. (2008). Structural insights into aberrant topological patterns of large-scale cortical networks in Alzheimer's disease, *Journal of Neuroscience* **28**, p. 4756.

Hernandez, V., Roman, J. E., Tomas, A. and Vidal, V. (2006). A survey of software for sparse eigenvalue problems, Tech. Rep. STR-6, Universidad Politécnica de Valencia, http://www.grycap.upv.es/slepc.

Higdon, R., Foster, N., Koeppe, R., DeCarli, C., Jagust, W., Clark, C., Barbas, N., Arnold, S., R.S. Turner, J. H. and Minoshima, S. (2004). A comparison of classification methods for differentiating fronto-temporal dementia from alzheimer's disease using FDG-PET imaging, *Stat Med* **23**, pp. 315–326.

Hodge, V. and Austin, J. (2004). A survey of outlier detection methodologies, *Artificial Intelligence Review* **22**, pp. 85–126.

Hoffmann, T., Chung, M., Dalton, K., Alexander, A., Wahba, G. and Davidson, R. (2004). Subpixel curvature estimation of the corpus callosum via splines and its application to autism, in *10th Annual Meeting of the Organization for Human Brain Mapping.*

Hoffmann-Ostenhof, M., Hoffmann-Ostenhof, T. and Nadirashvili, N. (1999). On the multiplicity of eigenvalues of the laplacian on surfaces, *Annals of Global Analysis and Geometry* **17**.

Holzrichter, M. and Oliveira, S. (1999). A graph based method for generating the Fiedler vector of irregular problems, *Parallel and Distributed Processing, Lecture Notes in Computer Science (LNCS)* **1586**, pp. 978–985.

Horak, D., Maletić, S. and Rajković, M. (2009). Persistent homology of complex networks, *Journal of Statistical Mechanics: Theory and Experiment* **2009**, p. P03034.

Horn, R. and Johnson, C. (1985). *Matrix Analysis* (Cambridge University Press, London).

Hosseinbor, P., Chung, M., Wu, Y.-C. and Alexander, A. (2011). Bessel Fourier orientation reconstruction: an analytical EAP reconstruction using multiple shell acquisitions in diffusion MRI, *Medical Image Computing and Computer-Assisted Intervention (MICCAI), Lecture Notes in Computer Science (LNCS)* **6892**, pp. 217–225.

Huang, S., Li, J., Sun, L., Liu, J., Wu, T., Chen, K., Fleisher, A., Reiman, E. and Ye, J. (2009). Learning brain connectivity of Alzheimer's disease from neuroimaging data, in *Proceedings of Neural Information Processing Systems Conference (NIPS)*, Vol. 22, pp. 808–816.

Huang, S., Li, J., Sun, L., Ye, J., Fleisher, A., Wu, T., Chen, K. and Reiman, E. (2010). Learning brain connectivity of Alzheimer's disease by sparse inverse covariance estimation, *NeuroImage* **50**, pp. 935–949.

Hurdal, M. K. and Stephenson, K. (2004). Cortical cartography using the discrete conformal approach of circle packings, *NeuroImage* **23**, pp. S119–S128.

Hutchinson, J. (1981). Fractals and self-similarity, *Indiana Univ. Math. J* **30**, pp. 713–747.

Jackowski, A., de Araujo, C., de Lacerda, A., de Jesus and Kaufman, J. (2009). Neurostructural imaging findings in children with post-traumatic stress disorder: Brief review, *Psychiatry and Clinical Neurosciences* **63**, pp. 1–8.

Janssen, P. and Stoica, P. (1988). On the expectation of the product of four matrix-valued Gaussianrandom variables, *IEEE Transactions on Automatic Control* **33**, pp. 867–870.

Jbabdi, S., Bellec, P., Toro, R., Daunizeau, J., Pélégrini-Issac, M. and Benali, H. (2008). Accurate anisotropic fast marching for diffusion-based geodesic tractography, *International Journal of Biomedical Imaging* **2008**, pp. 1–12.

Jerri, A. (1998). *The Gibbs phenomenon in Fourier analysis, splines and wavelet approximations* (Springer).

Jo, H., Lee, J.-M., Kim, J.-H., Shin, Y.-W., Kim, I.-Y., Kwon, J. and Kim, S. (2007). Spatial accuracy of fmri activation influenced by volume- and surface-based spatial smoothing techniques, *NeuroImage* **34**, pp. 550–564.

Johnson, S., Baxter, L., Susskind-Wilder, L., Connor, D., Sabbagh, M. and Caselli, R. (2004). Hippocampal adaptation to face repetition in healthy elderly and mild cognitive impairment, *Neuropsychologia* **42**, pp. 980–989.

Jolliffe, I. (2002). *Principal component analysis* (Springer verlag).

Jolliffe, I., Trendafilov, N. and Uddin, M. (2003). A modified principal component technique based on the LASSO, *Journal of Computational and Graphical Statistics* **12**, pp. 531–547.

Jones, D., Catani, M., Pierpaoli, C., Reeves, S., Shergill, S., O'Sullivan, M., Golesworthy, P., McGuire, P., Horsfield, M., Simmons, A., Williams, S. and Howard, R. (2006). Age effects on diffusion tensor magnetic resonance imaging tractography measures of frontal cortex connections in schizophrenia, *Human Brain Mapping* **27**, pp. 230–238.

Jones, P., Maggioni, M. and Schul, R. (2008). Manifold parametrizations by eigenfunctions of the Laplacian and heat kernels, *Proceedings of the National Academy of Sciences of the United States of America (PNAS)* **105**, pp. 1803–1808.

Jones, S., Buchbinder, B. and Aharon, I. (2000). Three-dimensional mapping of cortical thickness using Laplace's equation, *Human Brain Mapping* **11**, pp. 12–32.

Joshi, A., Shattuck, D. W., Thompson, P. M. and Leahy, R. M. (2009). A parameterization-based numerical method for isotropic and anisotropic diffusion smoothing on non-flat surfaces, *IEEE Transactions on Image Processing* **18**, pp. 1358–1365.

Joshi, S. (1998). *Large Deformation Diffeomorphisms and Gaussian Random Fields for Statistical Characterization of Brain Sub-Manifolds* (Ph.D. thesis. Washington University, St. Louis).

Joshi, S., Davis, B., Jomier, M. and Gerig, G. (2004). Unbiased diffeomorphic atlas construction for computational anatomy, *NeuroImage* **23**, pp. 151–160.

Joshi, S., Grenander, U. and Miller, M. (1997). The geometry and shape of brain sub-manifolds, *International Journal of Pattern Recognition and Artificial Intelligence: Special Issue on Processing of MR Images of the Human* **11**, pp. 1317–1343.

Joshi, S., Pizer, S., Fletcher, P., Yushkevich, P., Thall, A. and Marron, J. (2002). Multiscale deformable model segmentation and statistical shape analysis using medial descriptions, *IEEE Transactions on Medical Imaging* **21**, pp. 538–550.

Joshi, S., Wang, J., Miller, M., Van Essen, D. and Grenander, U. (1995). On the differential geometry of the cortical surface, *Vision Geometry IV, Vol. 2573, Proceedings of the SPIE's 1995 International Symposium on Optical Science, Engineering and Instrumentation* , pp. 304–311.

Kabani, N., Le Goualher, D., G. MacDonald and Evans, A. (2000). Measurement of cortical thickness using an automated 3-D algorithm: a validation study, *NeuroImage* **13**, pp. 375–380.

Kac, M. (1966). Can one hear the shape of a drum, *American Mathematical Monthly* **73**, pp. 1–23.

Kass, M., Witkin, A. and Terzopoulos, D. (1988). Snakes: active contour models, *International Journal of Computer Vision* **1**, pp. 321–331.

Kawohl, B. (1985). Rearrangements and convexity of level sets in PDE, *Lecture notes in mathematics* , 1150, pp. 1–134.

Kazi-Aoual, F., Hitier, S., Sabatier, R. and Lebreton, J. (1995). Refined approximations to permutation tests for multivariate inference, *Computational Statistics & Data Analysis* **20**, pp. 643–656.

Kelemen, A., Szekely, G. and Gerig, G. (1999). Elastic model-based segmentation of 3-d neuroradiological data sets, *IEEE Transactions on Medical Imaging* **18**, pp. 828–839.

Kendall, D. (1989). A survey of the statistical theory of shape, *Statistical Science* **4**, pp. 87–120.

Kennedy, D., O'Craven, K., Ticho, B., Goldstein, A., Makris, N. and Henson, J. (1999). Structural and functional brain asymmetries in human situs inversus totalis, *Neurology* **53**, pp. 1260–1265.

Kiebel, S., Poline, J.-P., Friston, K., Holmes, A. and Worsley, K. (1999). Robust smoothness estimation in statistical parametric maps using standardized residuals from the general linear model, *NeuroImage* **10**, pp. 756–766.

Kim, J., Singh, V., Lee, J., Lerch, J., Ad-Dab'bagh, Y., MacDonald, D., Lee, J., Kim, S. and Evans, A. (2005). Automated 3-D extraction and evaluation of the inner and outer cortical surfaces using a laplacian map and partial volume effect classification, *NeuroImage* **27**, pp. 210–221.

Kim, S., Koh, K., Lustig, M., Boyd, S. and Gorinevsky, D. (2008). An interior-point method for large-scale l_1-regularized least squares, *IEEE Journal of Selected Topics in Signal Processing* **1**, pp. 606–617.

Kim, S.-G., Chung, M., Hanson, J., Avants, B., Gee, J., Davidson, R. and Pollak, S. (2011). Structural connectivity via the tensor-based morphometry, in *The proceedings of IEEE International Symposium on Biomedical Imaging (ISBI)*, pp. 808–811.

Kim, S.-G., Chung, M., Schaefer, S., van Reekum, C. and Davidson, R. (2012a). Sparse shape representation using the laplace-beltrami eigenfunctions and its application to modeling subcortical structures, in *The proceedings of IEEE Computer Society Workshop on Mathematical Methods in Biomedical Image Analysis (MMBIA)*, pp. 25–32.

Kim, S.-G., Lee, H., Chung, M., Hanson, J., Avants, B., Gee, J., Davidson, R. and Pollak, S. (2012b). Agreement between the white matter connectivity based on the tensor-based morphometry and the volumetric white matter parcellations based on diffusion tensor imaging, in *The proceedings of IEEE International Symposium on Biomedical Imaging (ISBI)*, p. in press.

Kirby, M. (2000). *Geometric Data Analysis: An empirical approach to dimensionality reduction and the study of patterns* (John Wiley & Sons, Inc. New York, NY, USA).

Kishon, E., Hastie, T. and Wolfson, H. (1990). 3D curve matching using splines, in *Proceedings of the European Conference on Computer Vision*, pp. 589–591.

Koch, M., Norris, D. and Hund-Georgiadis, M. (2002). An investigation of functional and anatomical connectivity using magnetic resonance imaging, *NeuroImage* **16**, pp. 241–250.

Koh, E., Kim, T. and Cho, H. (2006). Mean curvature as a major determinant of β-sheet propensity, *Bioinformatics* **22**, p. 297.

Kollakian, K. (1996). Performance analysis of automatic techniques for tissue classification in magnetic resonance images of the human brain, Tech. Rep. Master's thesis, Concordia University, Montreal, Quebec, Canada.

Kolmogorov, A. and Fomin, S. (1970). *Introductory Real Analysis* (Dover Publications, Inc, New York).

Koren, Y. and Harel, D. (2002). A multi-scale algorithm for the linear arrangement problem, **2573**, pp. 296–309.

Kovacevic, N., Lobaugh, N., Bronskill, M., Levine, B., Feinstein, A. and Black, S. (2002). A robust method for extraction and automatic segmentation of brain images, *NeuroImage* **17**, pp. 1087–1100.

Kovačič, S. and Bajcsy, R. (1999). Multiscale/multiresolution representations, *Brain Warping* , pp. 45–65.

Kraina, A. and Castellanos, F. (2006). Brain development and ADHD, *Clinical Psychology Review* **26**, pp. 433–444.

Kreyszig, E. (1959). *Differential Geometry* (University of Toronto Press).

Kuperberg, G., Broome, M., McGuire, P., David, A., Eddy, M., Ozawa, F., Goff, D., West, W., Williams, S., van der Kouwe, A. *et al.* (2003). Regionally localized thinning of the cerebral cortex in schizophrenia, *Archives of General Psychiatry* **60**, pp. 878–888.

Kwapien, S. and Woyczynski, W. (1992). *Random Series and Stochastic Integrals: Single and Multiple*, Probability and Its Applications (Birkhauser).

Landau, L. and Lifshitz, E. (1989). *Fluid Mechanics*, 2nd edn. (Pagamon Press).

Lawson, C. and Hanson, R. (1974). *Solving Least Sqaures Problems* (Prentice-Hall).

Lazar, M., Weinstein, D., Tsuruda, J., Hasan, K., Arfanakis, K., Meyerand, M., Badie, B., Rowley, H., Haughton, V., Field, A., Witwer, B. and Alexander, A. (2003). White matter tractography using tensor deflection, *Human Brain Mapping* **18**, pp. 306–321.

Leadbetter, M., Lindgren, G. and Rootzén, H. (1982). *Extremes and Related Properties of Random Sequences and Processes* (Springer-Verlag, New York).

Lee, H., Chung, M., Kang, H., Kim, B.-N. and D.S., L. (2011a). Discriminative persistent homology of brain networks, in *IEEE International Symposium on Biomedical Imaging (ISBI)*, pp. 841–844.

Lee, H., Chung, M., Kang, H., Kim, B.-N. and Lee, D. (2011b). Computing the shape of brain networks using graph filtration and Gromov-Hausdorff metric, *MICCAI, Lecture Notes in Computer Science* **6892**, pp. 302–209.

Lee, H., Chung, M., Kang, H., Kim, B.-N. and Lee, D. (2011c). Persistent network homology from the perspective of dendrograms, .

Lee, H., Lee, D., Kang, H., Kim, B.-N. and Chung, M. (2011d). Sparse brain network recovery under compressed sensing, *IEEE Transactions on Medical Imaging* **30**, pp. 1154–1165.

Leemans, A., Sijbers, J., Backer, S. D., Vandervliet, E. and Parizel, P. (2006). Multiscale white matter fiber tract coregistration: A new feature-based approach to align diffusion tensor data, *Magnetic Resonance in Medicine* **55**, pp. 1414–1423.

Lehoucq, R., Sorensen, D. and Yang, C. (1998). *ARPACK Users' Guide: Solution of Large-Scale Eigenvalue Problems with Implicitly Restarted Arnoldi Methods* (SIAM Publications, Philadelphia).

Leow, A., Klunder, A., Jack, C., Toga, A., Dale, A., Bernstein, M., Britson, P., Gunter, J., Ward, C., Whitwell, J. *et al.* (2006). Longitudinal stability of MRI for mapping brain change using tensor-based morphometry, *NeuroImage* **31**, pp. 627–640.

Leow, A., Yanovsky, I., Chiang, M., Lee, A., Klunder, A., Lu, A., Becker, J., Davis, S., Toga, A. and Thompson, P. (2007). Statistical properties of Jacobian maps and the realization of unbiased large-deformation nonlinear image registration, *IEEE Transactions on Medical Imaging* **26**, pp. 822–832.

Lepore, N., Brun, C., Chiang, M., Chou, Y., Dutton, R., Hayashi, K., Lopez, O., Aizenstein, H., Toga, A., Becker, J. and Thompson, P. (2006). Multivariate statistics of the jacobian matrices in tensor based morphometry and their application to HIV/AIDS, *Lecture Notes in Computer Science* , pp. 191–198.

Lerch, J., Worsley, K., Shaw, W., Greenstein, D., Lenroot, R., Giedd, J. and Evans, A. (2006). Mapping anatomical correlations across cerebral cortex (MACACC) using cortical thickness from MRI, *NeuroImage* **31**, pp. 993–1003.

Lerch, J. P. and Evans, A. (2005). Cortical thickness analysis examined through power analysis and a population simulation, *NeuroImage* **24**, pp. 163–173.

Lester, A. and Simon, R. (1999). A survey of hierarchical non-linear medical image registration, *Pattern Recognition* **32**, pp. 129–149.

Leventon, M., Grimson, W. and Faugeras, O. (2000). Statistical shape influence in geodesic active contours, in *IEEE Conference on Computer Vision and Pattern Recognition (CVPR)*, Vol. 1, pp. 316–323.

Lévy, B. and Inria-Alice, F. (2006). Laplace-beltrami eigenfunctions towards an algorithm that " understands" geometry, in *IEEE International Conference on Shape Modeling and Applications, 2006*, p. 13.

Li, Y., Liu, Y., Li, J., Qin, W., Li, K., Yu, C. and Jiang, T. (2009). Brain Anatomical Network and Intelligence, *PLoS Computational Biology* **5**, 5, p. e1000395.

Lindeberg, T. (1994). *Scale-Space Theory in Computer Vision* (Kluwer Academic Publisher).

Lorensen, W. and Cline, H. (1987). Marching cubes: A high resolution 3D surface construction algorithm, in *Proceedings of the 14th annual conference on Computer graphics and interactive techniques*, pp. 163–169.

Luders, E., Narr, K., Thompson, P., Rex, D., Woods, R., DeLuca, J. L., H. and Toga, A. (2006a). Gender effects on cortical thickness and the influence of scaling, *Human Brain Mapping* **27**, pp. 314–324.

Luders, E., Thompson, P., Narr, K., Toga, A., Jancke, L. and Gaser, C. (2006b). A curvature-based approach to estimate local gyrification on the cortical surface, *NeuroImage* **29**, pp. 1224–1230.

MacDonald, J., Kabani, N., Avis, D. and Evans, A. (2000). Automated 3-D extraction of inner and outer surfaces of cerebral cortex from MRI, *NeuroImage* **12**, pp. 340–356.

Malladi, R. and Ravve, I. (2002). Fast difference schemes for edge enhancing Beltrami flow, in *Proceedings of Computer Vision-ECCV, Lecture Notes in Computer Science (LNCS)*, Vol. 2350, pp. 343–357.

Mallat, S. and Zhang, Z. (1993). Matching pursuits with time-frequency dictionaries, *IEEE Transactions on Signal Processing* **41**, pp. 3397–3415.

Mandelbrot, B. (1982). *The fractal geometry of nature* (Freeman).

Manes, F., Piven, J., Vrancic, D., Nanclares, V., Plebst, C. and Starkstein, S. (1999). An MRI study of the corpus callosum and cerebellum in mentally retarded autistic individuals, *Journal of Neuropsychiatry and Clinical Neurosciences* **11**, p. 470.

Marrelec, G., Kim, J., Doyon, J. and Horwitz, B. (2009). Largescale neural model validation of partial correlation analysis for effective connectivity investigation in functional MRI, *Human Brain Mapping* **30**, pp. 941–950.

Marrelec, G., Krainik, A., Duffau, H., Pélégrini-Issac, M., Lehéricy, S., Doyon, J. and Benali, H. (2006). Partial correlation for functional brain interactivity investigation in functional MRI, *NeuroImage* **32**, pp. 228–237.

Marsden, J. and Hughes, T. (1983). *Mathematical Foundations of Elasticity* (Dover Publications, Inc.).

Mather, M., Canli, T., English, T., Whitfield, S., Wais, P., Ochsner, K., Gabrieli, J. and Carstensen, L. (2004). Amygdala responses to emotionally valenced stimuli in older and younger adults, *Psychological Science* **15**, pp. 259–263.

McIntosh, A., bookstein, F., Haxby, J. and Grady, C. (1996). Spatial pattern analysis of functional brain images using partial least squares, *NeuroImage* **3**, pp. 143–157.

McIntosh, A. and Lobaugh, N. (2004). Partial least squares analysis of neuroimaging data: applications and advances, *NeuroImage* **23**, pp. 250–263.

McLeod, R. and Baart, M. (1998). *Geometry and Interpolation of Curves and Surfaces* (Cambridge University Press).

Mclntosh, A. and Gonzalez-Lima, F. (1994). Structural equation modeling and its application to network analysis in functional brain imaging, *Human Brain Mapping* **2**, pp. 2–22.

McMillan, A., Hermann, B., Johnson, S., Hansen, R., Seidenberg, M. and Meyerand, M. (2004). Voxel-based morphometry of unilateral temporal lobe epilepsy reveals abnormalities in cerebral white matter, *NeuroImage* **23**, pp. 167–174.

Mehta, S., Grabowski, T., Trivedi, Y. and Damasio, H. (2004). Evaluation of voxel-based morphometry for focal lesion detection in individuals, *NeuroImage* **20**, pp. 1438–1454.

Mémoli, F. (2008). Gromov-Hausdorff distances in Euclidean spaces, in *Workshop on Non-Rigid Shape Analysis and Deformable Image Alignment (CVPR workshop, NORDIA'08)*.

Meyer, M., Lee, H., Barr, A. and Desbrun, M. (2002). Generalized barycentric coordinates on irregular polygons, *Journal of Graphics Tools* **7**, pp. 13–22.

Meyer, Y. (2001). *Oscillating patterns in image processing and nonlinear evolution equations: the fifteenth Dean Jacqueline B. Lewis memorial lectures* (American Mathematical Society).

Miller, M., Banerjee, A., Christensen, G., Joshi, S., Khaneja, N., Grenander, U. and Matejic, L. (1997). Statistical methods in computational anatomy, *Statistical Methods in Medical Research* **6**, pp. 267–299.

Miller, M., Massie, A., Ratnanather, J., Botteron, K. and Csernansky, J. (2000). Bayesian construction of geometrically based cortical thickness metrics, *NeuroImage* **12**, pp. 676–687.

Milliken, J. and Edland, S. (2000). Mixed effect models of longitudinal alzheimer's disease data: a cautionary note, *Statist. Med.* **19**, pp. 1617–1629.

Milnor, J. (1973). *Morse Theory* (Princeton University Press).

Minshew, N. and Williams, D. (2007). The new neurobiology of autism: Cortex, connectivity, and neuronal organization, *Arch. Neurol.* , pp. 945–950.

Molenberghs, G. and Verbeke, G. (2005). *Models for Discrete Longitudinal Data* (Springer).

Mori, S., Crain, B., Chacko, V. and van Zijl, P. (1999). Three-dimensional tracking of axonal projections in the brain by magnetic resonance imaging, *Annals of Neurology* **45**, pp. 256–269.

Mori, S., Kaufmann, W., Davatzikos, C., Stieljes, Amodei, L., Fredericksen, K., Pearlson, G., Melhem, E., Solaiyappan, M., Raymond, G., Moser, H. and van Zijl, P. (2002). Imaging cortical association tracts in the human brain using diffusion-tensor-based axonal tracking, *Magnetic Resonance in Medicine* **47**, pp. 215–223.

Mori, S., Oishi, K., Jiang, H., Jiang, L., Li, X., Akhter, K., Hua, K., Faria, A., Mahmood, A., Woods, R. *et al.* (2008). Stereotaxic white matter atlas based on diffusion tensor imaging in an ICBM template, *NeuroImage* **40**, pp. 570–582.

Mori, S. and van Zijl, P. (2002). Fiber tracking: principles and strategies-a technical review, *NMR in Biomedicine* **15**, pp. 468–480.

Morozov, D. (2008). *Homological Illusions of Persistence and Stability* (Ph.D. thesis, Duke University).

Muller, H.-G. (2005). Functional modeling and classification of longitudinal data, *Scandinavian Journal of Statistics* **32**, pp. 223–240.

Mumford, D. and Shah, J. (1989). Optimal approximations by piecewise smooth functions and associated variational problems, *Comm. Pure Appl. Math* **42**, pp. 577–685.

Nacewicz, B., Dalton, K., Johnstone, T., Long, M., McAuliff, E., Oakes, T., Alexander, A. and Davidson, R. (2006). Amygdala volume and nonverbal social impairment in adolescent and adult males with autism, *Arch. Gen. Psychiatry* **63**, pp. 1417–1428.

Nadaraya, E. (1964). On estimating regression, *Theory Probab. Appl.* **9**, pp. 157–159.

Naiman, D. (1990). volumes for tubular neighborhoods of spherical polyhedra and statistical inference, *Ann. Statist.* **18**, pp. 685–716.

Nain, D., Styner, M., Niethammer, M., Levitt, J., Shenton, M., Gerig, G., Bobick, A. and Tannenbaum, A. (2007). Statistical shape analysis of brain structures using spherical wavelets, in *IEEE Symposium on Biomedical Imaging ISBI*.

Newman, M. (2003). The Structure and Function of Complex Networks, *SIAM Review* **45**, p. 167.

Newman, M., Barabasi, A. and Watts, D. (2006). *The structure and dynamics of networks* (Princeton University Press).

Newman, M., Strogatz, S. and Watts, D. (2001). Random graphs with arbitrary degree distributions and their applications, *Physical Review E* **64**, p. 26118.

Newman, M. and Watts, D. (1999). Scaling and percolation in the small-world network model, *Physical Review E* **60**, pp. 7332–7342.

Nichols, T. and Hayasaka, S. (2003). Controlling the familywise error rate in functional neuroimaging: a comparative review, *Stat Methods Med. Res.* **12**, pp. 419–446.

Nichols, T. and Holmes, A. (2002). Nonparametric permutation tests for functional neuroimaging: a primer with examples, *Human Brain Mapping* **15**, pp. 1–25.

Niethammer, M., Reuter, M., Wolter, F., Bouix, S., Peinecke, N., Koo, M. and Shenton, M. (2007). Global Medical Shape Analysis Using the Laplace-Beltrami Spectrum, *Lecture Notes in Computer Science* **4791**, p. 850.

O'Brien, R. and Muller, K. (1993). Unified power analysis for t-tests through multivariate hypotheses, *Applied analysis of variance in behavioral science* , pp. 297–344.

O'Donnell, L., Kubicki, M., Shenton, M., Dreusicke, M., Grimson, W. and Westin, C. (2006). A method for clustering white matter fiber tracts, *American Journal of Neuroradiology* **27**, pp. 1032–1036.

O'Donnell, L. and Westin, C. (2007). Automatic tractography segmentation using a high-dimensional white matter atlas, *IEEE Transactions on Medical Imaging* **26**, pp. 1562–1575.

Ohtake, Y., Belyaev, A. and Bogaevski, I. (2000). Polyedral surface smoothing with simultaneous mesh regularization, *Proceedings of Geometric Modeling and Processing. Theory and Applications* , pp. 229–237.

Osborne, M., Presnell, B. and Turlach, B. (2000). A new approach to variable selection in least squares problems, *IMA Journal of numerical analysis* **20**, pp. 389–404.

Osher, S. and Fedkiw, R. (2003). *Level set methods and dynamic implicit surfaces* (Springer Verlag).

Osher, S. and Sethian, J. (1988). Fronts propagating with curvature-dependent speed: algorithms based on Hamilton-Jacobi formulations, *Journal of computational physics* **79**, pp. 12–49.

Parker, G., Wheeler-Kingshott, C. and Barker, G. (2002). Estimating distributed anatomical connectivity using fast marching methods and diffusion tensor imaging, *IEEE Transactions on Medical Imaging* **21**, pp. 505–512.

Parker, J. (1996). *Algorithms for image processing and computer vision* (John Wiley & Sons, Inc. New York, NY, USA).

Paul, W. and Baschnagel, J. (1999). *Stochastic Processes from Physics to Finance* (Springer-Verlag, Berlin).

Paus, T., Zijdenbos, A., Worsley, K., Collins, D., Blumenthal, J., Giedd, J., Rapoport, J. and Evans, A. (1999). Structural maturation of neural pathways in children and adolescents: In vivo study, *Science* **283**, pp. 1903–1911.

Peng, J., Wang, P., Zhou, N. and Zhu, J. (2009). Partial correlation estimation by joint sparse regression models, *Journal of the American Statistical Association* **104**, pp. 735–746.

Penny, W., Stephan, K., Mechelli, A. and Friston, K. (2004). Comparing dynamic causal models, *NeuroImage* **22**, pp. 1157–1172.

Perona, P. and Malik, J. (1990). Scale-space and edge detection using anisotropic diffusion, *IEEE Trans. Pattern Analysis and Machine Intelligence* **12**, pp. 629–639.

Piekema, C., Kessels, R., Mars, R., Petersson, K. and Fernández, G. (2006). The right hippocampus participates in short-term memory maintenance of object-location associations, *NeuroImage* **33**, pp. 374–382.

Pinehiro, J. and Bates, D. (2002). *Mixed Effects Models in S and S-Plus*, 3rd edn. (Springer).

Piven, J., Arndt, S., Bailey, J. and Andreasen, N. (1996). Regional brain enlargement in autism: a magnetic resonance imaging study, *Journal of the American Academy of Child & Adolescent Psychiatry* **35**, pp. 530–536.

Piven, J., Bailey, J., Ranson, B. and Arndt, S. (1997). An MRI study of the corpus callosum in autism, *American Journal of Psychiatry* **154**, p. 1051.

Pizer, S., Fritsch, D., Yushkevich, P., Johnson, V. and Chaney, E. (1999). Segmentation, registration, and measurement of shape variation via image object shape, *IEEE Transactions on Medical Imaging* **18**, pp. 851–865.

Pizzagalli, D., Oakes, T., Fox, A., Chung, M., Larson, C., Abercrombie, H., Schaefer, S., Benca, R. and Davidson, R. (2004). Functional but not structural subgenual prefrontal cortex abnormalities in melancholia, *Molecular Psychiatry* **9**, pp. 393–405.

Plumbley, M. (2005). Geometry and homotopy for l_1 sparse representations, *Proceedings of SPARS* **5**, pp. 206–213.

Poline, J.-B. and Mazoyer, B. (1994). Analysis of individual brain activation maps using hierarchical description and multiscale detection, *IEEE Transactions on Medical Imaging* **13**, pp. 702–710.

Poline, J.-B., Worsley, K., Holmes, F. R., A.P. and Friston, K. (1995). Estimating smoothness in statistical parametric maps: Variability of p values, *Journal of Computer Assisted Tomography* **19**, pp. 788–796.

Pothen, A. and Fan, C. (1990). Computing the block triangular form of a sparse matrix, *ACM Transactions on Mathematical Software (TOMS)* **16**, p. 324.

Pujol, J., Vendrell, P., Junque, C., Martivilalta, J. and A., C. (1993). When does human brain development end? Evidence of corpus callosum growth up to adulthood, *Annals of Neurology* **34**, pp. 71–75.

Qiu, A., Bitouk, D. and Miller, M. (2006). Smooth functional and structural maps on the neocortex via orthonormal bases of the laplace-beltrami operator, *IEEE Transactions on Medical Imaging* **25**, pp. 1296–1396.

Qiu, A. and Miller, M. (2008). Multi-structure network shape analysis via normal surface momentum maps, *NeuroImage* **42**, pp. 1430–1438.

Quicken, M., Brechbuhler, C., Hug, J., Blattmann, H. and Szekely, G. (2000). Parameterization of closed surfaces for parametric surface description, *IEEE Computer Society Conference on Computer Vision and Pattern Recognition (CVPR)* , pp. 354–360.

Rajapakse, J., Giedd, J., DeCarli, C., Snell, J., McLaughlin, A., Vauss, Y., Krain, A., Hamburger, S. and Rapoport, J. (1996). A technique for single-channel mr brain tissue segmentation: Application to a pediatric sample, *Magnetic Resonance Imaging* **14**, pp. 1053–1065.

Ramsay, J. (2000). Differential equation models for satistical functions, *The Canadian Journal of Statistics* **28**, pp. 225–240.

Ramsay, J. and Silverman, B. (1997). *Functional Data Analysis* (Springer-Verlag).

Rao, C. and Toutenburg, H. (1999). *Linear Models:Least Squares and Alternatives* (Springer-Verlag).

Reuter, M. (2010). Hierarchical shape segmentation and registration via topological features of Laplace-Beltrami eigenfunctions, *International Journal of Computer Vision* **89**, pp. 287–308.

Reuter, M., Wolter, F.-E., Shenton, M. and Niethammer, M. (2009). Laplace-Beltrami eigenvalues and topological features of eigenfunctions for statistical shape analysis, *Computer-Aided Design* **41**, pp. 739–755.

Rice, S. (1944). Mathematical analysis of random noise, *Bell System Tech. J* **23**, pp. 282–332.

Riess, A., Abrams, M., Singer, H., Ross, J. and Denckla, M. (1996). Brain development, gender and iq in children: A volumetric imaging study, *Brain* **119**, pp. 1763–1774.

Robbins, S. (2003). Anatomical standardization of the human brain in euclidean 3-space and on the cortical 2-manifold. Tech. Rep. PhD thesis, School of Computer Science, McGill University, Montreal, Quebec, Canada.

Robert, C. and Casella, G. (2004). *Monte Carlo statistical methods* (Springer Verlag).

Robert, P. and Escoufier, Y. (1976). A unifying tool for linear multivariate statistical methods: the RV-coefficient, *Journal of the Royal Statistical Society. Series C (Applied Statistics)* **25**, pp. 257–265.

Rosenberg, S. (1997). *The Laplacian on a Riemannian Manifold* (Cambridge University Press).

Roy, S. (1953). On a heuristic method of test construction and its use in multivariate analysis, *Ann. Math. Statist.* **24**, pp. 220–238.

Rubinov, M. and Sporns, O. (2010). Complex network measures of brain connectivity: Uses and interpretations, *NeuroImage* **52**, pp. 1059–1069.

Rudin, W. (1991). *Functional Analysis* (McGraw-Hill).

Rusch, B., Abercrombie, H., Oakes, T., Schaefer, S. and Davidson, R. (2001). Hippocampal morphometry in depressed patients and control subjects: relations to anxiety symptoms, *Biological Psychiatry* **50**, pp. 960–964.

Rustamov, R. (2007). Laplace-Beltrami eigenfunctions for deformation invariant shape representation, in *Proceedings of the fifth Eurographics symposium on Geometry processing*, p. 233.

Sacan, O. O. F. H., A. and Wang, Y. (2007). Lfm-pro: A tool for detecting significant local structural sites in proteins, *Bioinformatics* **6**, pp. 709–716.

Sadiku, M. (1989). A simple introduction to finite element analysis of electromagnetic problems, *IEEE Transactions on Education* **32**, pp. 85–93.

Sadiku, M. (1992). *Numerical Techniques in Electromagnetics* (CRC Press).

Saffman, P. (1992). *Vortex Dynamics* (Cambridge University Press, New York).

Salmond, C., Ashburner, J., Vargha-Khadem, F., Connelly, A., Gadian, D. and Friston, K. (2002). Distributional assumptions in voxel-based morphometry, *NeuroImage* **17**, pp. 1027–1030.

Sapiro, G. (2001). *Geometric partial differential equations and image analysis* (Cambridge University Press).

Sato, Y., Nakajima, S., Shiraga, N., Atsumi, H., Yoshida, S., Koller, T., Gerig, G. and Kikinis, R. (1998). Three-dimensional multi-scale line filter for segmentation and visualization of curvilinear structures in medical images, *Medical Image Analysis* **2**, pp. 143–168.

Satterthwaite, F. (1946). An approximate distribution of estimates of variance components, *Biometrics* **2**, pp. 110–114.

Schmidt, V. and Spodarev, E. (2005). Joint estimators for the specific intrinsic volumes of stationary random sets, *Stochastic Processes and their Applications* **115**, pp. 959–981.

Ségonne, F., Pacheco, J. and Fischl, B. (2007). Geometrically accurate topology-correction of cortical surfaces using nonseparating loops, *IEEE Transactions on Medical Imaging* **26**, pp. 518–529.

Seo, S., Chung, M., Dalton, K. and Davidson, R. (2011a). Multivariate cortical shape modeling based on sparse representation, in *17th Annual Meeting of the Organization for Human Brain Mapping (HBM)*, p. 648.

Seo, S., Chung, M. and Voperian, H. (2011b). Mandible shape modeling using the second eigenfunction of the laplace-beltrami operator, in *Proceedings of SPIE Medical Imaging*, Vol. 7962, p. 79620Z.

Seo, S., Chung, M. and Vorperian, H. (2010). Heat kernel smothing using laplace-beltrami eigenfunctions, in *Medical Image Computing and Computer-Assisted Intervention – MICCAI 2010, Lecture Notes in Computer Science*, Vol. 6363, pp. 505–512.

Sethian, J. (2002). *Level Set Methods and Fast Marching Methods: Evolving Interfaces in Computational Geometry, Fluid Mechanics, Computer Vision and Material Science* (Cambridge University Press).

Shattuck, D. and Leahy, R. (2001). Automated graph-based analysis and correction of cortical volume topology, *IEEE Transactions on Medical Imaging* **20**, pp. 1167–1177.

Shen, L. and Chung, M. (2006). Large-scale modeling of parametric surfaces using spherical harmonics, in *Third International Symposium on 3D Data Processing, Visualization and Transmission (3DPVT)*.

Shen, L., Ford, J., Makedon, F. and Saykin, A. (2004). surface-based approach for classification of 3d neuroanatomical structures, *Intelligent Data Analysis* **8**, pp. 519–542.

Shen, L., Saykin, A., Chung, M., Huang, H., Ford, J., Makedon, F., McHugh, T. and Rhodes, C. (2006). Morphometric analysis of genetic variation in hippocampal shape in mild cognitive impairment: Role of an il-6 promoter polymorphism, in *Life Science Society Computational Systems Bioinformatics Conference.*

Shi, Y., Lai, R., Krishna, S., Sicotte, N., Dinov, I. and Toga, A. (2008a). Anisotropic Laplace-Beltrami eigenmaps: Bridging Reeb graphs and skeletons, in *Computer Vision and Pattern Recognition (CVPR) Workshop on Mathematical Methods in Biomedical Image Analysis (MMBIA), IEEE Computer Society Conference on*, pp. 1–7.

Shi, Y., Lai, R., Krishna, S., Sicotte, N., Dinov, I. and Toga, A. W. (2008b). Anisotropic Laplace-Beltrami eigenmaps: Bridging Reeb graphs and skeletons, in *Proceedings of Mathematical Methods in Biomedical Image Analysis (MMBIA)*, pp. 1–7.

Shinkareva, S., Ombao, H., Sutton, B., Mohanty, A. and Miller, G. (2006). Classification of functional brain images with a spatio-temporal dissimilarity map, *NeuroImage* **33**, pp. 63–71.

Siegmund, D. and Worsley, K. (1996). Testing for a signal with unknown location and scale in a stationary gaussian random field, *Annals of Statistics* **23**, pp. 608–639.

Silvester, P. and Ferrari, R. (1983). *Finite Elements for Electrical Engineers* (Cambridge University Press).

Singh, G., Memoli, F., Ishkhanov, T., Sapiro, G., Carlsson, G. and Ringach, D. (2008). Topological analysis of population activity in visual cortex, *Journal of Vision* **8**, pp. 1–18.

Sled, J., Zijdenbos, A. and Evans, A. (1988). A nonparametric method for automatic correction of intensity nonuniformity in mri data, *IEEE Transactions on Medical Imaging* **17**, pp. 87–97.

Small, C. (1996). *The Statistical Theory of Shape* (Springer, New York).

Smith, R. (1989). Extreme value analysis of environmental time series: an application to trend detection in ground-level ozone, *Statistical Science* **4**, pp. 367–377.

Smith, S. (2002). Fast robust automated brain extraction, *Human Brain Mapping* **17**, pp. 143–155.

Sochen, N., Kimmel, R. and Malladi, R. (1998). A general framework for low level vision, *IEEE Transactions on Image Processing* **7**, pp. 310–318.

Song, C., Havlin, S. and Makse, H. (2005). Self-similarity of complex networks, *Nature* **433**, pp. 392–395.

Sporns, O., Tononi, G. and Edelman, G. (2000). Theoretical neuroanatomy: relating anatomical and functional connectivity in graphs and cortical connection matrices, *Cerebral Cortex* **10**, p. 127.

Sporns, O., Tononi, G. and Kotter, R. (2005). The human connectome: a structural description of the human brain, *PLoS Computational Biology* **1**.

Sporns, O. and Zwi, J. (2004). The small world of the cerebral cortex, *Neuroinformatics* **2**, pp. 145–162.

Staempfli, P., Jaermann, T., Crelier, G., Kollias, S., Valavanis, A. and Boesiger, P. (2006). Resolving fiber crossing using advanced fast marching tractography based on diffusion tensor imaging, *NeuroImage* **30**, pp. 110–120.

Staib, L. and Duncan, J. (1996). Model-based deformable surface finding for medical images, *IEEE Transactions on Medical Imaging* **15**, pp. 720–731.

Stakgold, I. (2000). *Boundary value problems of mathematical physics* (Society for Industrial Mathematics).

Stevens, C. (1995). *The six core theories of modern physics* (The MIT Press).

Stevens, C. (2003). *Introduction to Linear Algebra, 3rd edition* (Wellesley-Cambridge Press).

Stratemann, S. A., Huang, J. C., Maki, K., Hatcher, D. C. and Miller, A. J. (2010). Evaluating the mandible with cone-beam computed tomography, *American Journal of Orthodontics and Dentofacial Orthopedics* **137**, pp. S58–S70.

Styner, M., Gerig, G., Joshi, S. and Pizer, S. (2003). Automatic and robust computation of 3D medial models incorporating object variability, *International Journal of Computer Vision* **55**, pp. 107–122.

Styner, M., Oguz, I., Xu, S., Brechbuhler, C., Pantazis, D., Levitt, J., Shenton, M. and Gerig, G. (2006). Framework for the statistical shape analysis of brain structures using spharm-pdm, in *Insight Journal, Special Edition on the Open Science Workshop at MICCAI*.

Sullivan, E., Marsh, L. and Pfefferbaum, A. (2005). Preservation of hippocampal volume throughout adulthood in healthy men and women. *Neurobiology of Aging* **26**, p. 1093.

Swayze 2nd, V., Andreasen, N., Alliger, R., Yuh, W. and Ehrhardt, J. (1992). Subcortical and temporal structures in affective disorder and schizophrenia: a magnetic resonance imaging study. *Biological psychiatry* **31**, pp. 221–240.

Talairach, J. and Tournoux, P. (1988). Co-planar stereotactic atlas of the human brain: 3-dimensional proportional system. an approach to cerebral imaging, *Thieme, Stuttgart* .

Tang, B., Sapiro, G. and Caselles, V. (1999). Direction diffusion, in *The Proceedings of the Seventh IEEE International Conference on Computer Vision*, pp. 2:1245–1252.

Tasdizen, T., Whitaker, R., Burchard, P. and Osher, S. (2006). Geometric surface smoothing via anisotropic diffusion of normals, in *Geometric Modeling and Processing*, pp. 687–693.

Taubin, G. (1995). Curve and surface smoothing without shrinkage, in *The Proceedings of the Fifth International Conference on Computer Vision*, pp. 852–857.

Taubin, G. (2000). Geometric Signal Processing on Polygonal Meshes, in *EURO-GRAPHICS*.

Taylor, J. and Worsley, K. (2007). Detecting sparse signals in random fields with an application to brain mapping, *Journal of the American Statistical Association* **102**, pp. 913–928.

Taylor, J. and Worsley, K. (2008). Random fields of multivariate test statistics, with applications to shape analysis, *Annals of Statistics* **36**, pp. 1–27.

Tench, C., Morgan, P., Blumhardt, L. and Constantinescu, C. (2002). Improved white matter fiber tracking using stochastic labeling, *Magn. Res. Med.* **48**, pp. 677–683.

Thirion, J.-P. and Calmon, G. (1999). Deformation analysis to detect quantify active lesions in 3d medical image sequences, _IEEE Transactions on Medical Imaging_ **18**, pp. 429–441.

Thomaz, C., Boardman, J., Counsell, S., Hill, D., Hajnal, J., Edwards, A., Rutherford, M., Gillies, D. and Rueckert, D. (2006). A whole brain morphometric analysis of changes associated with preterm birth, in _SPIE Medical Imaging 2006: Image Processing_, Vol. 6144, pp. 1903–1910.

Thompson, D. (1961). _On Growth and Form_ (Cambridge University Press, New York).

Thompson, P., Cannon, T., Narr, K., van Erp, T., Poutanen, V., Huttunen, M., Lonnqvist, J., Standertskjold-Nordenstam, C., Kaprio, J., Khaledy, M. _et al._ (2001). Genetic influences on brain structure, _Nature Neuroscience_ **4**, pp. 1253–1258.

Thompson, P., Giedd, J., Woods, R., MacDonald, D., Evans, A. and Toga, A. (2000). Growth patterns in the developing human brain detected using continuum-mechanical tensor mapping, _Nature_ **404**, pp. 190–193.

Thompson, P., Hayashi, K., de Zubicaray, G., Janke, A., Rose, S., Semple, J., Herman, D., Hong, M., Dittmer, S., Doddrell, D. and Toga, A. (2003). Dynamics of gray matter loss in alzheimer's disease, _J. Neuroscience_ **23**, pp. 994–1005.

Thompson, P. and Toga, A. (1996). A surface-based technique for warping 3-dimensional images of the brain, _IEEE Transactions on Medical Imaging_ **15**, pp. 1–16.

Thompson, P. and Toga, A. (1999). Anatomically driven strategies for high-dimensional brain image warping and pathology detection. _Brain Warping_, pp. 311–336.

Thompson, P. M., MacDonald, D., Mega, M. S., Holmes, C. J., Evans, A. C. and Toga, A. W. (1997). Detection and mapping of abnormal brain structure with a probabilistic atlas of cortical surfaces, _Journal of Computer Assisted Tomography_ **21**, pp. 567–581.

Thottakara, P., Lazar, M., Johnson, S. and Alexander, A. (2006). Probabilistic connectivity and segmentation of white matter using tractography and cortical templates, _NeuroImage_ **29**, pp. 868–878.

Tibshirani, R. (1996). Regression shrinkage and selection via the LASSO, _Journal of the Royal Statistical Society. Series B (Methodological)_ **58**, pp. 267–288.

Timm, N. and Mieczkowski, T. (1997). _Univariate and multivariate general linear models : theory and applications using SAS software_ (SAS Publishing).

Timsari, B. and Leahy, R. (2000). An optimization method for creating semi-isometric flat maps of the cerebral cortex, in _The Proceedings of SPIE, Medical Imaging_.

Tlusty, T. (2007). A relation between the multiplicity of the second eigenvalue of a graph laplacian, courant's nodal line theorem and the substantial dimension of tight polyhedral surfaces, _Electrnoic Journal of Linear Algebra_ **16**, pp. 315–24.

Toga, A. (1999). _Brain Warping_ (Academic Press).

Toga, A. and Thompson, P. (2003). Mapping brain asymmetry, _Nature Reviews Neuroscience_ **4**, pp. 37–48.

Tohka, J., Zijdenbos, A. and Evans, A. (2004). Fast and robust parameter estimation for statistical partial volume models in brain MRI, *NeuroImage* **23**, pp. 84–97.

Tuch, D. (2004). Q-ball imaging, *Magnetic Resonance in Medicine* **52**, pp. 1358–1372.

Tzourio-Mazoyer, N., Landeau, B., Papathanassiou, D., Crivello, F., Etard, O., Delcroix, N., Mazoyer, B. and Joliot, M. (2002). Automated anatomical labeling of activations in spm using a macroscopic anatomical parcellation of the mni mri single-subject brain, *NeuroImage* **15**, pp. 273–289.

Vailant, M., Qiu, A., Glaunes, J. and Miller, M. (2007). Diffeomorphic metric surface mapping in subregion of the superior temporal gyrus, *NeuroImage* **34**, pp. 1149–1159.

Vallet, B. and Lévy, B. (2008). Spectral geometry processing with manifold harmonics, *Computer Graphics Forum* **27**, pp. 251–260.

Vidal, C., DeVito, T., Hayashi, K., Drost, D., Williamson, P., Craven-Thuss, B., Herman, D., Sui, Y., Toga, A., Nicolson, R. and Thompson, P. (2003). Detection and visualization of corpus callosum deficits in autistic children using novel anatomical mapping algorithms, in *Proc. International Society for Magnetic Resonance in Medicine*.

Vilanova, A., Berenschot, G. and van Pul, C. (2004). DTI visualization with streamsurfaces and evenly-spaced volume seeding, in *VisSym04 Joint Eurographics-IEEETCVG Symposium on Visualization, Conference Proceedings*, pp. 173–182.

Wahba, G. (1990). *Spline models for observational data* (SIAM, New York).

Walhovd, K., Westlye, L., Amlien, I., Espeseth, T., Reinvang, I., Raz, N., Agartz, I., Salat, D., Greve, D., Fischl, B. *et al.* (2009). Consistent neuroanatomical age-related volume differences across multiple samples, *Neurobiology of Aging* .

Wang, F.-Y. (1997). Sharp explict lower bounds of heat kernels, *Annals of Probability* **24**, pp. 1995–2006.

Wang, L., Swank, J., Glick, I. E., Gado, M. H., Miller, M. I., Morris, J. C. and Csernansky, J. (2003). Changes in hippocampal volume and shape across time distinguish dementia of the alzheimer type from healthy aging, *NeuroImage* **20**, pp. 667–682.

Wang, S. and Chung, M. (2005). Parameterization and classification of closed anatomical curves, *Department of Statistics, University of Wisconsin-Madison, Technical Report* **1113**.

Wang, Z. and Vemuri, B. (2005). DTI segmentation using an information theoretic tensor dissimilarity measure, *IEEE Transactions on Medical Imaging* **24**, pp. 1267–1277.

Warfield, S., Robatino, A., Dengler, J., Jolesz, F. and Kikinis, R. (1999). Brain warping, .

Watson, G. (1964). Smooth regression analysis, *Sankhyā: The Indian Journal of Statistics, Series A* **26**, pp. 359–372.

Watts, D. and Strogatz, S. (1998). Collective dynamics of 'small-world' networks *Nature* **393**, 6684, pp. 440–442.

Wilbraham, H. (1848). On a certain periodic function, *Cambridge and Dublin Math. Journal* **3**, pp. 198–201.

Wilk, M. and Gnanadesikan, R. (1968). Probability plotting methods for the analysis for the analysis of data, *Biometrika* **55**, p. 1.

Witelson, S. (1985). The brain connection: the corpus callosum is larger in left-handers, *Science* **229**, p. 665.

Witelson, S. (1989). Hand and sex differences in the isthmus and genu of the human corpus callosum: a postmortem morphological study, *Brain* **112**, p. 799.

Witkin, A. (1983). Scale-space filtering, in *Int. Joint Conference on Artificial Intelligence*, pp. 1019–1021.

Wood, Z., Hoppe, H., Desbrun, M. and Schröder, P. (2004). Removing excess topology from isosurfaces, *ACM Transactions on Graphics (TOG)* **23**, pp. 190–208.

Worlsey, K., Poline, J.-B., Vandal, A. and Friston, K. (1995). Test for distributed, non-focal brain activations, *NeuroImage* **2**, pp. 173–181.

Worsley, K. (1994). Local maxima and the expected euler characteristic of excursion sets of $\chi 2$, f and t fields. *Advances in Applied Probability.* **26**, pp. 13–42.

Worsley, K. (1996). *An unbiased estimator for the roughness of a multivariate Gaussian random field: Technical Report* (Department of Mathematics and Statistics, McGill University).

Worsley, K. (2003). Detecting activation in fmri data. *Statistical Methods in Medical Research.* **12**, pp. 401–418.

Worsley, K., Andermann, M., Koulis, T., MacDonald, D. and Evans, A. (1999). Detecting changes in nonisotropic images, *Human Brain Mapping* **8**, pp. 98–101.

Worsley, K., Cao, J., Paus, T., Petrides, M. and Evans, A. (1998). Applications of random field theory to functional connectivity, *Human Brain Mapping* **6**, pp. 364–7.

Worsley, K., Charil, A., Lerch, J. and Evans, A. (2005a). Connectivity of anatomical and functional MRI data, in *2005 IEEE International Joint Conference on Neural Networks, 2005. IJCNN'05. Proceedings*, Vol. 3, pp. 1534–1541.

Worsley, K., Chen, J., Lerch, J. and Evans, A. (2005b). Comparing functional connectivity via thresholding correlations and singular value decomposition, *Philosophical Transactions of the Royal Society B: Biological Sciences* **360**, p. 913.

Worsley, K., Evans, A., Marrett, S. and Neelin, P. (1992). A three-dimensional statistical analysis for CBF activation studies in human brain, *Journal of Cerebral Blood Flow and Metabolism* **12**, pp. 900–900.

Worsley, K., Marrett, S., Neelin, P. and Evans, A. (1996a). Searching scale space for activation in pet images, *Human Brain Mapping* **4**, pp. 74–90.

Worsley, K., Marrett, S., Neelin, P., Vandal, A., Friston, K. and Evans, A. (1996b). A unified statistical approach for determining significant signals in images of cerebral activation, *Human Brain Mapping* **4**, pp. 58–73.

Worsley, K., Taylor, J., Carbonell, F., Chung, M., Duerden, E., Bernhardt, B., Lyttelton, O., Boucher, M. and Evans, A. (2009). SurfStat: A Matlab toolbox for the statistical analysis of univariate and multivariate surface and volumetric data using linear mixed effects models and random field theory, *NeuroImage* **47**, p. S102.

Worsley, K., Taylor, J., Tomaiuolo, F. and Lerch, J. (2004). Unified univariate and multivariate random field theory, *NeuroImage* **23**, pp. S189–195.

Wright, I. C., McGuire, P. K., Poline, J.-B., Travere, J. M., Murray, R. M., Frith, C. D., Frackowiak, R. S. J. and Friston, K. J. (1995). A voxel-based method for the statistical analysis of gray and white matter density applied to schizophrenia. *NeuroImage* **2**, pp. 244–252.

Wu, C. (1983). On the convergence properties of the EM algorithm, *The Annals of Statistics* **11**, pp. 95–103.

Wu, Y.-C. and Alexander, A. (2007). Hybrid diffusion imaging, *NeuroImage* **36**, pp. 617–629.

Xie, X., Chung, M. and Wahba, G. (2006). Magnetic resonance image segmentation with thin plate spline thresholding, in *Technical Report 1105, University of Wisconsin, Department of Statistics*.

Xu, Y., Valentino, D., Scher, A., Dinov, I., White, L., Thompson, P., Launer, L. and Toga, A. (2008). Age effects on hippocampal structural changes in old men: the haas, *NeuroImage* **40**, pp. 1003–1015.

Yaglom, A. (1987). *Correlation Theory of Stationary and Related Random Functions Vol. I: Basic Results* (Springer-Verlag).

Yezzi, A. and Prince, J. (2001). A PDE approach for measuring tissue thickness, in *IEEE Computer Society Conference on Computer Vision and Pattern Recognition (CVPR)*, Vol. 1, pp. I–87.

Yezzi, A. and Prince, J. (2003). An Eulerian PDE approach for computing tissue thickness, *IEEE Transactions on Medical Imaging* **22**, pp. 1332–1339.

Yoruk, E., Acar, B. and Bammer, R. (2005). A physical model for DT-MRI based connectivity map computation, *Lecture Notes in Computer Science* **3749**, p. 213.

Yotter, R. A., Dahnke, R. and Gaser, C. (2009). Topological correction of brain surface meshes using spherical harmonics, in *Medical Image Computing and Computer-Assisted Intervention – MICCAI 2009, Lecture Notes in Computer Science*, Vol. 5762 (Springer), pp. 125–132.

Young, M. (1992). Objective analysis of the topological organization of the primate cortical visual system, *Nature* **358**, pp. 152–155.

Yu, P., Grant, P., Qi, Y., Han, X., Segonne, F., Pienaar, R., Busa, E., Pacheco J., Makris, N., Buckner, R. *et al.* (2007). Cortical Surface Shape Analysis Based on Spherical Wavelets, *IEEE Transactions on Medical Imaging* **26**. p. 582.

Yushkevich, P., Zhang, H., Simon, T. and Gee, J. (2007). Structure-specific statistical mapping of white matter tracts using the continuous medial representation, in *IEEE 11th International Conference on Computer Vision (ICCV)*, pp. 1–8.

Zalesky, A. and Fornito, A. (2009). A DTI-derived measure of cortico-cortical connectivity, *IEEE Transactions on Medical Imaging* **27**, pp. 1023–1036.

Zalesky, A., Fornito, A., Harding, I., Cocchi, L., Y"ucel, M., Pantelis, C. and Bullmore, E. (2010). Whole-brain anatomical networks: Does the choice of nodes matter? *NeuroImage* **50**, pp. 970–983.

Zhang, H., Avants, B., Yushkevich, P., Woo, J., Wang, S., McCluskey, L., Elman, L., Melhem, E. and Gee, J. (2007a). High-dimensional spatial normalization of diffusion tensor images improves the detection of white matter differences: An example study using amyotrophic lateral sclerosis, *IEEE Transactions on Medical Imaging* **26**, pp. 1585–1597.

Zhang, H., van Kaick, O. and Dyer, R. (2007b). Spectral methods for mesh processing and analysis, in *EUROGRAPHICS*, pp. 1–22.

Zhang, H., van Kaick, O. and Dyer, R. (2010). Spectral mesh processing, *Computer Graphics Forum* **29**, pp. 1865–1894.

Zhang, H., Yushkevich, P., Alexander, D. and Gee, J. (2006). Deformable registration of diffusion tensor MR images with explicit orientation optimization, *Medical Image Analysis* **10**, pp. 764–785.

Zhu, H., Ibrahim, J., Tang, N., Rowe, D., Hao, X., Bansal, R. and Peterson, B. (2007). A statistical analysis of brain morphology using wild bootstrapping, *IEEE Transactions on Medical Imaging* **26**, pp. 954–966.

Zhu, L. and Jiang, T. (2004). Parameterization of 3D brain structures for statistical shape analysis, in *Medical Imaging 2004: Image Processing, Proc. SPIE*, Vol. 5370, pp. 1254–1261.

Zijdenbos, A., Jimenez, A. and Evans, A. (1998). Pipelines: Large scale automatic analysis of 3D brain data sets, *NeuroImage* **7S**, p. 783.

Zipunnikov, V., Caffo, B., Yousem, D., Davatzikos, C., Schwartz, B. and Crainiceanu, C. (2011a). Functional principal components model for high-dimensional brain imaging, *NeuroImage* **58**, pp. 772–784.

Zipunnikov, V., Greven, S., Caffo, B., Reich, D. and Crainiceanu, C. (2011b). Longitudinal high-dimensional data analysis, *Johns Hopkins University, Dept. of Biostatistics Working Papers* .

Zomorodian, A. (2001). *Computing and Comprehending Topology: Persistence and Hierarchical Morse Complexes* (Ph.D. Thesis, University of Illinois, Urbana-Champaign).

Zomorodian, A. (2009). *Topology for computing, Cambridge Monographs on Applied and Computational Mathematics*, Vol. 16 (Cambridge University Press, Cambridge).

Zomorodian, A. and Carlsson, G. (2005). Computing persistent homology, *Discrete and Computational Geometry* **33**, pp. 249–274.

Zou, H., Hastie, T. and Tibshirani, R. (2006). Sparse principal component analysis, *Journal of computational and graphical statistics* **15**, pp. 265–286.

Index